Beeson: I can only postulate that some eosinophilotactic factor is being produced as the initial event. Histocytosis X is a completely mysterious disease.

White: I am impressed by the large number of new factors you mentioned which attract eosinophils. Where does C5a stand now? Is this just a general granulocyte chemotactic factor?

Beeson: Other complement fractions have been shown to have some effect but C5a seems to be the strongest chemotactic factor.

White: It is not particularly specific for eosinophils; it also attracts granulocytes.

Beeson: In the Boyden chamber, yes. Neutrophils come through, but C5a seems to have a preferential attraction for eosinophils.

Gowans: What is the latest information on how lymphocytes tell the bone marrow to make more eosinophils? Is the idea that large T lymphocytes or their progeny migrate into the bone marrow and exert their effect locally?

Beeson: Spry (1970) looked with labelled large lymphocytes. They were found in bone marrow, but not preferentially. We put a large number of thoracic duct lymphocytes in a millipore chamber in the peritoneum of a rat. This appeared to stimulate eosinophilia in a normal rat, as if the lymphocytes were liberating a lymphokine, but we could never find it in the blood in a sufficient quantity to be recognizable.

Gowans: Do you find increased numbers of T lymphocytes in the bone marrow in cases where there is either a profound eosinophilia, or an accumulation of eosinophils in the tissues?

Beeson: We have never looked for evidence of that.

Davies: How would one look for T lymphocytes in human bone marrow?

Pepys: There are considerable problems in demonstrating T lymphocytes in human tissue satisfactorily, since T cells in cryostat sections seem no longer to bind sheep erythrocytes. However, T cells have been stained with anti-T cell antibodies in sections of human gut and liver (Husby *et al.* 1975; Strickland *et al.* 1975; Meuwissen *et al.* 1976). Specific anti-T serum could therefore be used on smears of bone marrow cells, or cell suspensions from bone marrow might be prepared and tested for other human T cell markers.

Rosen: There are no E rosetting cells or PHA-responsive cells in human bone marrow (Geha *et al.* 1974).

Seligmann: You would probably need to exsanguinate the subject in order to be sure you were dealing with bone marrow cells!

Pepys: I would like to draw attention to the possible connection between the T-cell mediation of eosinophilia and the T-cell dependence of IgE antibody production. We have looked at the effect of complement depletion in mice on the induction of IgE antibody production (Pepys *et al.* 1976, 1977; Pepys 1976). Mice primed at six weeks of age with alum-ovalbumin produced neither IgE antibody nor eosinophilia, but, after a booster dose of antigen four weeks later, they formed high titres of IgE anti-ovalbumin antibody and developed a considerable but transient eosinophilia. The eosinophilia was greatest at the peak of the IgE response. Animals which were depleted of complement for four days or so at the time of priming failed to produce IgE antibody after the booster and also did not develop eosinophilia. Since *in vivo* complement depletion suppresses T-dependent antibody responses without affecting T cell activation and activity (Pepys 1976; Rumjanek *et al.* 1976), this suggests that the T dependence of eosinophilia may reflect the T dependence of IgE antibody production, rather than a direct effect of T cells or a T cell lymphokine.

The mechanisms by which IgE antibody might mediate eosinophilia are not clear, but IgE-dependent antigen-specific mast cell and basophil degranulation release the eosinophil chemotactic factor of anaphylaxis (ECF-A) and other active substances. It is not known whether ECF-A or other mast cell products can stimulate eosinopoiesis as well as local eosinophil accumulation, but this is being studied (K. F. Austen, personal communication).

Beeson: Judged by studies done in Japan and elsewhere, one does not always find an elevated level of IgE in parasitic infestations (Takenaka *et al.* 1975).

Gowans: Dr Beeson made a distinction between agents that attract eosinophils into tissues and agents which tell the bone marrow to make more of them. They are not necessarily the same.

Lachmann: Dr Rosen, do children who are agammaglobulinaemic but have normal T cell function develop eosinophilia in response to parasitic infection?

Rosen: They do, and children with severe combined immunodeficiency who have no T cells also develop marked eosinophilia: it is one of the characteristics of the disease. But I cannot be certain that it is not due to transplacental passage of maternal T cells.

Davies: One should remember the example of the polymorph where, as Blanden and his colleagues have shown, certain kinds of neutrophilic infiltrations induced by pox viruses are T cell-dependent in the broad sense that an animal that has no T cells, or only a few, will not get granulocytosis (Blanden 1974). On the other hand, the *E. coli*-induced granulocytosis (Walls *et al.* 1971) is completely thymus-independent, in that an animal with no T cells will develop if anything a slightly better granulocytosis. Thus no firm statement can be made about the neutrophil, as it has many functional properties, some of which are T cell-dependent, and others not.

Ferguson: In humans with graft-versus-host disease after bone marrow transplantation, blood eosinophilia is a constant and striking finding. Presumably that is a thymus-dependent reaction.

Rosen: It is.

Vaerman: I recall that the major protein of the granules of eosinophils is very rich in sulphydryl groups.

Beeson: Gleich *et al.* (1974) describe it as a very basic protein that is rich in SH groups. The possibilities of ways in which this material, which is unique to eosinophils, may affect the functioning of other cells are many, and this is one of the exciting areas for future research.

Lachmann: The reaction of heparin and highly basic compounds like protamine has been shown by Gewurz and his colleagues (Rent *et al.* 1975) to be strongly complement-activating. This has tended to be regarded rather as a pharmacological reaction, but one can picture that a heparin molecule from the mast cell reacting with a highly basic protein from the eosinophil in the extravascular space may also be able to recruit the complement system in inflammatory reactions where this occurs.

Brandtzaeg: If I may revert to Dr Mayrhofer's experiments with regard to the mast cell's potential for producing IgE (pp. 155–175), there are mucosal mast cells in normal intestine in fair numbers. Could the sections be incubated with serum from infected animals?

Mayrhofer: One could try that, or attempt to show concentration of IgE into mast cells *in vivo* after intravenous infusion of myeloma IgE. I have not done either.

Soothill: Dr Mayrhofer, can you give us an idea of how much IgE you are talking about in these tissues? It looks a lot in the micrographs. When a child develops allergy he becomes positive to prick tests before we can detect IgE in his serum. We postulated that all the IgE being made is taken up on the mast cells. I would like to have some idea how much IgE the mast cells take up and how long it stays.

Mayrhofer: I don't know the answer to that. The binding of IgE to the surface of skin mast cells sensitizes them maximally for antigen-induced degranulation for a week or ten days and then the sensitivity wanes over the course of weeks. I do not know how much IgE is present in these mucosal mast cells, except that their fluorescence is roughly comparable to that of the IgE-secreting plasma cells found in the mesenteric lymph nodes of infested animals.

Vaerman: Ishizaka & Ishizaka (1975) have claimed that mast cells are able to fix about 10^6 molecules of IgE when fully saturated with myeloma protein.

Soothill: If we know how many cells, we can calculate the amount per gram of tissue.

Vaerman: The affinity of basophils or mast cells for IgE was very high.

Lachmann: I am worried about the idea that IgE passively taken up by mast cells is then excreted, in view of the findings that IgE binding to mast cells persists, certainly in the skin, for weeks and that its affinity appears to be so high. Are you suggesting either that whole mast cells come out, or that there is some proteolytic process stripping the IgE from the cell surface?

Mayrhofer: I can see fluorescent mast cells between the epithelial cells of the gut and the respiratory tract. It is possible that these cells are merely shed into the secretions, liberating their IgE by autolysis or the action of digestive enzymes. However, if the IgE is actually contained in the cytoplasm, it seems possible that it might be released along with histamine and heparin when the cell encounters antigen.

White: It seems that Dr Mayrhofer has described a very particular mast cell. How do such cells relate to so-called globule leucocytes? They have been regarded as spent mast cells. Do you see eosinophils around globule leucocytes?

Beeson: Yes. Mann (1969) has beautiful pictures of five or six eosinophils around the degranulated mast cell.

Mayrhofer: The evidence that mucosal mast cells become globule leucocytes is not direct. The two cell types have similar staining properties. Globule leucocytes tend to contain less amines (Miller & Walshaw 1972) and under the electron microscope they tend to have more empty vacuoles than mast cells lying in the lamina propria (Murray *et al.* 1968) and for these reasons may be cells that have discharged some of their contents. However, there is no direct evidence that mast cells migrate from the lamina propria into the epithelium.

There is a third cell in the intestine, whose relationship with the two other types mentioned above is also unknown. Globule leucocytes are described in the epithelium of the crypts and the bases of villi, with very few near the villi tips. However, if one looks at the gut of normal rats, there are cells in the epithelial layer of the villus, extending to the tips, which look like intraepithelial lymphocytes but which contain small numbers of Alcian-blue positive granules. The origin and fate of these cells is quite unknown.

Vaerman: Sometimes one sees eosinophils which phagocytose granules from the mast cells that have liberated these granules, and it has been said that this phagocytosis activates the eosinophil, which then liberates its factors, especially the arylsulphatase for the neutralization of SRS-A from the mast cell.

Beeson: This may be similar to the phenomenon that Shelley (1962) described of how to detect drug sensitivity by special stains of peripheral blood. He said one could find degranulated basophils as evidence of an immunological reaction going on.

Lachmann: Would anyone like to suggest what the physiological function of IgE is, particularly in the gut where all these IgE-containing cells are found?

Ogilvie: The original hypothesis suggested by Barth *et al.* (1966) that IgE has a 'gate-opening' role still holds. There is no evidence against the idea that a function of IgE is to increase the passage of other immunoglobulins across the mucosal surface. There is evidence from other parasite systems that an anaphylactic reaction can sometimes exacerbate other immune responses. The classic example in helminths is the so-called 'self-cure' where, if an animal carrying a high burden of certain nematodes suddenly takes in a large secondary burden of that parasite, the previously established worm burden disappears within twenty-four hours. This reaction has all the characteristics of an immediate hypersensitivity reaction. In this situation, however, you do not always get protection, because very often the secondary load of parasites which apparently triggers the expulsion of those worms already in the host then takes the place of the expelled population.

Booth: That is an interesting contrast to what happens to bacteria in the gut. If you have an existing bacterial load which is non-adherent, for example in the stagnant loop syndrome, and you put in a particular strain, it is eliminated very quickly by the resident population (S. Tabagchali & S. L. Gorbach, unpublished observations).

Soothill: Dr Ogilvie, are you saying that you think self-cure may be mediated by IgE, but that you are not too sure how useful it is? I think that you have previously suggested that it is useful, but not an IgE effect.

Ogilvie: Unfortunately there are two quite different types of worm rejection, both of which have been described as a 'self-cure' reaction, but only one of them reflects the development of resistance to reinfection. What is known as classical self-cure was first described by Stoll in 1929 and in more detail by Stewart (1953) in sheep and it is in this situation that an incoming secondary infection may induce an anaphylactic reaction which expels established worms without inducing protection to further infection, as just described. Unfortunately, some authors also describe the termination of a *Nippostrongylus* infection as a 'self-cure' reaction too. In this case there is protection because the immunity generated during this process is very strong and long-lasting; the rats are immune for months. It is in this last mechanism that it has not yet proved possible to demonstrate a role for IgE antibodies.

Booth: How similar are parasites in the gut in terms of antigenicity? Are there large numbers of different antigenic determinants in different organisms, or in one particular parasite load are they all derived from the same original parasite so that they are all antigenically identical?

Ogilvie: In one particular parasite load, worms would not be derived from a single worm; in general, worms do not multiply within their host as bacteria, viruses and protozoa do. Different worm species have many antigens in common (Capron *et al.* 1968) and in fact it has proved difficult to detect species-specific antigens, so that even now serological tests for helminth parasites are incapable of identifying a worm infection as far as the species level.

White: One wonders how far the proper 'self-cure' reaction in *Haemonchus* infestation is an effective contribution to immunity. Is it associated with inflammation in the gut wall?

Ogilvie: Yes; inflammation does occur in *Haemonchus* infection.

References

ALLEN, J. R. (1973) Tick resistance: basophils in skin reactions of resistant guinea pigs. *Int. J. Parasitol. 3*, 195-200

BARTH, E. E. E., JARRETT, W. F. A. & URQUHART, G. M. (1966) Studies on the mechanism of the self-cure reaction in rats infected with *Nippostrongylus brasiliensis*. *Immunology 10*, 459-464

BLANDEN, R.V. (1974) T cell response to viral and bacterial infection. *Transplant. Rev. 19*, 56-88

BUTTERWORTH, A. E., STURROCK, R. F., HOUBA, V., MAHMOUD, A. A. F., SHER, A. & REES, P. H. (1975) Eosinophils as mediators of antibody-dependent damage to schistosomula. *Nature (Lond.) 256*, 727-729

BUTTERWORTH, A. E., COOMBS, R. R. A., GURNER, B. W. & WILSON, A. B. (1976) Receptors for antibody-opsonic adherence on the eosinophils of guinea pigs. *Int. Arch. Allergy Appl. Immunol. 51*, 368

CAPRON, A., BIGUET, J., VERNES, A. & AFCHAIN, D. (1958) Structure antigénique des helminthes. Aspects immunologiques des relations hôte-parasite. *Pathol. Biol. 16*, 121-138

CONNELL, J. T. (1968) Morphological changes in eosinophils in allergic disease. *J. Allergy 41*, 1-9

GEHA, R. S., GATIEN, J. G., PARKMAN, R., CRAIN, J. D., ROSEN, F. S. & MERLER, E. (1974) Discontinuous density gradient analysis of human bone marrow: presence of alloantigen-responsive, PHA-unresponsive cells in normal bone marrow; absence of B lymphocytes in the bone marrow of patients with X-linked agammaglobulinemia. *Clin. Immunol. Immunopathol. 2*, 404-415

GLEICH, G. J., LOEGERING, D. A., KUEPPERS, F., BAJAJ, S. P. & MANN, K. G. (1974) Physiochemical and biological properties of the major basic protein from guinea pig eosinophil granules. *J. Exp. Med. 140*, 313-332

HIGASHI, G. I. & CHOWDHURY, A. B. (1970) *In vitro* adhesion of eosinophils to infective larvae of *Wuchereria bancrofti*. *Immunology 19*, 65-84

HSÜ, S. Y. L., HSÜ, H. F., PENICK, G. D., LUST, G. L. & OSBORNE, J. W. (1974) Dermal hypersensitivity to schistosome cercariae in rhesus monkeys during immunization and challenge. I. Complex hypersensitivity reactions of a well-immunized monkey during the challenge. *J. Allergy Clin. Immunol. 54*, 339-349

HSÜ, S. Y. L., HSÜ, H. F., PENICK, G. D., LUST, G. L., OSBORNE, J. W. & CHENG, H. F. (1975) Mechanism of immunity to schistosomiasis: histopathologic study of lesions elicited in rhesus monkeys during immunization and challenge with cercariae of *Schistosoma japonicum*. *J. Reticuloendothel. Soc. 18*, 167-185

HUBSCHER, T. (1975) Role of the eosinophil in the allergic reactions. II. Release of prostaglandins from human eosinophilic leukocytes. *J. Immunol. 114*, 1389-1393

HUSBY, G., STRICKLAND, R. G., CALDWELL, J. L. & WILLIAMS, R. C., Jr (1975) Localization of T- and B- cells and alpha fetoprotein in hepatic biopsies from patients with liver disease. *J. Clin. Invest. 56*, 1198-1209

ISHIZAKA, T. & ISHIZAKA, K. (1975) Biology of immunoglobulin E. Molecular basis of reaginic hypersensitivity. *Prog. Allergy 19*, 60-121

MAHMOUD, A. A. F., WARREN, K. S. & PETERS, P. A. (1975a) A role for the eosinophil in acquired resistance to *Schistosoma mansoni* infection as determined by anti-eosinophil serum. *J. Exp. Med.* 142, 805-814

MAHMOUD, A. A. F., WARREN, K. S. & GRAHAM, R. C., JR (1975b) Anti-eosinophil serum and the kinetics of eosinophilia in *Schistosomiasis mansoni*. *J. Exp. Med.* 142, 560-573

KATER, L. A., GOETZL, E. J. & AUSTEN, K. F. (1976) Isolation of human eosinophil phospholipase D. *J. Clin. Invest.* 57, 1173-1180

MANN, P. R. (1969) An electron-microscope study of the relations between mast cells and eosinophil leucocytes. *J. Pathol.* 98, 183-186

MEUWISSEN, S. G. M., FELTKAMP-VROOM, T. M., BRUTEL DE LA RIVIÈRE, A., VON DEM BORNE, A. E. G. KR. & TYTGAT, G. N. (1976) Analysis of the lympho-plasmacytic infiltrate in Crohn's disease with special reference to identification of lymphocyte subpopulations. *Gut* 17, 770-780

MILLER, H. R. P. & WALSHAW, R. (1972) Immune reactions in mucous membranes. IV. Histochemistry of intestinal mast cells during helminth expulsion in the rat. *Am. J. Pathol.* 69, 195-206

MURRAY, M., MILLER, H. R. P. & JARRETT, W. F. H. (1968) The globule leukocyte and its derivation from the subepithelial mast cell. *Lab. Invest.* 19, 222-234

PEPYS, M. B. (1976) Role of complement in the induction of immunological responses. *Transplant. Rev.* 32, 93-120

PEPYS, M. G. & BUTTERWORTH, A. E. (1974) Inhibition by C3 fragments of C3-dependent rosette formation and antigen-induced lymphocyte transformation. *Clin. Exp. Immunol.* 18, 273-282

PEPYS, M. B., WANSBROUGH-JONES, M. H., MIRJAH, D. D., DASH, A. C., BRIGHTON, W. D., HEWITT, B. E., BRYANT, D. E. W., PEPYS, J. & FELDMANN, M. (1976) Complement in the induction of IgA and IgE antibody production. *J. Immunol.* 116, 1746

PEPYS, M. B., BRIGHTON, W. D., HEWITT, B. E., BRYANT, D. E. W. & PEPYS, J. (1977) Complement in the induction of IgE antibody production. *Clin. Exp. Immunol.*, in press

RENT, R., ERTEL, N., EISENSTEIN, R. & GEWURZ, H. (1975) Complement activation by interaction of polyanions and polycations. I. Heparin-protamine induced consumption of complement. *J. Immunol.* 114, 120-124

RUMJANEK, V. M., BRENT, L. & PEPYS, M. B. (1976) Cell-mediated immunological responsiveness in mice decomplemented with Cobra venom factor. *Immunology*, in press

SARAN, R. (1973) Cytoplasmic vacuoles of eosinophils in tropical pulmonary eosinophilia. *Am. Rev. Resp. Dis.* 108, 1283-1295

SCHRIBER, R. A. & ZUCKER-FRANKLIN, D. (1975) Induction of blood eosinophilia by pulmonary embolization of antigen-coated particles: the relationship to cell-mediated immunity. *J. Immunol.* 114, 1348-1353

SHELLEY, W. B. (1962) Adventures with the basophil. *J. Invest. Dermatol.* 39, 277-280

SPRY, C. J. F. (1970) Eosinophil production. Thesis submitted for the D. Phil. degree, University of Oxford, Chapter 6

STEWART, D. F. (1963) Studies on resistance of sheep to infestation with *Haemonchus contortus* and *Trichostrongylus* spp. and on the immunological reactions of the sheep exposed to infestation. V. The nature of the 'self-cure' phenomenon. *Aust. J. Agric. Res.* 4, 100-117

STOLL, N. R. (1929) Studies with *Haemonchus contortus*. I. Acquired resistance of hosts under natural reinfection conditions out of doors. *Am. J. Hyg.* 10, 384-418

STRICKLAND, R. G., HUSBY, G., BLACK, W. C. & WILLIAMS, R. C., JR (1975) Peripheral blood and intestinal lymphocyte subpopulations in Crohn's disease. *Gut* 16, 847-853

TAI, P. C. & SPRY, C. J. F. (1976) Studies on blood eosinophils. I. Patients with a transient eosinophilia. *Clin. Exp. Immunol.* 24, 415-422

TAKENAKA, T., OKUDA, M., KUBO, K. & UDA, H. (1975) Studies on interrelations between eosinophilia, serum IgE and tissue mast cells. *Clin. Allergy*, 5, 175-180

WALLS, R. S., BASTEN, A., LEUCHARS, E. & DAVIES, A. J. S. (1971) Contrasting mechanisms for eosinophilic and neutrophilic leucocytoses. *Br. Med. J.* 3, 157-159

Genetic and nutritional variations in antigen handling and disease

J. F. SOOTHILL

Department of Immunology, Institute of Child Health, London

Abstract Low function (deficiency), within the 'normal range', of each of five immunity functions is associated with immunopathological disease, and/or defective antigen handling. These are probably genetically determined, either polygenic or single gene, but environmental factors such as diet influence them greatly, and the vulnerability may be especially great in the newborn period. The relevant systems are those involved in the immune elimination of antigen (antibody and macrophages) and those possibly involved in the immune exclusion of antigen (IgA, the alternative pathway of complement, and cilial action). The gut has an especially complicated role in antigen-handling, and feeding influences its capacity to do so. Eczema was prevented by a regimen of neonatal antigen avoidance, which was largely breast-feeding, and it is likely that other immunopathological diseases result from antigen contact during periods of malnutrition. The mechanisms of such effects are likely to be complicated, but adjustment of the environment to suit the genetically vulnerable, particularly in the newborn period, can lead to the prevention of disease.

When immunity mechanisms react with antigen in the tissue, damage occurs, but usually antigen is eliminated and the reaction is terminated. The high incidence of immunopathological diseases in patients with immunodeficiency led to the concept that the mechanism which causes the damage may in itself be normal, but may be overstimulated by excessive antigen contact, because another mechanism had failed to eliminate or exclude the antigen (Soothill 1976a). This contrasts with the more orthodox theory that such disease results from primary overactivity of the damaging mechanism. There is now considerable evidence to support this view, and it leads to quite different approaches to prevention and treatment.

MECHANISMS OF ANTIGEN EXCLUSION

Antigen exclusion is particularly important in the gut, but it also occurs in the

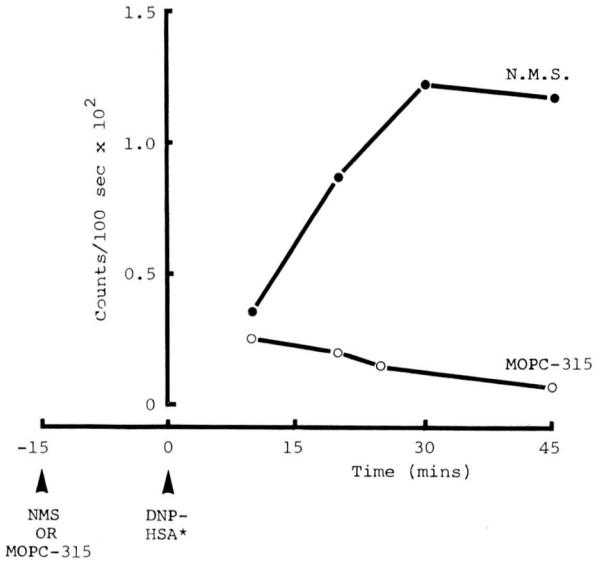

FIG. 1. Radioactivity in the serum of two rats injected into the trachea with ^{125}I-labelled DNP-HSA (DNP-HSA*) at time 0. Fifteen minutes previously the rats had received (also by intratracheal injection) either mouse serum containing MOPC-315 IgA myeloma protein (○) or normal mouse serum (●).

respiratory tract and skin. Though the skin and mucus membrane barriers (cell layer, cilia and mucus) are the main mechanisms, the adaptive immune response plays a part. Lippard et al. (1936) showed that when a child first drinks cow's milk (at whatever age), first cow's milk antigen and then antibody to cow's milk is detected in his blood. This change could be an effect of either immune exclusion or immune elimination of absorbed antigen, but Walker et al. (1972) have shown by studies with everted gut sacs that the effect is partly one of immune exclusion. Extracts of gut wall will produce the effect (André et al. 1974) but the precise mechanism is not established in the gut; IgA, the immunoglobulin principally secreted in the mucus, can achieve immune exclusion in the respiratory tract (Stokes et al. 1975) (Fig. 1) but it is likely that other antibodies can do so too.

MECHANISMS OF IMMUNE ELIMINATION

Antigen is eliminated by antibody, complement and phagocytes, and it is likely that defective function of one of these, primary (genetic) or secondary, could lead to defective elimination.

TABLE 1

'Immunodeficiency' within the normal range (>5% of the population) which contributes to vulnerability to immunopathological disease

Antigen specificity	Mechanism	Deficiency	Environmental influence
Specific?	IR genes?	HLA-related	–
Non-specific	Antigen exclusion	IgA(transient)	Infant feeding, birth season
		Complement (alternative pathway)	Infant feeding?, birth season?
	Antigen elimination	Low affinity antibody	Nutrition, infection
		Macrophage clearing (PVP)	Nutrition, infection
		Cystic fibrosis gene	

COMMON IMMUNODEFICIENCY UNDERLYING IMMUNOPATHOLOGY

Most of the recognized immunodeficiency diseases are rare and inherited by single abnormal genes, but these are a minority of the real problem. Immunopathology is so common (e.g. the highly familial phenomenon of atopy occurs in 16% of British children [Godfrey & Griffiths 1976]), that the variation underlying it is probably polygenic. We have studied the variation of certain immunity functions, selected because poor function would lead to defective antigen handling, and/or immunopathology. In Table 1 five such functions are listed, poor function of which occurs in more than 1 in 20 of the population (i.e. within the 'normal range'). These defects, whether of the adaptive immunity mechanisms or not, are all non-specific, in contrast to the IR (immune response) gene theory of Benacerraf & McDevitt (1972) which has led to the search for linkage between certain immunopathological diseases and certain HLA types. There is another fundamental contrast between these two approaches. Most of the systems that we are studying can be strongly influenced by environmental factors, so prevention is possible, whereas we cannot change our HLA type.

In a prospective study of the development of allergy in infants of allergic parents we showed that the development of infantile eczema and positive prick tests to common antigens was preceded by transient IgA deficiency (Fig. 2) (Taylor et al. 1973; Soothill et al. 1976). Perhaps the allergy results from defective antigen exclusion by IgA, perhaps from another immunodeficiency associated with but independent of IgA, or perhaps from differences of gut flora (see below, p. 231). However it works, since the deficiency is transient it is possible that avoidance of the damaging environment in the brief period of

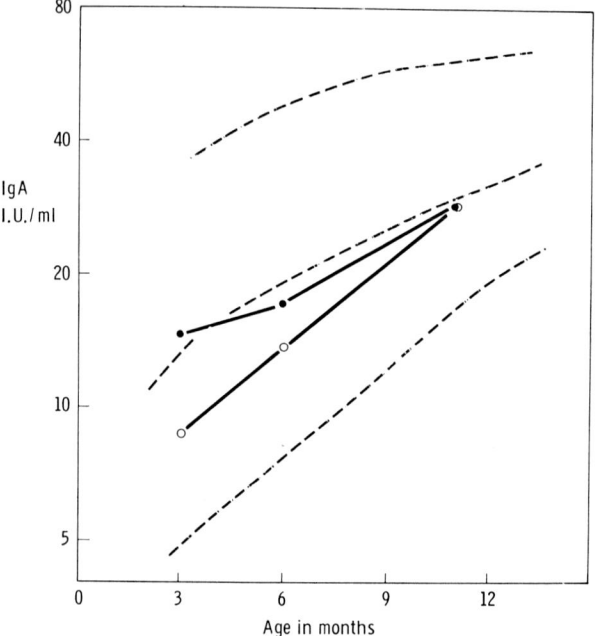

FIG. 2. Log mean values of serum IgA during the first year of life in infants of reaginic parents. ○, those with evidence of atopy. ●, those without. Means ± 2 s.D. for healthy British children reported by Hobbs (1970) are approximately indicated.

deficiency, and therefore of presumed vulnerability, might prevent disease; the results of a prospective study of this are encouraging for the prevention of eczema (preliminary results quoted by Soothill 1976a). If IgA works by activating the alternative pathway of complement, it is not surprising that a defect of opsonization for yeast phagocytosis (Miller *et al.* 1968), related to defective activation of the alternative pathway of complement (Soothill & Harvey 1976a), is associated with allergy (Soothill & Harvey 1976b). It was first thought to be rare, but we find this function defective in about 5% of the population and it contributes considerably to recurrent infection. The defect appears to be inherited in an unusual dominant way, and most affected individuals have only minor symptoms, so it is likely that environment can influence the effects greatly, perhaps particularly in the neonatal period. The effects of the defect, including severe diarrhoea, can be greatly improved by plasma infusion. The other surface defect, also resulting from a single gene defect, is heterozygosity for the cystic fibrosis gene, which includes again about 5% of people. Their sera have a factor which disrupts ciliary function, so we thought that this might be associated with defective antigen clearance, and so allergy. The incidence of allergy is significantly raised (Warner *et al.* 1976), confirming the importance of surface antigen handling in immunopathology, though the nature of this defect does not point to preventive treatment.

Though it is possible that defective antigen elimination may underly the high incidence of immunopathology in patients with defects of individual complement components, none are common enough to be included in our list of defects within the 'normal range'; it is possible, however, that the defect in the alternative pathway of complement may operate at this level, rather than by immune exclusion. We have established two such systems in mice at other stages of the process, which are interrelated but perhaps partly independent. Inbred mice strains differ in the affinity of their antibody response to unadjuvantized soluble protein antigens on an antigen non-specific basis (Soothill & Steward 1971), and this is related to their capacity for immune elimination of antigen (Alper *et al.* 1972) (Fig. 3). Breeding suggests that this characteristic is transmitted by polygenic inheritance (Katz & Steward 1975). This is a different system of variation from the polygenically inherited variation of titre of agglutinating antibody, demonstrated by Biozzi *et al.* (1975) by genetic selection; it is uncertain how much variation in agglutinating antibody response there is in unselected individuals, but presumably it does vary. It is interesting that the low responders in this system survive longer than the high responders.

Animals making low affinity antibody with antigen in saline, produce high affinity antibody and achieve effective immune elimination when immunized with antigen in adjuvant (Fig. 3), so we suspected that the relevant function is the cooperation system—presumably macrophages and/or T lymphocytes. Carbon clearance and blockade studies confirmed this link (Passwell *et al.* 1974*a*) and a new macrophage function test, the clearance of polyvinyl pyrrolidone (PVP), showed identical ranking with affinity of antibody (Morgan & Soothill 1975) (Fig. 4). Though, for each strain, immunized mice clear PVP faster than immunized mice, an immunized CBA mouse clears PVP no faster than an unimmunized Ajax mouse, and the effect of immunization on the latter is far greater (Fig. 5). A method of measuring antibody affinity suitable for applying to man has still to be developed, but PVP clearance can be measured in man, and such differences are found.

So genetically determined differences in antigen exclusion and elimination exist, and some which can be tested are related to immunopathological disease. It is likely that all are, and that they contribute to local gut damage produced by any of the mechanisms listed by Coombs & Gell (1975). This theory would anticipate their participating together, which indeed they do. There is evidence that gut damage may be mediated by IgE, by complement activation (Matthews & Soothill 1970), and perhaps by cell-mediated responses (see Ferguson &

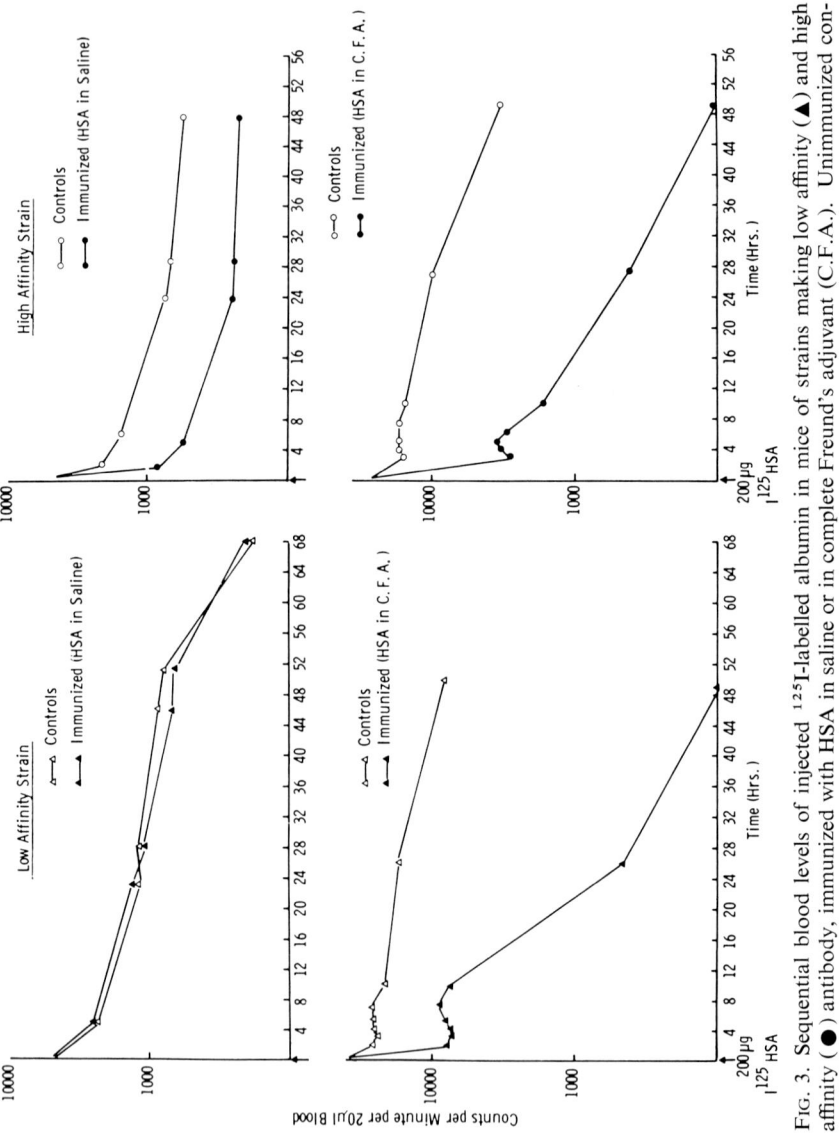

FIG. 3. Sequential blood levels of injected ^{125}I-labelled albumin in mice of strains making low affinity (▲) and high affinity (●) antibody, immunized with HSA in saline or in complete Freund's adjuvant (C.F.A.). Unimmunized controls of the same strains are shown (△, ○).

MacDonald, this volume pp. 305–319). Dissemination of absorbed food antigens or complexes also leads to distant damage (e.g. eczema). The normal mechanism of avoiding such damage may be not only effective immune exclusion and

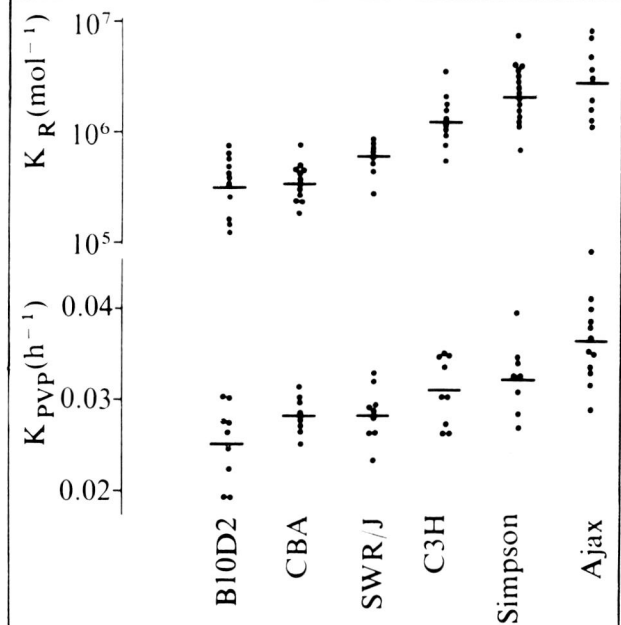

FIG. 4. Clearance of polyvinyl pyrrolidone (K_{PVP}) in mice of six inbred strains, compared with affinity (K_R) of antibody for HSA.

elimination of antigen, but also the partial tolerance sometimes induced by eating antigen (Chase 1946; Thomas & Parrott 1974). Disease would be expected to result from defects in any of these functions.

ALIMENTARY INFLUENCES ON ANTIGEN HANDLING

We undertook our study of the role of transient IgA deficiency and of artificial feeding in the development of childhood allergy with the immune exclusion hypothesis in mind, but there are many other possibilities. Perhaps the transient IgA deficiency parallels a transient deficiency of suppressor T cells, or might lead to an uncontrolled, relatively adverse flora which might affect the response to swallowed antigens in a relatively immunodeficient child. The faeces of breast-fed infants grow mainly bifidobacteria, and those of bottle-fed babies mainly *Escherichia coli*. Perhaps *E. coli* growth is more uncontrolled and adherent to the mucosa of the relatively IgA-deficient infant than that of the healthy infant, so that damage is done, and endotoxin gets in, to adjuvantize

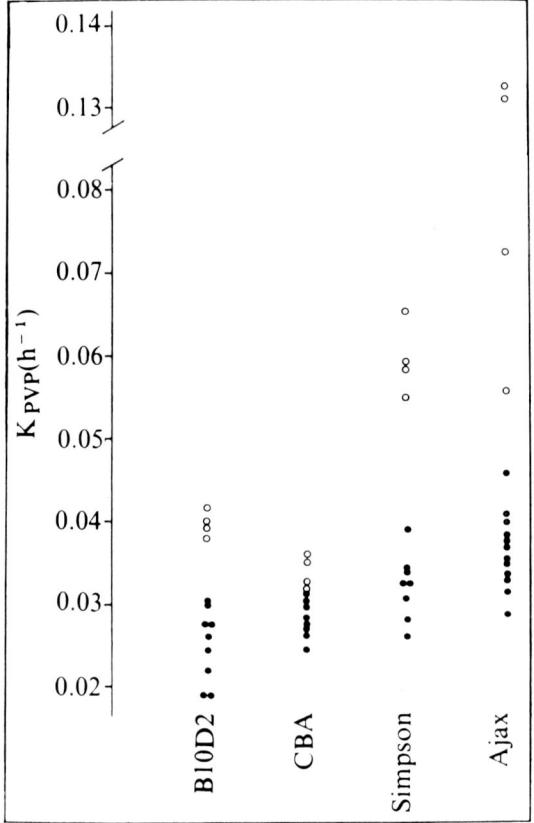

FIG. 5. Clearance of polyvinyl pyrrolidone (K_{PVP}) in normal mice (●) and mice immunized with 1 µg PVP (○).

absorbed swallowed antigens. The development of allergy in the infants with the opsonizing defect may result from any of these systems, or they may fail to activate the alternative pathway of complement by endotoxin, and therefore to eliminate it quickly too.

Apart from damage to the genetically vulnerable individual by suboptimal early feeding, there are other ways in which feeding can influence the relevant immunity functions. Many immunity mechanisms are defective in malnutrition (Chandra 1976; Soothill 1976b). Isocaloric protein or individual amino acid deprivation reduces the affinity of antibody (Passwell et al. 1974b), and the macrophage function, as measured by PVP clearance (Coovadia & Soothill 1976) (Fig. 6). The effect of protein malnutrition on macrophages is rapidly reversed by refeeding, as is the transferrin deficiency—also of immu-

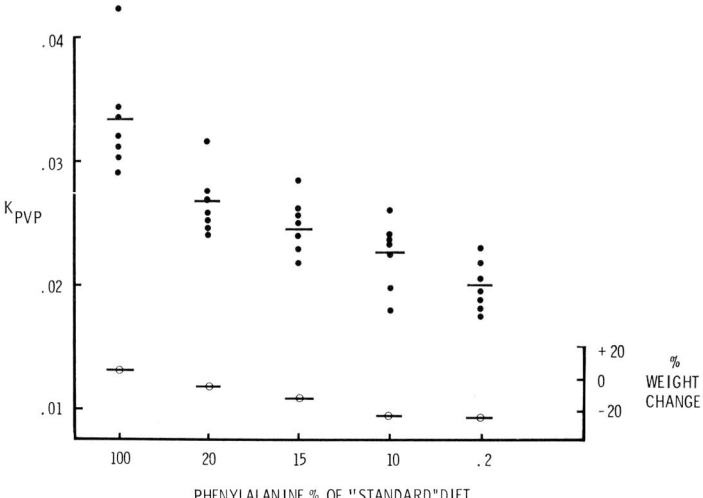

FIG. 6. Effect of dietary phenylalanine restriction on polyvinyl pyrrolidone clearance (K) and weight change in male Ajax mice.

nological significance (Antia *et al.* 1968). But the T cell deficiency persists for years (Chandra 1976), and may well influence cooperation in the antibody response, and so immune elimination of antigen. We are at present investigating another possible sustained effect of transient malnutrition on antigen handling. Animals genetically prone to produce low affinity antibody to antigen in saline produce high affinity antibody when their primary immunization is with antigen in adjuvant (Soothill & Steward 1971): if they are given antigen in saline first, they continue to make low affinity antibody even after subsequent administration of antigen in adjuvant—the 'doctrine of original sin' (Steward *et al.* 1974). We are investigating whether first contact with antigen at a time of protein deprivation has a long-term effect on the affinity of the antibody response to it, even after a return to a normal diet. If it is so, it has important implications for infant feeding, and possibly for the effects of secondary malnutrition due to gut disease.

IMPLICATIONS FOR GUT DISEASE AND ALIMENTARY ALLERGY

It is likely, therefore, that variation in the capacity to exclude or eliminate food antigens occurs, and that it contributes to both local and generalized disease. The incidence of allergy to foods is uncertain, and the only definite basis for diagnosis is the three-fold cycle of remission and exacerbation with withdrawal and reintroduction of the food described by Goldman (1976), which is not always applicable. Food allergy is particularly a problem in young children, who often grow out of it (presumably by the deficient mechanism maturing), and contributes to such very common symptoms as eczema, diarrhoea and infantile failure to thrive, though it is not known how often this occurs.

The role of primary malnutrition in a wide range of infections is recognized, and it probably contributes to immunopathological disease too. But demonstrated sensitization to food antigens is not necessarily damaging. Chandra (1976) has shown a high incidence of precipitating antibodies to cow's milk antigens in the sera of children with kwashiorkor, and they get better if fed cow's milk. Presumably, though exclusion was defective as a result of secondary immunodeficiency, elimination was adequate. But it is likely that in the genetically predisposed, damage might occur. Perhaps as well as malaria and other infections, malnutrition contributes to the high incidence of nephritis in developing countries, and better feeding will prevent much of it before malaria eradication is possible. The same factors could operate for absorbed food antigens.

Secondary malnutrition in chronic gut disease leading to defective antigen handling in the genetically predisposed could contribute to the distant manifestations of inflammatory bowel disease—arthritis, vasculitis, and so on—as well as the development of anti-food antibodies (Taylor & Truelove 1961). But the complexity of such hypotheses is illustrated by the problem of ulcerative colitis. Acheson & Truelove (1961) reported that patients with ulcerative colitis had been on artificial feeding in infancy at a time when this was unusual, but this was later discounted when their hypothesis of cow's milk allergy, based on the detection of anti-milk antibody, became less clear, when it was shown that such patients have antibodies to many food antigens. It is possible that the food antibodies are an irrelevant effect of both primary and secondary defects of immune exclusion of antigen, and that the disease results from a damaging gut flora becoming established in an infant with transient relative immunodeficiency, whose gut flora was poorly controlled because of artificial feeding in infancy. Perhaps a damaging cross-reacting auto-allergic sensitization, such as that described by Perlmann et al. (1967), occurs as a result of a poorly controlled *E. coli* flora, due to artificial feeding in an infant with transient immunodeficiency. Since immunodeficiency is associated with so many effects, the pathogenetic mechanism causative in each particular disease cannot be established retrospectively. Only prospective studies such as ours in infantile allergy (Taylor et al. 1973; Soothill et al. 1976; Soothill 1976a) can answer the questions and establish how to prevent the diseases. Since I think that infant feeding underlies so many chronic late effects, we intend to look for these, as well as the more acute effects of infantile allergy and infection, in a large prospective study that we are planning.

References

ACHESON, E. D. & TRUELOVE, S. C. (1961) Early weaning in the aetiology of ulcerative colitis. *Br. Med. J. 2*, 924

ALPERS, J. H., STEWARD, M. W. & SOOTHILL, J. F. (1972) Differences in immune elimination in inbred mice. The role of low affinity antibody. *Clin. Exp. Immunol. 12*, 121

ANDRÉ, C., LAMBERT, R., BAZIN, H. & HEREMANS, J. F. (1974) Interference of oral immunization with the intestinal absorption of heterologous albumin. *Eur. J. Immunol. 4*, 701

ANTIA, A. V., MCFARLANE, H. & SOOTHILL, J. F. (1968) Serum siderophilin in kwashiorkor. *Arch. Dis. Child. 43*, 459

BENACERAFF, B. & MCDEVITT, H. O. (1972) Histocompatibility-linked immune response genes. *Science (Wash. D.C.) 175*, 273

BIOZZI, G., STIFFEL, C., MOUTON, D. & BOUTHILLIER, Y. (1975) Selection of lines of mice with high and low antibody responses to complex immunogens, in *Immunogenetics and Immunodeficiency* (Benacerraf, B., ed.), p. 215, Medical & Technical Publishing Co. Ltd, Lancaster

CHANDRA, R. K. (1976) Immunological consequences of malnutrition including fetal growth retardation, in *Food and Immunology (Swedish Nutrition Foundation Symposium XIII)*, Almqvist & Wiksell International, Stockholm, in press

CHASE, M. W. (1946) Inhibition of experimental drug allergy by prior feeding of the sensitizing agent. *Proc. Soc. Exp. Biol. Med. 61*, 257

COOMBS, R. R. A. & GELL, P. G. H. (1975) Classification of allergic reactions responsible for clinical hypersensitivity and disease, in *Clinical Aspects of Immunology* (Gell, P. G. H., Coombs, R. R. A. & Lachmann, P. J., eds.), Blackwell, Oxford

COOVADIA, H. M. & SOOTHILL, J. F. (1976) The effect of amino acid restricted diets on the clearance of ^{125}I-labelled polyvinyl pyrrolidone in mice. *Clin. Exp. Immunol. 23*, 562

FERGUSON, A. & MACDONALD, T. T. (1977) Effects of local delayed hypersensitivity on the small intestine, this volume, pp. 305-319

GODFREY, R. C. & GRIFFITHS, M. (1976) The prevalence of immediate positive skin tests to *Dermatophagoides pteronyssinus* and grass pollen in schoolchildren. *Clin. Allergy 6*, 79

GOLDMAN, A. S. (1976) Food allergy in infancy with special emphasis on cow's milk allergy, in *Food and Immunology (Swedish Nutrition Foundation Symposium XIII)*, Almqvist & Wiksell International, Stockholm, in press

HOBBS, J. R. (1970) Simplified radial immunodiffusion. *Assoc. Clin. Pathol. Broadsheet no. 68*

KATZ, F. E. & STEWARD, M. W. (1975) The genetic control of antibody affinity in mice. *Immunology 29*, 543

LIPPARD, V. W., SCHLOSS, O. M. & JOHNSON, P. A. (1936) Immune reactions induced in infants by intestinal absorption of incompletely digested cow's milk proteins. *Am. J. Dis. Child. 51*, 562

MATTHEWS, T. S. & SOOTHILL, J. F. (1970) Complement activation after milk feeding in children with cow's milk allergy. *Lancet 2*, 893

MILLER, M. E., SEALS, J., KAYE, R. & LEVITSKY, L. C. (1968) A familial plasma-associated defect of phagocytosis: a new cause of recurrent bacterial infection. *Lancet 2*, 60

MORGAN, A. G. & SOOTHILL, J. F. (1975) The relationship between macrophage clearance of PVP and affinity of anti-protein antibody response in inbred mouse strains. *Nature (Lond.) 254*, 711

PASSWELL, J. H., STEWARD, M. W. & SOOTHILL, J. F. (1974a) Inter mouse strain differences in macrophage function, and its relationship to antibody response. *Clin. Exp. Immunol. 17*, 159

PASSWELL, J. H., STEWARD, M. W. & SOOTHILL, J. F. (1974b) The effects of protein malnutrition on macrophage function and the amount and affinity of antibody response. *Clin Exp. Immunol. 17*, 491

PERLMANN, P., HAMMARSTRÖM, S., LAGERCRANTZ, R. & CAMPBELL, D. (1967) Auto-antibodies to colon in rats and human ulcerative colitis: a cross-reactivity with *E. coli* O14 antigen. *Proc. Soc. Exp. Biol. Med. 125*, 975

SOOTHILL, J. F. (1976a) Some intrinsic and extrinsic factors predisposing to allergy. *Proc. R. Soc. Med. 69*, 439

SOOTHILL, J. F. (1976b) Immunodeficiency, allergy and infant feeding, in *Food and Immunology (Swedish Nutrition Foundation Symposium XIII)*, Almqvist & Wiksell International, Stockholm, in press

SOOTHILL, J. F. & HARVEY, B. A. M. (1976a) A defect of the alternative pathway of complement. *Clin. Exp. Immunol.*, in press

SOOTHILL, J. F. & HARVEY, B. A. M. (1976b) Defective opsonization. A common immunity deficiency. *Arch. Dis. Child. 51*, 91

SOOTHILL, J. F. & STEWARD, M. W. (1971) The immunopathological significance of the heterogeneity of antibody affinity. *Clin. Exp. Immunol. 9*, 193

SOOTHILL, J. F., STOKES, C. R., TURNER, M. W., NORMAN, A. P. & TAYLOR, B. (1976) Predisposing factors and the development of reaginic allergy in infancy. *Clin. Allergy, 6*, 305

STEWARD, M. W., GAZE, S. E. & PETTY, R. E. (1974) Low affinity antibody production in mice—a form of immunological tolerance? *Eur. J. Immunol. 4*, 751

STOKES, C. R., SOOTHILL, J. F. & TURNER, M. W. (1975) Immune exclusion is a function of IgA. *Nature (Lond.) 255*, 745

TAYLOR, K. B. & TRUELOVE, S. C. (1961) Circulating antibodies to milk proteins in ulcerative colitis. *Br. Med. J. 2*, 924

TAYLOR, B., NORMAN, A. P., ORGEL, H. A., STOKES, C. R., TURNER, M. W. & SOOTHILL, J. F. (1973) Transient IgA deficiency and pathogenesis of infantile atopy. *Lancet 2*, 111

THOMAS, H. C. & PARROTT, D. M. V. (1974) The induction of tolerance to soluble protein antigen by oral administration. *Immunology 27*, 631

WALKER, W. A., ISSELBACHER, K. J. & BLOCH, K. J. (1972) Intestinal uptake of macromolecules: effect of oral immunization. *Science (Wash. D.C.) 177*, 608

WARNER, J. O., NORMAN, A. P. & SOOTHILL, J. F. (1976) Cystic fibrosis heterozygosity in the pathogenesis of allergy. *Lancet 1*, 990

Discussion

André: I have some data on transient IgA deficiency in adult allergy. It is known that infection of the gut with *Giardia lamblia* results in a reduction in IgA synthesis by the plasma cells associated with a reduction in the number of IgA plasmocytes in jejunal lamina propria and in the external secretion of IgA (Popović *et al.* 1974). I confirmed that fact in five patients (C. André, unpublished work 1975), using Dr Brandtzaeg's method (Brandtzaeg *et al.* 1974), and observed that in such patients there is a decrease in the density of IgA plasma cells and an increase in the density of IgE plasma cells. After treatment, the number of IgA cells increased and that of IgE cells decreased. One of these patients was suffering from asthma and after treatment for *Giardia lamblia*, this trouble disappeared.

Brandtzaeg: I did not know about this general phenomenon of *Giardia* suppressing local IgA production. I have only had the opportunity to look at one case and the gut of this patient was crowded with IgA-producing cells.

Evans: According to your hypothesis, Professor Soothill, would you not expect a variation in the incidence of hay fever according to birth date? Presumably if a child is born after the antigen has gone he is not exposed to it until he is about a year old.

Soothill: Table 1 (p. 227) did in fact claim an effect of birth season. It is apparently not pollen that matters but dermatophagoides (Soothill *et al.* 1976). There is variation of incidence of allergy with birth date and if you want to avoid allergy, and are an allergic family, take the contraceptive pill for Christmas and the New Year! Allergy is most likely with birth in September and October. Is this an effect of early contact with dermatophagoides or is it an effect of meeting respiratory syncytial virus at the time of the physiological trough in IgG, at three months? I don't know, but whatever the mechanism, using the pill at the right time would reduce the incidence of the disease.

Brandtzaeg: There are two questions in relation to the mechanism of antigen exclusion by IgA. In your patients with transient IgA deficiency, you apparently think that there is a strict relation between serum IgA, which you measure, and secretory IgA.

Soothill: The concentration of secretory IgA at three months was not related to the subsequent development of allergy, but secretory IgA levels rise more quickly than those of serum IgA and I believe we should have measured it in the first few days of life. From the clinical point of view, I do not mind what the mechanism is. The point is that the deficiency preceded the illness. Is it IgA deficiency which matters or is the transient IgA deficiency related to another transient deficiency, perhaps of a suppressor T cell population, for example? That is an equally good explanation of the phenomenon. I am not committed to the immune exclusion hypothesis as an explanation of the phenomenon; but we have shown that allergy follows, and therefore presumably results from immunodeficiency, and that the effect of that deficiency can be manipulated by appropriate handling, namely breast-feeding.

Brandtzaeg: There are data indicating that rather mature intestinal IgA levels are reached as soon as 1–2 months of age (Haneberg & Aarskog 1975).

Soothill: Yes. We probably just looked too late.

Brandtzaeg: On the model of immune exclusion in mice in the respiratory tract, you specified IgA, but I think you indicated that IgG may do the same thing. The specific feature of IgA is that it gets out, to do the job.

Soothill: Exactly. We are interested in what IgA does because it is in the right place. It *can* achieve this exclusion; whether it is important, I do not know.

André: I have used the same experimental model in the gut of BALB/c mice as you use in the respiratory tract of the rat (Stokes *et al.* 1975). The absorption of DNP-conjugated ^{125}I-labelled human serum albumin was measured *in vivo* and *in vitro* on everted gut sacs. MOPC-315 IgA myeloma protein which binds to DNP prevents the absorption *in vivo* as it does *in vitro* when used at equivalence. Forty-fold less MOPC-315 than equivalence interferes with the absorption of DNP-albumin *in vitro* but not *in vivo*. I wonder if better results could be obtained *in vivo* by using secretory myeloma protein. The efficiency and resistance of MOPC-315 protein would be different in the respiratory tract, where you don't have proteolytic enzymes.

Soothill: We chose the easy route first; E. C. Swarbrick & C. R. Stokes are struggling with the gut now. I am encouraged that you can produce these effects. They think that they can too, but they have found the dose problem a real one.

Pepys: What do you think about Dr André's idea that IgA might mediate tolerance and that might be its role rather than simple immune exclusion (André *et al.* 1975)?

Soothill: I am very happy with that idea, but it does not make any difference to my pursuit, as a physician, of avoiding adverse contact with antigens in the vulnerable period. There are many possible explanations. I am merely using the low serum IgA as a marker for the deficiency.

White: You described work with mice that have a deficient function of their macrophages. You stated that the graded affinity of the antibody can be corrected by adjuvant. Do you mean Freund's complete adjuvant, and is it therefore the mycobacteria that correct the defect?

Soothill: Freund's complete or incomplete adjuvants work, and so does pertussis vaccine.

White: So it does not depend on mycobacteria. The difference between a simple antigen injection and Freund's incomplete adjuvant is I imagine due to long stimulation.

Soothill: You find macrophages in the site of the granuloma, however. We turned to measuring the macrophage function because we felt that the adjuvant was probably giving the macrophages the strongest encouragement.

White: Could I turn it round the other way? You are looking at a mouse which you regard as 'deficient'. Can I suggest that the mouse producing the high affinity antibody is deficient? If you give a long-continued antigenic stimulus, this then corrects the deficiency in avidity. In other words, the normal immune response produces a limited stimulation of the animal, since feedback mechanisms come in to stop the process and you would normally produce low affinity antibodies.

Soothill: It is known that the immune response matures. We gave four doses of antigen at weekly intervals, and bled the mice two weeks later. We looked at it over a considerable variation of time. The affinity of the antibody increases and the antibody disappears. This is a widely recognized phenomenon, so I do not fully understand your point.

White: I am suggesting that your mice correspond to Biozzi's low-responder mice (Biozzi *et al.* 1971), which also are regarded as being macrophage-deficient. This means that they produce antibodies for a short period of time, but such poor producers were the more successful survivors under natural conditions. You could regard them as the animals with more efficient feedback mechanisms, which stop antibody production.

Soothill: This interpretation is possible, but I think unlikely, since the poor macrophage function is clearly a 'deficiency' and dietary protein deprivation reduces macrophage function and affinity of antibody—it can hardly be expected to improve a response. I think that antigen elimination is a main function of antibody, and the low-affinity responders are certainly poor at this. And the combined effect is a big one. In all the animals we immunized with polyvinyl pyrrolidone, the clearance was increased. But even an immunized CBA mouse (a slow clearance strain) clears PVP less quickly than an unimmunized Ajax mouse. In the immunized Ajax mouse the clearance goes right up.

White: Do you see differences in the shape of the immune response between your low and high macrophage function groups?

Soothill: If by 'shape' you mean the duration of precipitating or agglutinating antibody, we have not measured this since they are only poorly related to the amount of antibody (Abt) and affinity. Abt is not obviously related to affinity.

White: In Biozzi's system, the low macrophage function group produce a lower level of antibody for a shorter period of time, whereas in the strain with high macrophage function, he found a high and prolonged antibody production.

Soothill: Biozzi selected on two systems: on the agglutination function of antibody, which is related both to the amount of antibody and to affinity, and on the clearance of carbon particles. You are talking about the former, selection for agglutination.

Lachmann: Katz & Steward (1976) have shown that the genetic control of the affinity and of the quantity of antibody made by mice are distinct, so they are selecting for different genetic parameters. On the other hand, Professor White is right, because in Biozzi's system the mice producing high antibody titres survive less long.

Lehner: Are you suggesting that there is a cause-and-effect relationship between the increased affinity in the mice and the increased macrophage processing? This may of course be due to another cause, because one could envisage an increase in macrophage processing increasing the antibody titre but not in the same sense increasing the affinity of these antibodies.

Soothill: Titre does not give a precise description of antibody response, but agglutination titre depends partly on affinity, so I do not quite understand your distinction. I am suggesting that the high affinity response to antigen in saline results from active and efficient macrophage function, optimally presenting antigen to B cells.

Lehner: In order to get increased affinity, you presumably select out, as Andersson (1970) has suggested, cells secreting high affinity IgG antibody. How do macrophages do this?

Soothill: I don't know, but I gave you the information we have so far. As I described, manipulation, hormonal, nutritional, or by blockade, affects antibody affinity and macrophage clearance together, and you can lower the affinity of the antibody response by blockading the macrophages.

Cebra: Did you look at the IgG1:IgG2 antibody ratio ordinarily produced in these strains to your injected antigens? Secondly, in transient IgA deficiencies in children, have the effects of B cell mitogens in possibly stimulating the maturation of IgA plasma cells from peripheral blood lymphocytes been examined?

Soothill: This has been done in patients with no detectable serum IgA and normal numbers of lymphocytes with surface IgA (Cooper *et al.* 1971). We haven't done this in the transient cases. I have assumed it would work. We have not looked at the G1:G2 ratios.

Rosen: The transient cases have normal IgA fluorescent B cells. I don't know that anyone has stimulated them with B mitogens.

Cebra: Is there an effect on clonal expression caused by suppression of the IgA cells such that IgE cells may proliferate out and express their product to a greater extent than usual? Do you think that there is some reciprocal relationship of IgA to IgE antibody expression?

Soothill: It is attractive to link these two ideas, but we have not pursued this.

Porter: Is the diarrhoea you mentioned associated with nutritional antigens or is it due to bacterial involvement?

Soothill: I don't know. Dr Rosen will be referring to the problems of diarrhoea and immunodeficiency. It is a major feature in these children with defective yeast opsonization, but it is still essentially unexplained.

Porter: You claimed that giving plasma spontaneously cleared up the diarrhoea.

Soothill: Yes, it is a very impressive effect. And both functions are restored—the opsonization of yeasts and the activation of complement by inulin.

References

ANDERSSON, B. (1970) Studies on the regulation of avidity at the level of the single antibody forming cell. The effect of antigen dose and time after immunization. *J. Exp. Med. 132*, 77-88

ANDRÉ, C., HEREMANS, J. F., VAERMAN, J. P. & CAMBIASO, C. L. (1975) A mechanism for the induction of immunological tolerance by antigen feeding: antigen–antibody complexes. *J. Exp. Med. 142*, 1509-1519

BIOZZI, G., MOUTON, D., BOUTHILLIER, Y., DECREUSEFOND, C. & STIFFEL, C. (1971) Cytodynamique de la réponse immunologique chez 2 lignées de souris 'bonne' et 'mauvaise' productrices d'anticorps. *Ann. Inst. Pasteur (Paris) 121*, 690

BRANDTZAEG, P., BAKLIEN, K., FAUSA, O. & HOEL, P. S. (1974) Immunohistochemical characterization of local immunoglobulin formation in ulcerative colitis. *Gastroenterology 66*, 1123-1136

COOPER, M. D., LAWTON, A. R. & BOCKMAN, D. E. (1971) Agammaglobulinaemia with B lymphocytes. *Lancet 1*, 757

HANEBERG, B. & AARSKOG, D. (1975) Human fecal immunoglobulins in healthy infants and children, and in some with diseases affecting the intestinal tract and the immune system. *Clin. Exp. Immunol. 22*, 210-222

KATZ, F. E. & STEWARD, M. W. (1976) Studies on the genetic control of antibody affinity. The independent control of antibody levels and affinity in Biozzi mice. *J. Immunol. 117*, 477

POPOVIĆ, O., PENDIĆ, B., PALJM, A., ANDREJEVIĆ, M. & TRPKOVIĆ, D. (1974) Giardiasis. Local immune defense and responses. *Eur. J. Clin. Invest. 4*, 380 (abstr.)

SOOTHILL, J. F., STOKES, C. R., TURNER, M. W., NORMAN, A. P. & TAYLOR, B. (1976) Predisposing factors and the development of reaginic allergy in infancy. *Clin. Allergy, 6*, 235

STOKES, C. R., SOOTHILL, J. F. & TURNER, M. W. (1975) Immune exclusion is a function of IgA. *Nature (Lond.) 255*, 745-746

Gastrointestinal complications of immunodeficiency syndromes

AUBREY J. KATZ and FRED S. ROSEN

Department of Medicine, Children's Hospital Medical Center and Department of Pediatrics, Harvard Medical School, Boston

Abstract Patients with B cell deficiency have a high incidence of prolonged *Giardia lamblia* infection of the gastrointestinal tract that causes symptoms of malabsorption with villus flattening. The changes are reversible with therapy directed against *Giardia*. There is a high incidence of pernicious anaemia in patients with agammaglobulinaemia. Those with abnormal B lymphocytes tend to develop lymphoid nodular hyperplasia. Gastrointestinal disease is rare in boys with X-linked agammaglobulinaemia when compared with adults with the 'acquired' or common variable form of the disease. T cell deficiency results in intractable diarrhoea and monilial infection of the gastrointestinal tract.

The primary immunodeficiency diseases are a prolix collection of syndromes which cannot be readily classified on the basis of aetiology, genetics or any other factor. It has appeared suitable and workable to classify these syndromes on the basis of their respective T or B cell deficiencies. The working classification of the World Health Organization Committee on primary immunodeficiencies is given in Table 1. The association between immunodeficiency and gastrointestinal abnormalities is well known and sheds light on the role of the immune system in maintaining normal gastrointestinal function. The gastrointestinal disorders which have been described in association with the primary immunodeficiency syndromes are listed in Table 2. It is obvious from this list that most of the abnormalities of the gastrointestinal tract occur in patients with common variable agammaglobulinaemia. Among these patients 20–50% develop gastrointestinal disease. On the other hand it is extremely rare to encounter gastrointestinal complications in X-linked agammaglobulinaemia. Of all the B cell abnormalities, gastrointestinal disease is thus seen most frequently, but not exclusively, in those patients with common variable agammaglobulinaemia.

TABLE 1

Primary immunodeficiency disorders

Type	Suggested cellular defect			Inheritance		
	B cells (Circulating Ig-bearing B lymphocytes)		T cells	X-linked	Autosomal recessive	Other[a]
	Absent or very low	Easily detectable or increased				
X-linked agammaglobulinaemia	×	(×)[b]		×		
Thymic hypoplasia			×			×
Severe combined immunodeficiency	×	×	×	×	×	×
with dysostosis	×	?	×		×	
with ADA[c] deficiency	×		×		×	
with generalized haematopoietic hypoplasia	×		×		×	
Selective Ig deficiency						
IgA deficiency	?	×	(×)			×
Others		?				×
X-linked immunodeficiencies—increased IgM	×			×		
Immunodeficiency with ataxia telangiectasia	×		×		×	
Immunodeficiency with thrombocytopenia and eczema (Wiskott-Aldrich syndrome)			×	×		
Immunodeficiency with thymoma	×		×			×
Immunodeficiency with normal or hypergammaglobulinaemia	×	×	(×)			×
Transient hypogammaglobulinaemia of infancy		×				×
Variable immunodeficiencies (largely unclassified and very frequent)	×	×	(×)		(×)	×

[a] Implies multifactorial or unknown genetic basis or no genetic basis.
[b] Some cases with circulating B lymphocytes without detectable surface Ig have been found.
[c] Adenosine deaminase.

TABLE 2

Primary immunodeficiencies and gastrointestinal disease

Immunodeficiency syndrome	Gastrointestinal disorder
1. X-linked agammaglobulinaemia	Unusual
2. X-linked immunodeficiency with increased IgM	Gastrointestinal malignancy
3. Transient hypogammaglobulinaemia of infancy	Diarrhoea
4. Selective IgA deficiency	5% develop gastrointestinal disease, mainly gluten-sensitive enteropathy; isolated reports of inflammatory bowel disease
5. Secretory IgA deficiency	Intestinal candidiasis
6. Common variable agammaglobulinaemia	Giardiasis (most common) Lymphoid nodular hyperplasia Atrophic gastritis leading to pernicious anaemia Bacterial overgrowth Disaccharidase deficiency 'Flat villus' lesion (not gluten-sensitive)
7. Thymic hypoplasia	Moniliasis
8. Severe combined immunodeficiency	Chronic diarrhoea; usually idiopathic, occasionally salmonella or *E. coli*
9. Ataxia telangiectasia	Increased α-fetoprotein Reticuloendothelial malignancy
10. Wiskott-Aldrich syndrome	Increased incidence of malignancy

A persistent and constant finding amongst patients with T cell deficiency is intractable diarrhoea. Almost all patients with profound T cell deficiency develop intractable, watery diarrhoea, frequently caused by salmonella or shigella or enteropathogenic *Escherichia coli*. In patients in whom the T cell deficiency has been corrected by bone marrow or thymic transplants there has been a prompt cessation of the diarrhoea. The reversal of diarrhoea by the establishment of T cell chimaerism seems to indicate the importance of T cells in preventing this gastrointestinal catastrophe. In our discussion of gastrointestinal disease we follow the anatomical arrangement of the gastrointestinal tract, rather than discussing the gastrointestinal complications of each disease entity.

GASTROINTESTINAL ABNORMALITIES ASSOCIATED WITH IMMUNE DEFICIENCY

1. Oral cavity and oesophagus

Stomatitis and oesophagitis secondary to moniliasis, herpes simplex and cytomegalovirus commonly occur in patients with T cell deficiency. *Candida albicans* is perhaps the most common pathogen in patients with severe combined immunodeficiency.

2. Stomach

The association between pernicious anaemia and agammaglobulinaemia has been well described (Twomey *et al.* 1970; Conn *et al.* 1968; Gelfand *et al.* 1972). Patients with pernicious anaemia and hypogammaglobulinaemia differ from those with classical Addisonian pernicious anaemia. They develop their symptoms at a much earlier age than patients with Addisonian pernicious anaemia. Antibodies to intrinsic factor, parietal cells and thyroglobulin, which are well described in patients with classical pernicious anaemia, are not found, and this provides evidence that circulating antibodies may play no role in the development of pernicious anaemia. A complete absence of plasma cells is noted in gastric mucosal biopsies, as compared to the abundant numbers of plasma cells in patients with atrophic gastritis with Addisonian pernicious anaemia. Many agammaglobulinaemic patients with pernicious anaemia also have diarrhoea or malabsorption. Gelfand *et al.* (1972) reported identical twins with pernicious anaemia and hypogammaglobulinaemia. Despite the absence of antibodies to intrinsic factor, cell-mediated hypersensitivity to intrinsic factor was shown in a macrophage inhibition factor (MIF) assay. An increased incidence of gastric carcinoma is also reported in agammaglobulinaemic patients (Hermans & Huizenga 1972).

3. Small bowel

A. *Giardia lamblia.* Infestation with *Giardia lamblia* is by far the most common gastrointestinal abnormality in patients with common variable immunodeficiency (Fig. 1). *Giardia lamblia* was first discovered by Antoni Van Leeuwenhoek in 1681 when he recovered it from his own stool. Giardiasis has been well described in association with malabsorption but the mechanism of malabsorption is unclear. Some authors (Hoskins *et al.* 1967) have described marked mucosal changes characterized by villus flattening in immunologically

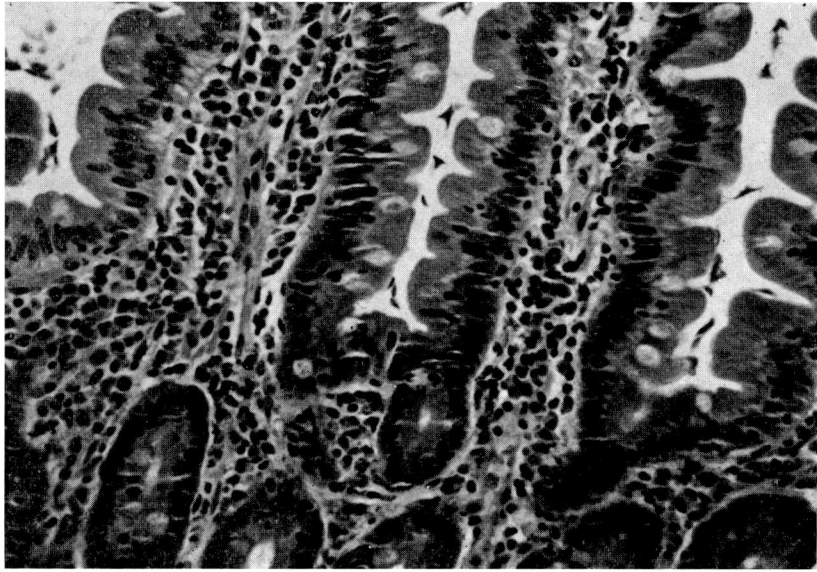

FIG. 1. View of the jejunum from a patient with common variable immunodeficiency. *Giardia lamblia* organisms are abundantly evident in the crypts. No villus abnormality is noted. × 120.

normal patients, while Brandborg *et al.* (1967) and Morecki & Parker (1967) have described mucosal invasion by the parasite with normal villus structure. Erlandsen & Chase (1974) have shown with electron microscopy studies that *Giardia* attaches to the microvillus border of the mucosal cell and that the subsequent abnormalities may be a result of direct injury to the microvillus border in combination with mechanical blockade of the mucosal surface. In patients with normal immunological function *Giardia* does not usually cause marked villus flattening although inflammation of the lamina propria is usually evident. In immunodeficient patients, however, Ament *et al.* (1973) have demonstrated a patchy intestinal lesion with varying degrees of villus flattening (Figs. 2 and 3). Treatment with metronidazole or atabrine has resulted in complete reversal of the villus lesion with alleviation of symptoms in most patients. Thus it would appear that there is a difference in the effect of *Giardia* infestation on the intestinal mucosa between immunodeficient and immunologically competent patients. It should also be stressed that the diagnosis of *Giardia lamblia* infection of the intestinal tract cannot be made easily on examination of the stool; the stool is far less revealing than examination of the duodenal fluid, mucosal imprinting and intestinal biopsy for the definitive diagnosis of giardiasis.

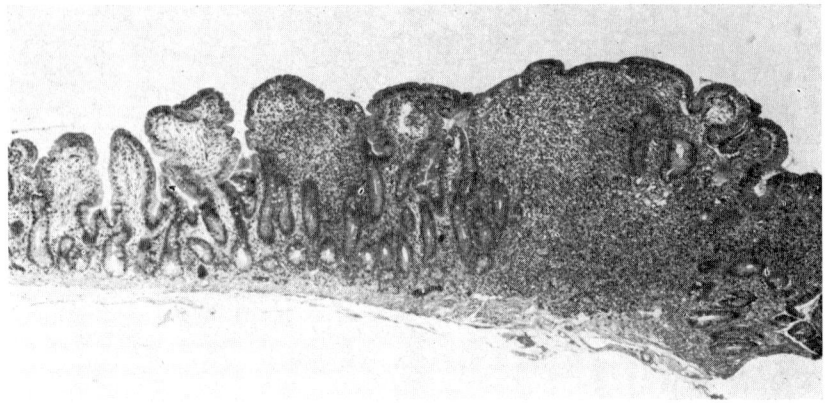

Fig. 2. Patchy villus flattening in the jejunum from a patient with common variable immunodeficiency. No evidence of giardiasis. × 27.

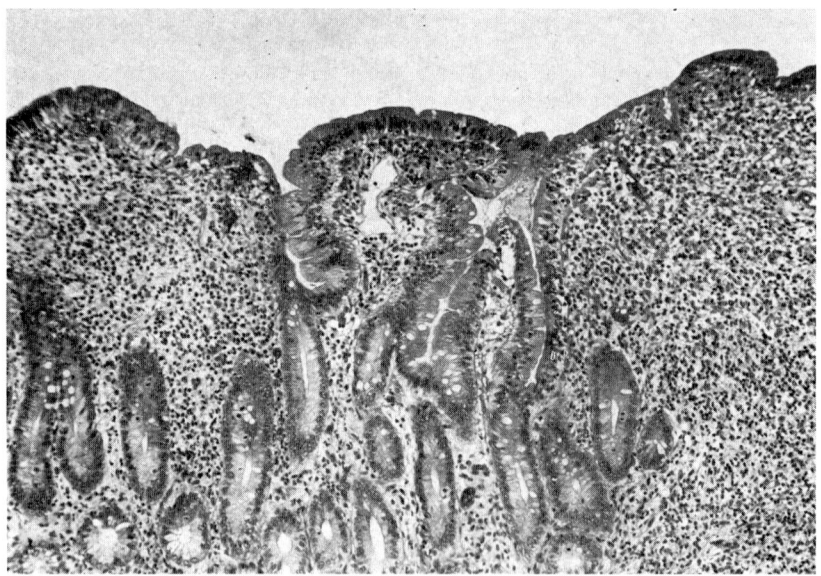

Fig. 3. High-power view of area of villus flattening from the jejunum of a patient with common variable immunodeficiency. Although there are abundant lymphocytes in the lamina propria, no plasma cells are seen. × 133.

B. *Lymphoid nodular hyperplasia.* Nodular lymphoid hyperplasia in the small intestine is associated with immunoglobulin deficiency states (Hermans et al. 1966) (Fig. 4). It is often associated with other gastrointestinal mani-

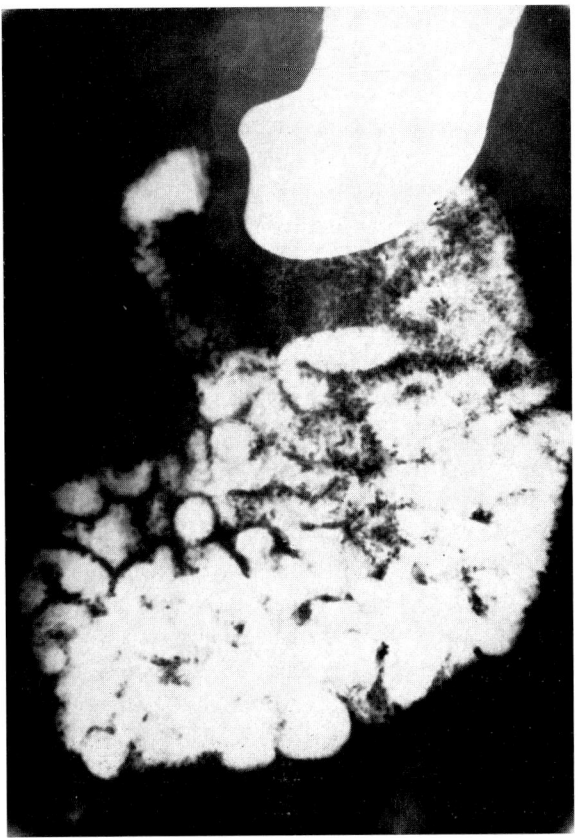

Fig. 4. An X-ray of the small bowel of a patient with common variable immunodeficiency showing nodular lymphoid hyperplasia extensively throughout the bowel.

festations of immunodeficiency, most notably giardiasis. There is a marked heterogeneity in B cell number in patients with acquired or common variable agammaglobulinaemia. In 19 patients with acquired agammaglobulinaemia, Geha et al. (1974) found markedly depressed numbers of circulating B cells in four patients, normal numbers in ten patients and an increase in number in five patients. The latter patients, with an increased number of B cells, had prominent lymph nodes with microscopical evidence of germinal centre hyperplasia. All patients with nodular lymphoid hyperplasia and agammaglobulinaemia have B cells, and the lymphoid hyperplasia of the intestinal tract is not encountered in agammaglobulinaemic patients without B lymphocytes. In the X-linked form of agammaglobulinaemia, where there is almost always complete absence of B cells in the bone marrow and peripheral blood (Geha et al. 1973), no patients have been described with nodular lymphoid hyperplasia of the intestinal tract. Lymphoid hyperplasia of the terminal ileum is a normal finding in children and young adults and lymphoid nodular hyperplasia of the large bowel is a rare finding not associated with agammaglobulinaemia.

C. *Villus flattening.* There are many known causes of villus flattening in addition to that seen in gluten-sensitive enteropathy. In primary immunodeficiency the most common cause of villus flattening is giardiasis (Ament *et al.* 1973). Selective IgA deficiency in association with villus flattening as originally described by Crabbé & Heremans (1967) is a gluten-sensitive lesion, whereas villus flattening associated with common variable agammaglobulinaemia is not usually due to gluten sensitivity. In gluten-sensitive enteropathy (coeliac sprue) serum and mucosal immunoglobulin changes have been extensively described. The serum IgA concentration is elevated during the active phase and serum IgM is low (Hobbs & Hepner 1968). These values return to normal on gluten restriction. Intestinal mucosal studies by Falchuk & Strober (1974) have revealed increased IgA and IgM values which return to normal on gluten withdrawal. In patients with selective IgA deficiency and gluten-sensitive enteropathy, immunofluorescent studies have revealed increased IgM-producing cells in the lamina propria, probably a compensatory mechanism for the lack of IgA. It is extremely important to realize that none of the patients with IgA deficiency and gluten-sensitive enteropathy has been subjected to a gluten challenge to see whether the lesion is reproducible. This step is essential for the diagnosis of gluten sensitivity, as many types of the 'flat gut lesion' will respond to gluten withdrawal.

An *in vitro* organ culture model of gluten-sensitive enteropathy has been described in which the surface epithelial cells of jejunal biopsies of patients with active disease improve after 24 hours of incubation in a gluten-free environment. This improvement is inhibited in the presence of gluten protein (Falchuk *et al.* 1974). The addition of corticosteroids to the medium completely abolishes the inhibitory effect of gluten. We are now using this model to investigate the 'flat gut lesion' in patients with agammaglobulinaemia. Preliminary observations in two patients with villus flattening and agammaglobulinaemia reveal that the lesion improves in a gluten-free environment, and this improvement is not inhibited by the addition of gluten to the medium. We have as yet not had the opportunity to study the mucosa of a patient with IgA deficiency and gluten-sensitive enteropathy.

D. *Bacterial overgrowth.* Although significant numbers of aerobic and anaerobic organisms are present in the proximal jejunum of patients with agammaglobulinaemia (Parkin et al. 1972; Ament et al. 1973) there appears to be little or no correlation with the severity of the gastrointestinal symptoms and prolonged antibiotic therapy has not been of value. Many of these patients with bacterial overgrowth have achlorhydria and atrophic gastritis and some have pernicious anaemia.

In immunocompetent individuals, gastric acidity and intestinal motility are important factors in preventing bacterial overgrowth. The mechanism of steatorrhoea in this instance appears to be related to bile salt deconjugation and/or direct mucosal damage. The presence of achlorhydria in these patients probably predisposes to bacterial overgrowth, but why no clinically significant symptomatology occurs is unknown.

E. *Disaccharidase deficiency.* Disaccharidase deficiency with villus flattening has been described in a number of patients with immunodeficiency (Dubois et al. 1970). In this series, however, no evidence of giardiasis was found, which is unusual. Ament et al. (1973) found four cases with abnormal lactose tolerance tests—three patients with common variable immunodeficiency and one infant with infantile X-linked agammaglobulinaemia, all of whom responded to lactose withdrawal. That the association between disaccharidase deficiency and primary immunodeficiency is specific remains to be clarified; it seems possible that most cases of disaccharidase deficiency in these conditions are secondary to mucosal disease.

4. Large bowel disease

Colonic or rectal disease is unusual in patients with immunodeficiency. There have been isolated reports of ulcerative colitis and Crohn's disease, and one case of gluten-sensitive enteropathy and ulcerative colitis has been described (Falchuk & Falchuk 1975).

5. Dissociation of intestinal and circulating B lymphocytes

Broom et al. (1975) and McClelland et al. (1976) have reported finding B lymphocytes in intestinal biopsies of patients with common variable immunodeficiency who have no circulating B lymphocytes. B cells with surface immunoglobulin, and *in vitro* synthesis and secretion of immunoglobulin by these cells, have been demonstrated. The pathophysiological importance of these findings is not clear at the moment, but they may explain differences among patients in their susceptibility to giardiasis and other gastrointestinal complications.

6. Liver disease

The association between immunodeficiency and liver disease of any kind is rarely reported in the literature. We have observed four patients with X-linked agammaglobulinaemia with persistent hepatitis B antigenaemia, with no development of chronic hepatitis. Three patients with the Wiskott-Aldrich syndrome developed hepatitis B antigenaemia but none developed chronic hepatitis or the carrier state. The natural history of hepatitis B in immunodeficient patients needs to be studied further in view of increasing evidence that the persistence of hepatitis B antigen and the subsequent development of chronic liver disease is related to abnormalities in immune function.

7. Gastrointestinal malignancy

It has been established that there is an increased incidence of neoplasia in patients with immune deficiency. Thirteen of 110 patients with immune deficiency seen at the National Institutes of Health over a period of less than ten years developed malignant tumours (Waldmann et al. 1972). Lymphoreticular malignancy is the commonest type of neoplasia found in these patients.

The development of lymphoma and leukaemia has been reported in patients with X-linked agammaglobulinaemia and we have three brothers with sex-linked agammaglobulinaemia, all of whom developed B cell lymphomas at 10–16 years of age in the terminal ileum. None of them had any evidence of gastrointestinal involvement before the malignancy developed. In common variable hypogammaglobulinaemia lymphoreticular malignancies are also common, and there is a considerable incidence of gastric carcinoma. Gastrointestinal malignancy occurs in association with nodular lymphoid hyperplasia in a high percentage of patients who develop cancer. Ten per cent of patients with ataxia telangiectasia have been reported to develop malignancy, usually of the lymphoid tissue. The Wiskott-Aldrich syndrome is characterized by a very high incidence of malignant disease, also usually of reticular endothelial tissue. It is of interest to note that in patients with intestinal lymphangiectasia who have protein-losing enteropathy, lymphopenia and consequent abnormalities in cellular immunity, three of 50 patients developed malignancy, two, lymphoma and one, reticular cell sarcoma of the stomach (Waldmann et al. 1972). In patients with immunodeficiency with helper IgM the gastrointestinal tract, including the liver and gall bladder, become infiltrated with IgM-bearing cells. The infiltrate can undergo malignant degeneration and has been fatal in several cases.

8. Protein-losing enteropathy

Studies of labelled plasma proteins have allowed the demonstration of excessive gastrointestinal protein loss as a major pathophysiological disorder leading to hypoproteinaemia and hypogammaglobulinaemia. This condition has been described in association with over 80 disorders. Some of these disorders are also associated with lymphopenia. A classical example of this type is intestinal lymphangiectasia. Many patients with agammaglobulinaemia and gastrointestinal disease also have gastrointestinal protein loss and therefore it may be difficult to differentiate them from patients with protein-losing enteropathy alone.

SPECIFIC IMMUNE DEFICIENCY SYNDROMES

Selective IgA deficiency

Selective IgA deficiency occurs in one in 500–700 of the general population. The majority of these cases occur spontaneously, but there is an increased incidence in families with hypogammaglobulinaemia. Many of these patients may be asymptomatic or develop recurrent upper respiratory infections. In a review of 205 patients Ammann & Hong (1971) reported a high incidence of autoimmune disease but only ten patients had gastrointestinal disease, eight of whom had gluten-sensitive enteropathy and two, inflammatory bowel disease. It would thus appear that patients who lack both serum IgA and IgM have a much higher incidence of gastrointestinal disease than patients with selective IgA deficiency. Bienenstock (1975) has demonstrated that under special conditions IgM antibodies may become associated with secretory piece and assume similar characteristics to IgA in secretions. This may explain the protective effect of IgM in selective IgA deficiency and the relative paucity of gastrointestinal disease.

ACKNOWLEDGEMENTS

This work was supported by grants FR128 and AI05877 of the US Public Health Service.

References

AMENT, M. E., OCHS, H. D. & DAVIS, S. D. (1973) Structure and function of the gastrointestinal tract in primary immunodeficiency syndromes. A study of 39 patients. *Medicine* 52, 227
AMMANN, A. J. & HONG, R. (1971) Selective IgA deficiency. Presentation of 30 cases and a review of the literature. *Medicine 50*, 223-236
BIENENSTOCK, J. (1975) The local immune response. *Am. J. Vet. Res. 36*, 488

BRANDBORG, L. L., TANKERSLEY, C. B., GOTTLIEB, S. et al. (1967) Histological demonstration of mucosal invasion by *Giardia lamblia* in man. *Gastroenterology 52*, 143-150

BROOM, B. C., DE LA CONCHA, E. G., WEBSTER, A. D. B. et al. (1975) Dichotomy between immunoglobulin synthesis by cells in gut and blood of patients with hypogammaglobulinemia. *Lancet 2*, 253-256

CONN, H. O., BINDER, H. & BURNS, B. (1968) Pernicious anemia and immunologic deficiency. *Ann. Intern. Med. 68*, 603-612

CRABBÉ, P. A. & HEREMANS, J. F. (1967) Selective IgA deficiency with steatorrhea. *Am. J. Med. 42*, 319-326

DUBOIS, R. S., ROY, C. C., FULGINITI, V. A. et al. (1970) Disaccharidase deficiency in children with immunology deficits. *J. Paediatr. 76*, 377

ERLANDSEN, S. L. & CHASE, D. A. (1974) Morphological alteration in the microvillus border of villous epithelial cells produced by intestinal microorganisms. *Am. J. Clin. Nutr. 27*, 1277-1286

FALCHUK, K. R. & FALCHUK, Z. M. (1975) Selective immunoglobulin A deficiency, ulcerative colitis and gluten sensitive enteropathy. A unique association. *Gastroenterology 69*, 503-506

FALCHUK, Z. M., GEBHARD, R. L., SESSOMS, C. et al. (1974) An *in vitro* model of gluten-sensitive enteropathy. *J. Clin. Invest. 53*, 487-500

FALCHUK, Z. M. & STROBER, W. (1974) Gluten-sensitive enteropathy. Synthesis of antigliadin antibody *in vitro*. *Gut 15*, 947

GEHA, R. S., ROSEN, F. S. & MERLER, E. (1973) Identification and characterization of subpopulations of lymphocytes in human peripheral blood after fractionation on discontinuous gradients of albumin: the cellular defect in X-linked agammaglobulinemia. *J. Clin. Invest. 52*, 1726-1734

GEHA, R. S., SCHNEEBERGER, E., MERLER, E. et al. (1974) Heterogeneity of 'acquired' or common variable agammaglobulinemia. *N. Engl. J. Med. 291*, 1-6

GELFAND, E. W., BERKEL, A. I., GODWIN, H. A. et al. (1972) Pernicious anemia, hypogammaglobulinemia and altered lymphocyte reactivity. *Clin. Exp. Immunol. 11*, 187-199

HERMANS, P. E. & HUIZENGA, K. A. (1972) Association of gastric carcinoma with idiopathic late-onset immunoglobulin deficiency. *Ann. Intern. Med. 76*, 605-609

HERMANS, P. E., HUIZENGA, K. A., HOFFMAN, H. N. et al. (1966) Dysgammaglobulinemia associated with nodular lymphoid hyperplasia of the small intestine. *Am. J. Med. 40*, 78-89

HOBBS, J. R. & HEPNER, G. W. (1968) Deficiency of IgM in coeliac disease. *Lancet 1*, 217

HOSKINS, L. C., WINAVER, S. J., BROITMAN, S. A. et al. (1967) Clinical giardiasis and intestinal malabsorption. *Gastroenterology 53*, 265-279

MCCLELLAND, D. B. L., SHEARMAN, D. J. C. & VAN FURTH, R. (1976) Synthesis of immunoglobulin and secretory component by gastrointestinal mucosa in patients with hypogammaglobulinaemia or IgA deficiency. *Clin. Exp. Immunol. 25*, 103-111

MORECKI, R. & PARKER, J. G. (1967) Ultrastructural studies of the human *Giardia lamblia* and subjacent jejunal mucosa in a subject with steatorrhea. *Gastroenterology 52*, 151-164

PARKIN, D. M., MCCLELLAND, D. B. L., O'MOORE, R. R. et al. (1972) Intestinal bacterial flora and bile salt studies in hypogammaglobulinaemia. *Gut 13*, 182

TWOMEY, J. J., JORDAN, P. H., LAUGHTER, A. H. et al. (1970) Gastric disorder in immunoglobulin deficient patients. *Ann. Intern. Med. 72*, 499-504

WALDMANN, T. A., STROBER, W. & BLAESE, R. M. (1972) Immunodeficiency disease and malignancy. *Ann. Intern. Med. 77*, 605-628

Discussion

Ferguson: I have had the impression that diarrhoea is not a feature where a patient or animal has T cell deficiency but normal antibody production. This has certainly been my experience from one child with thymic aplasia, and a substantial number of patients with Hodgkin's disease and impaired cell-mediated immunity. I thought that it was when T cell deficiency was combined with antibody deficiency that the severe diarrhoeal syndrome occurred.

Rosen: That is not completely true. Children without T cells have severe diarrhoea, whether or not they have B cells. The term 'combined immunodeficiency' was coined because most of these children lack T and B cells, but some have B cells. It is not clear whether those who have B cells make antibody, but the presence or absence of B cells does not alter the severe diarrhoea.

Pierce: I am interested in the influence that T or B cell deficiency may have in predisposing children to infection with specific types of diarrhoea-causing organisms. I would expect invasive organisms, such as viruses, shigellae, salmonellae and invasive *Escherichia coli*, to predominate as causes of diarrhoea in children with T cell deficiency, since T cells presumably contribute to defence mechanisms within the mucosa. I would also expect non-invasive pathogens, such as *Vibrio cholerae* and enterotoxigenic *E. coli*, to cause disease in children with B cell deficiency, since antibody appears to be a major means of defending the mucosal surface. However, you say that diarrhoea is uncommon in B cell deficiency. Since the non-invasive enteropathogens such as *V. cholerae* or enterotoxigenic strains of *E. coli* are not very prevalent in the USA your patients may not be encountering them and thus may not be revealing their susceptibility. Is it known whether persons with only B cell deficiency have more trouble with diarrhoea in underdeveloped countries where these enteropathogens are more common, or whether pure B cell deficiency is a rare disorder in those parts of the world because they do not survive infancy?

Rosen: I cannot answer that. I suspect such children do not survive in the tropics.

Lachmann: There is evidence in rabbits that to get diarrhoea from shigella organisms you need an allergic response to the organism itself in the first place (Matsumura 1962). If you are not capable of mounting the response the infection may, I suppose, destroy the bowel altogether, but you might not get the typical diarrhoea syndrome.

Pierce: I have always thought that the dysentery syndrome was due to invasion of the colon, while the diarrhoeal syndrome is now thought to be due to an effect of enterotoxin on the small bowel with resultant water and electrolyte secretion.

Booth: Could I make a comment on selective IgA deficiency and coeliac disease? Another way of looking at the data is to see how many coeliac disease cases in a big series are IgA deficient, which gives a better picture to compare with your one in five hundred of the normal population who have selective IgA deficiency and many who may be completely asymptomatic. The figure in my own series of about 200 patients is that one in fifty coeliac patients is IgA deficient. There clearly is an association but I do not know what it means.

Secondly, there is a report from Cambridge and my department of a pair of identical twins (Lewkonia *et al.* 1976). We showed that they were discordant: one was IgA-deficient and the other was not.

Rosen: The genetics of IgA deficiency is not clear. There is all kinds of conflicting information about its inheritance. It has been said to be inherited as a dominant; it has also been said to be X-linked, and even an autosomal recessive. The only convincing evidence is that of van Loghem (1974) that the inheritance of the defect is not linked to the Am locus, which is a structural gene for IgA corresponding to the Gm locus of IgG.

Booth: This presumably implies something environmental that switches on IgA production in the neonate. I have always assumed that the antigenic stimulus must be bacterial, in that this 'switch on' does not happen in the germ-free animal, who is receiving normal dietary antigens.

Rosen: It can certainly be switched on *in utero* in natural infection with syphilis or *Toxoplasma* or cytomegalovirus.

Porter: Husband & McDowell (1975) have done some work in the fetal lamb, giving *E. coli* antigens *in utero*. As early as fifteen days before parturition IgA cells were seen in the lamina propria. IgM cells predominated at birth. Germ-free animals certainly show no response. We have maintained pigs for up to six weeks in the germ-free state without the appearance of IgA.

Rosen: The normal human newborn can be looked on as a germ-free animal. There are a normal number of B cells in cord blood, by fluorescence and erythrocyte-rosetting markers.

Gowans: You mentioned a class of B cell deficient patients whose B cells do not respond to T cell signals and who develop nodular hyperplasia of lymphoid tissue. Is there anything wrong with them clinically? How are they picked up?

Rosen: They are susceptible to pyogenic infections, like other people with agammaglobulinaemia. They usually present with respiratory infection. In our hands, with the tetanus toxoid system we cannot get these patients' T cells to activate their own B cells, *in vitro*, but some of them have a striking germinal centre hyperplasia, in Peyer's patches and lymph nodes.

Pepys: Most of the patients whom we see with nodular lymphoid hyperplasia are referred to us with undiagnosed diarrhoea. We find that they have common variable immunodeficiency. Many are not infected with *Giardia* and don't respond to metronidazole therapy. We have not had any autopsies so we do not know whether the nodules are in Peyer's patches, but they are far more frequent than the lymphoid aggregates found in the normal intestine. One can find two in one peroral jejunal biopsy. Some of the cells in these nodules have been shown *in vitro* to have B cell markers (M. B. Pepys & A. C. Dash, unpublished work).

Booth: You can find them all over the colon too, so it is not limited to the small intestine. It might not be a Peyer's patch phenomenon.

Seligmann: Do you imply that in your experience, Dr Rosen, most immunodeficient patients with nodular intestinal hypoplasia have enlarged peripheral lymph nodes with giant follicles and that, conversely, patients with enlarged peripheral nodes have nodular intestinal hypoplasia? This is not our experience.

Rosen: In some cases they are associated.

Soothill: The hyperplasia is not necessarily in the gastrointestinal tract, and it can be startling. It may be looked upon as a tumour. Clinically, it is important to make the distinction. I have protected several patients from dangerous anticancer treatment: where respiratory obstruction results, such minor local treatment as low dose X-ray will clear it, and they do fine.

On the question of *Giardia lamblia*, we have looked for it in many immunodeficient children with diarrhoea, largely the common variable type, and have only occasionally found it. I have put some patients on to metronidazole therapy because of the report that it may affect for instance bacteroides, and some of the patients in whom we have not found *Giardia lamblia* in faeces or biopsy have apparently improved with the treatment, so I am concerned with the clear identity of these phenomena.

Rosen: I think any pathologist used to these things can tell the difference. There is an age difference distribution of *Giardia lamblia*. What were the ages of your patients? That could explain the difference.

Soothill: These were mainly children aged 4–14 years.

Booth: Can we ask the parasite immunologists why these patients should specifically get this parasitic infection and nothing else?

Ogilvie: Nothing is known. The only intestinal protozoan parasites that have been studied in any detail immunologically are the coccidea.

Booth: Is it fair to say that *Giardia* is a more anaerobic parasite than any other?

Ogilvie: I don't think one can answer that.

Davies: Is this parasite causing any harm, or is it just there?

Rosen: You can get a sprue-like syndrome from it—malabsorption, diarrhoea, weight loss and steatorrhoea. If you treat with metronidazole or atabrine all these symptoms disappear.

Evans: Does the bowel recover as well?

Rosen: The villous flattening is not commonly seen but when it is, it goes away with the treatment.

Ferguson: We have evidence that the enteropathy associated with *Giardia* infection is due to the immune response, and I shall touch on this point later (p. 315). In normal people there probably is an immune response to *Giardia* which involves both antibodies and T cells. In hypogammaglobulinaemic individuals, the blocking or modulating properties of antibody will be absent, thus allowing enhanced or excessive T cell response and T cell-induced enteropathy. We have seen this in an antibody-deficient mouse model. *Giardia* infection has measurable but small effects on mucosal architecture in normal mice, but in antibody-deficient animals, giardiasis causes villous atrophy and crypt hyperplasia (A. Ferguson, G. Paul & T. T. MacDonald, unpublished 1976).

Davies: In that case if you treated the T cells, presumably the disease would also be cured.

Rosen: That would be rather drastic, however.

Davies: You are using Flagyl, an imidazole compound which is almost certainly active against lymphocytes as well as against the parasite. One has no real precedent for treating a parasitic infection in an immunosuppressed patient.

Brandtzaeg: Is there any information on T cell function in coeliac disease patients with selective IgA deficiency?

Rosen: I am not aware of any information.

Bienenstock: Ogra *et al.* (1975) have described a recent and retrospective study of cot death and an apparent deficiency of secretory component, and other cases have been reported (Strober *et al.* 1976). They are not all the same diseases, but one can't leave the subject of immunodeficiency without considering secretory component deficiency.

Rosen: Strober's case, which presented clinically with *Monilia* enteritis, had a normal serum IgA level, a low number of IgA-bearing cells or synthesizing cells in the gut, and a very small amount of secretory IgM, which is relevant to the earlier discussion of the role of secretory piece and the homing of B cells. Dr Brandtzaeg raised some valid objections to that report, since no biosynthetic studies had been done of secretory piece (p. 101).

Soothill: The terms cot death, or sudden infant death syndrome, describe the children who die suddenly in the first year of life from no clear cause, a surprisingly frequent event. There is doubt whether this is a disease, or a syndrome. It has been suggested that it is an immunopathological phenomenon. Such evidence includes the work of Robin Coombs and Mavis Gunther on the high incidence of anti-cow's milk antibody in the children (Parish *et al.* 1960). Ogra *et al.* (1975) reported that post-mortem tracheal washings and immunofluorescence studies of the bronchial mucus membrane were deficient either in secretory IgA deficiency or in secretory piece, or both. I believe that others have looked in a similar way and not found this.

Bienenstock: The important point was that Ogra suggested, on the basis of immunofluorescent studies of the presence of anti-viral antibody, that respiratory syncytial virus antigen was present in those patients, and that perhaps the defence mechanisms of the mucosa had allowed another antigen in, and that was the cause of the sudden death.

Soothill: The observation of viral antigens, especially RSV, is a confirmation of the work of Gardiner (1974) in the UK, who supplied Ogra with the antisera. How it links with the possible secretory piece deficiency and IgA deficiency is not yet clear.

Lachmann: I think it is fair to say that there are still as many hypotheses about the aetiology of cot deaths as there are groups working on it!

Bienenstock: I am simply interested in the question of secretory component in immunodeficiency, because therein would lie clues to the functioning of IgA at the mucosal surface.

Brandtzaeg: There was a comment in *The Lancet* on Ogra's report by Williams *et al.* (1976). They made salivary gland extracts from ten cot death patients. They found secretory component in all of them. Incidentally, virus infection of the glandular epithelium may reduce secretory component synthesis. Ogra's finding might be secondary to the effects of a virus infection. With regard to Strober's report, another similar case was published by the same group describing a 52-year-old male, as I discussed (p. 101), but in both cases neither immunofluorescence nor synthetic studies of secretory component were made. However, a finding in both these patients was a 20-fold increase of the IgM level in the intestinal secretions. This was not commented on by the authors. It seems similar to what happens in selective IgA deficiency. Perhaps there was a true glandular secretion of IgM with bound secretory component. This possibility was apparently not investigated.

Soothill: Turner *et al.* (1975) reported raised IgE levels and IgE antibodies to dermatophagoides and other inhaled antigens in a group of children who died suddenly. Buried in their data was the fact that they were also IgA deficient in a way absolutely superimposable on the data in our prospective study of the development of allergy. This has encouraged me to believe that there is some truth in the idea of immunodeficiency underlying sudden death in infancy, but allergy and susceptibility to viral infection may both be independent effects of immunodeficiency, and which causes the death is still not clear (Turner & Soothill 1975). I have more confidence in Turner's information than in many other reports because it was a large series systematically run. We are running a comparable series in the UK at the moment.

Seligmann: Are there any documented cases where there is lack of or an extremely low level of secretory IgA with normal or almost normal serum

IgA? Since it has been claimed that such a situation can occur, some of you may have seen such cases.

As a comment, you can see intestinal nodular hyperplasia in patients with selective IgA deficiency, which is interesting in respect of the way IgA-committed cells home into Peyer's patches.

Rosen: I have not seen any cases of absent secretory IgA with serum IgA present, but this has been reported. IgA-deficient patients have B cells bearing surface IgA.

André: A young man studied by Dr J. P. Revillard and myself in Lyons was completely agammaglobulinaemic. When we used immunofluorescence to look for plasma cells in his bone marrow, we found absolutely no plasma cells; there were some in the lamina propria. He doesn't secrete any immunoglobulin in saliva or in intestinal secretions.

Pepys: Both we (M. B. Pepys & A. C. Dash, unpublished work) and others (Broom *et al.* 1975) have made the same observation in a number of patients with common variable immunodeficiency, some of whom have low levels of immunoglobulin in the serum and secretions, but have apparently normal staining of populations of plasma cells in the lamina propria. So they have immunoglobulin-containing plasma cells which don't seem to secrete, at least at the same rate as in normal individuals.

Booth: There seem to be several types of selective IgA deficiency. There are some with no IgA cells. The more common type seems to have just a few. In other cases there is an antibody to the IgA and the IgA-secreting cells are normal.

Brandtzaeg: Savilahti (1973) showed a relationship between serum IgA levels and secretory IgA cells in the lamina propria. He found that serum IgA levels have to be less than 20% of normal before there is a change in the intestinal immunocyte population. The best sign of what is happening there is that the proportion of IgM cells increases. With regard to the immunoglobulin-secreting cells in the lamina propria of hypogammaglobulinaemic patients, Dr Pepys, when you say that there sometimes are apparently normal cell populations do you mean numerically normal?

Pepys: We have not counted, but we have a number of patients with common variable immunodeficiency, low serum immunoglobulin levels and normal-looking lamina propria plasma cell populations.

Ferguson: McClelland *et al.* (1976) have compared immunoglobulin synthesis by *in vitro* cultured intestinal biopsies and the numbers of plasma cells detected by immunofluorescence in the same specimens. They studied patients with hypogammaglobulinaemia and found considerably more immunoglobulin synthesis by biopsy fragments than would be anticipated from the numbers of immunoglobulin-containing cells there. They suggest that some of the intestinal lymphoid cells can synthesize but cannot secrete or store immunoglobulins.

References

BROOM, B. C., DE LA CONCHA, E. G., WEBSTER, A. D. B., LOEWI, G. & ASHERSON, G. L. (1975) Dichotomy between immunoglobulin synthesis by cells in gut and blood of patients with hypogammaglobulinaemia. *Lancet 2*, 253-256

GARDINER, P. S. (1974) The role of viruses in SIDS, in *SIDS 1974* (Robinson, R. R., ed.), Canadian Foundation for Study of Infant Deaths

HUSBAND, A. J. & MCDOWELL, G. H. (1975) Local and systemic immune responses following oral immunisation of foetal lambs. *Immunology 29*, 1019-1028

LEWKONIA, R. M., GAIRDNER, D. & DOE, W. F. (1976) IgA deficiency in one of identical twins. *Br. Med. J. 1*, 311-313

MCCLELLAND, D. B. L., SHEARMAN, D. J. C. & VAN FURTH, R. (1976) Synthesis of immunoglobulin and secretory component by gastrointestinal mucosa in patients with hypogammaglobulinaemia or IgA deficiency. *Clin. Exp. Immunol. 25*, 103-111

MATSUMURA, T. (1962) Studies on bacterial cross allergic reaction as the basis of natural sensitization by intestinal flora. *Gunma J. Med. Sci. 11*, 4

OGRA, P. L., OGRA, S. S. & COPPOLA, P. R. (1975) Secretory component and sudden-infant-death syndrome. *Lancet 2*, 387-390

PARISH, W. E., BARRETT, A. M., COOMBS, R. R. A., GUNTHER, M. & CAMPS, F. E. (1960) Hypersensitivity to milk and sudden death in infancy. *Lancet 2*, 1106

SAVILAHTI, E. (1974) *See* Workshop on secretory immunoglobulins, in *Progress in Immunology II*, vol. 1 (Brent, L. & Holborow, J., eds.), pp. 238-243, North-Holland, Amsterdam

STROBER, W., KRAKAUER, R., KLAEVEMAN, H. L., REYNOLDS, H. Y. & NELSON, D. L. (1976) Secretory component deficiency: a disorder of the IgA immune system. *N. Engl. J. Med. 294*, 351-356

TURNER, K. J. & SOOTHILL, J. F. (1975) Sudden-infant-death syndrome and immunodeficiency. *Lancet 2*, 917

TURNER, K. J., BALDO, B. A. & HILTON, J. M. N. (1975) IgE antibodies to *D. pteronyssinus. Asp. fumigatus* and β-lactoglobulin in sudden infant death syndrome. *Br. Med. J. 1*, 357

VAN LOGHEM, E. (1974) Familial occurrence of isolated IgA deficiency associated with antibodies to IgA. Evidence against a structural gene defect. *Eur. J. Immunol. 4*, 57-60

WILLIAMS, A. L., HOSKING, C. S. & WAKEFIELD, E. (1976) Secretory component and sudden infant death. *Lancet 1*, 485-486

Immunobiology and pathogenesis of alpha chain disease

MAXIME SELIGMANN

Laboratory of Immunochemistry and Immunopathology (INSERM U 108), Research Institute on Blood Diseases, Hôpital Saint-Louis, Paris

Abstract Alpha chain disease, the most frequent of the heavy chain diseases, is a proliferative disorder of B lymphoid cells involving primarily the small intestine and mesenteric nodes. The characteristic immunoglobulin, whose detection by immunochemical techniques may present some difficulties, consists of incomplete α chains devoid of light chains. The deleted portion of the α chain is located in the Fd segment and involves both the variable and first constant domains. In both of two proteins for which structural data are available, normal sequence resumes at the beginning of the hinge region. The absence of L chains is due to a failure of synthesis. Alpha chain disease appears to proceed in two stages. The early stage is characterized by a possibly non-malignant diffuse and extensive plasma cell infiltration which may be reversible after administration of antibiotics. The later stage is characterized by overt neoplasia (immunoblastic lymphoma). The socio-geographic distribution of the digestive form of alpha chain disease shows a clear predilection for underprivileged populations living in areas with a high degree of infestation by intestinal pathogens which play presumably a crucial role in the pathogenesis of the disease.

Alpha chain disease is a proliferative disorder of B lymphoid cells affecting mainly young patients and involving primarily the IgA secretory system, in which plasma cells produce a population of immunoglobulin (Ig) molecules consisting of incomplete α chains devoid of light chains. Since the first description of this new immunoglobulin abnormality (Seligmann *et al.* 1968) in a young Syrian patient affected with malabsorption and diffuse plasmacytic infiltration of the small intestine (Rambaud *et al.* 1968), more than 100 cases have been recognized to our knowledge. Alpha chain disease is thus the most frequent of the heavy chain diseases. In three of these patients alpha chain disease was apparently confined to the respiratory tract (Stoop *et al.* 1971; Faux *et al.* 1973; Florin-Christensen *et al.* 1974). All the other patients were affected with the digestive form of the disease which is mainly localized in the small intestine and the mesenteric lymph nodes. We wish to discuss here some of the basic problems raised by this condition, many of which are closely related to the subject of this symposium.

The main methods used for the immunochemical (Seligmann et al. 1969, 1971), cellular (Seligmann et al. 1969; Buxbaum & Preud'homme 1972) and structural (Wolfenstein-Todel et al. 1974) studies have been previously described in detail.

NATURE OF IMMUNOGLOBULIN ABNORMALITY

The diagnosis of alpha chain disease (α-CD) relies entirely upon the detection of the pathological protein. In half of the 80 cases studied in our laboratory, the α-CD protein was not noticeable on the serum electrophoregram. When detectable by electrophoresis, it showed an abnormal broad band usually in the $\alpha 2$ or β region. The diagnosis is usually suspected or established by the immunoelectrophoretic analysis of the serum of these patients. In many cases the protein abnormality has escaped detection by routine immunoelectrophoresis using polyvalent antiserum to normal human serum, and analysis with monospecific antisera to IgA is essential. The abnormal component usually gives an abnormal precipitin line either extending from the $\alpha 1$ globulins to the slow $\beta 2$ region or showing a faster electrophoretic mobility than normal IgA. However, in a few patients the α-CD protein had a slow electrophoretic mobility. The anomalous component does not of course precipitate with antisera to light chains. It should however be emphasized that this lack of precipitation with anti-κ and anti-λ antisera is not a sufficient criterion for the diagnosis of α-CD since a number of IgA myeloma proteins, even though they contained light chains (mainly λ chains), failed to precipitate with most such antisera. We have found that selected antisera to IgA which contain antibodies related to the conformational specificity of the Fab region—i.e. precipitating only with α- and light chains combined—are very useful for the diagnosis of α-CD by immunoelectrophoresis or the Ouchterlony technique. The immunoselection plate method of Rádl has also been used (Doe et al. 1972). In all doubtful cases the pathological protein should be purified, reduced and alkylated, and the lack of light chains should be demonstrated directly.

The striking and unexpected electrophoretic heterogeneity of these presumably monoclonal α-CD proteins is certainly due in part to the heterogeneity of their N-terminal sequences, as discussed below. It may also be related to two other features, the high carbohydrate content of most α-CD proteins and their high tendency to polymerize. Indeed on ultracentrifugation α-CD proteins appear to consist of dimers with a 3-4S sedimentation constant and, in most instances, of larger polymers of various sizes. J chain was found in all purified α-CD proteins so far studied.

The concentration of the α-CD protein in the urine is usually very low. In most patients, however, it could be detected in concentrated urine and had the same electrophoretic and immunochemical characteristics as that in the serum. Bence-Jones proteinuria was never found. The pathological protein was also found in significant amounts in jejunal fluid, in patients with the digestive form of the disease, as expected from the involvement of the intestine, whereas the secretory IgA in the parotid saliva of these patients was normal.

The serum levels of normal IgA, IgG and IgM molecules are usually depressed. These decreases are not solely due to a protein-losing enteropathy, as shown by the disproportionate depression of serum Ig levels relative to the serum albumin concentration. Deficiencies of humoral immunity as well as cellular immunity have been demonstrated in a few patients. No functional tests of the secretory immune system have been performed in these patients to our knowledge.

The molecular weight of the monomeric polypeptide subunit of various α-CD proteins was found to vary between 29 000 and 34 000. The length of these chains is thus more than half but less than three-quarters of that of normal α1 heavy chains. Antigenic analysis and chemical studies indicated that the entire Fc fragment was present in α-CD proteins, that their C-terminus was identical with that of normal α1 chains and that the heavy-light peptide was missing. The hinge region was shown to be present in all eight proteins so far studied. In view of these results and of the molecular weight data, the missing portion of the chain is located in the Fd segment and involves both the V_H and C_1 regions.

The N-terminal sequences of several α-CD proteins were shown to be heterogeneous. Even for those proteins with a single N-terminal amino acid, marked heterogeneity became apparent after two steps in degradation. Attempts to obtain the N-terminal sequence on an automated sequencer were unsuccessful. The N-terminal residues were different from those found in any of the subgroups of the variable regions of normal heavy chains. The most likely explanation of this heterogeneity is that it is the consequence of a limited intracellular proteolysis occurring after synthesis. The fact that the N-terminal residues found in the seven proteins studied were valine and/or isoleucine suggests that the degradation stops at this level for some reason, which could possibly be enzyme specificity, steric hindrance or the presence of a carbohydrate moiety. An analogous limited intracellular post-synthetic proteolysis of the NH2-terminus of an incomplete protein has been described for a non-sense mutant of alkaline phosphatase produced by *Escherichia coli* (Natori & Garen 1970).

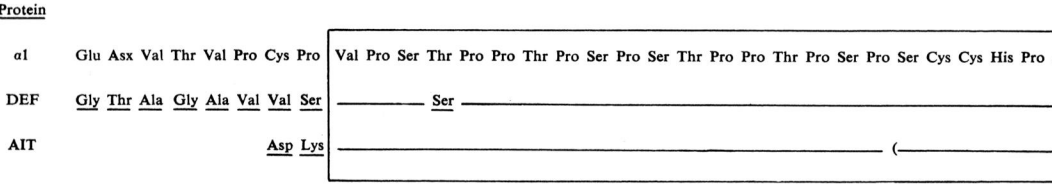

FIG. 1. Comparison of the hinge region of a myeloma α1 chain and of α-CD proteins DEF and AIT. Identical residues are in the box. Non-homologous residues are underlined. Line in the box indicates the sequence identical to that shown in the top peptide. (From Wolfenstein et al. 1975).

The demonstration of a large internal deletion in a γ-heavy chain disease protein (Frangione & Milstein 1969) led us to postulate that in α-CD we were dealing with a similar primary deletion followed and obscured by a secondary limited proteolysis (Seligmann et al. 1971). This hypothesis has been supported to some extent by biosynthetic and structural studies but has not yet been completely proved. Structural studies were performed in Dr Franklin's laboratory and in our laboratory on two α-CD proteins, DEF and AIT (Wolfenstein-Todel et al. 1974, 1975). The amino acid sequence of the hinge region of these two proteins, compared with that of a normal α1 chain, is shown in Fig. 1. Normal synthesis resumes in both proteins at a valine residue in the hinge region just preceding a segment which contains a partially duplicated fragment and the inter-heavy chain disulphide bonds. Starting with this valine residue at position 9, and with the exception of a substitution of threonine for serine at residue 12 of protein DEF, the sequence is completely identical to that of a normal α1 chain. It is of interest that this valine residue at position 9 of this tryptic hinge peptide could represent the counterpart of glutamine at position 216 of γ chains, the site where normal synthesis resumes in several γ-CD proteins with internal deletions (Frangione & Franklin 1973; Franklin & Frangione 1975). Fig. 1 indicates that the first eight residues of the tryptic peptide of protein DEF and the first two residues of the peptide of protein AIT differ from the sequence which normally precedes the valine in α1 chains. These short segments were thought to correspond to the variable region. If this assumption proves to be correct, the primary defect in these α-CD proteins would be an internal deletion encompassing most of the V_H and C_{H1} domains. It is, however, not excluded that the segment preceding the valine which marks the beginning of the normal sequence is not a portion of the normal V region but rather corresponds to an unusual repair of broken DNA or to a non-cleaved polypeptide (? precursor; ? viral genome). It appears therefore essential to obtain N-terminal sequences of several α-CD proteins, despite the heterogeneity which precluded success in previous attempts.

All 60 α-CD proteins which have been typed so far in our laboratory belong to the α1 subclass. The absence of a single case of α2 heavy chain disease in this series is probably not accidental since 10% of the normal serum IgA and 30% of the normal secretory IgA molecules belong to the α2 subclass (Grey *et al.* 1968). The fact that all the molecules of α-CD protein in a given patient belong to only one IgA subclass and the finding of a single amino acid substitution in position 12 of protein DEF (Fig. 1) (which could however possibly represent an allotypic difference) strongly suggest that α-CD proteins are monoclonal. However, this assumption cannot be confirmed because an essential criterion for monoclonality, namely structural homogeneity of the variable region, could not be demonstrated. All attempts to raise individually specific ('idiotypic') antibodies to several α-CD proteins have failed in our laboratory.

CELLULAR STUDIES

Cultures of jejunal biopsy specimens from α-CD patients in medium containing ^{14}C-labelled amino acids have established that the α-CD protein is synthesized *in vitro* by the proliferating cells. Radio-immunoelectrophoretic analysis of protein synthesized *in vitro* by cells teased from mesenteric nodes also demonstrated the production of labelled α-CD proteins. Immunofluorescent studies of intestinal mucosa and mesenteric nodes revealed variable and sometimes weak staining in the cytoplasm of cells composing the cellular infiltrate. No membrane-bound immunoglobulin was usually detectable on the surface of α-CD protein-synthesizing cells.

Biosynthetic studies with *in vitro* labelling excluded the possibility of the synthesis of a normal-size α chain followed by intracellular degradation to a smaller fragment after its release from the ribosomes (Buxbaum & Preud'homme 1972).

Immunofluorescent studies failed to detect any light chain production in the cells which secrete α-CD proteins. No free labelled light chains were found at radio-immunoelectrophoretic analysis of proteins synthesized *in vitro* by intestinal or mesenteric node proliferating cells. This failure of light chain synthesis has been confirmed by biosynthetic studies of nascent Ig subunits in such patients. The possibility remains, however, that the light chain is transcribed but not translated. Studies looking for the presence or absence of its messenger are warranted, since Cowan *et al.* (1974) have detected an inactive light chain messenger RNA in a non-secreting variant of a mouse myeloma which contained an abnormally short heavy chain and failed to synthesize light chain.

NATURAL HISTORY OF ALPHA CHAIN DISEASE

The natural history of α-CD is probably of utmost importance but is not yet fully elucidated. Its spontaneous course may be continuous but often proceeds as exacerbations separated by more or less complete and prolonged improvements. The main clinical features of the digestive form of α-CD are markedly uniform: severe malabsorption syndrome, chronic diarrhoea with steatorrhoea, abdominal pains, vomiting, massive loss of weight, finger clubbing.

The most important characteristic of α-CD is that the disease appears to proceed in two stages. The early stage is characterized by a diffuse and extensive plasma cell infiltration of the entire length of the small intestine, particularly in the upper part. Multiple biopsies taken during laparotomy or with a peroral capsule show a massive infiltration of the lamina propria by round cells which belong mostly to the plasma cell series, as confirmed by electron microscopy. The plasma cell infiltration causes wide separation and sparsity of the crypts and obliteration of the villous architecture without significant impairment of the integrity of the surface epithelium. In some instances the infiltrate extends to the deep submucosa. Mesenteric lymph nodes very often show the same cellular infiltrate which may lead to an obliteration of the normal architecture. In the absence of therapy, there is progressive deterioration usually culminating in frank malignancy with immunoblastic tumours which may lead to obstruction, intussusception or perforation of the small intestine. The lymphoma cells may form single or multiple circumscribed tumours. In some of these cases, the characteristic plasma cell infiltration of α-CD might not be recognized if intestinal biopsies were not performed at a site distant from the tumours. Noticeably, at any stage of the growth of the lymphoma, mesenteric lymph nodes show usually a higher degree of malignancy than the intestinal wall.

Patients with well-documented initial status and adequate long-term follow-up are still scarce. In two patients who were regularly followed in Paris until death, it was possible to observe the progressive passage from the mature plasmacytic proliferation of α-CD to overt malignant lymphomas (Bognel et al. 1972; Galian et al. 1977). Foci of large malignant cells first appeared in the deep mucosa and submucosa of the gut and all transitional forms between these cells and the plasma cells were observed.

Alpha chain disease is clearly a disease of the gut-associated lymphoid system. The extensive plasma cell infiltration almost always remains confined to the enteromesenteric area. Involvement of the large intestine or stomach is rare. Hepatosplenomegaly is usually not observed. Peripheral lymphadenopathy is a very rare sign. Abdominal lymphangiography may reveal in some patients an involvement of the retroperitoneal lymph nodes. Even at the second stage, dissemination of the immunoblastic tumours outside the abdomen is a rare and late event of the disease.

Whether the plasmacytic phase of α-CD is 'pre-malignant' is open to question. The hypothesis of a benign process seems unlikely in those patients with high and rising serum levels of the pathological protein, if its monoclonal nature is confirmed. This explanation is also unlikely when the plasma cell proliferation penetrates deeply into the submucosa and possibly muscularis propria, or completely disorganizes the architecture of the mesenteric nodes and shows atypical forms with an admixture of large 'immunoblastic' cells. This pleomorphic invasive proliferation probably represents the early stage of the malignant lymphoma. However, in most cases, the plasma cells of the infiltrate appear to be mature, well-differentiated with scarce mitoses. This does not necessarily militate against malignancy since in other malignant lymphoproliferative disorders such as chronic lymphocytic leukaemia and Waldenström's macroglobulinaemia the proliferating cells are normal in appearance. Karyotypic studies of plasma cells taken from the intestinal infiltrate during the 'benign' phase may help to resolve this question. The truly benign nature of α-CD at its initial stage is a real possibility since apparently complete remission of the disease was achieved in several patients treated only with oral antibiotics (Rogé et al. 1970; Monges et al. 1975; Rambaud et al. 1976; B. Ramot, personal communication). Disappearance of the α-CD protein from the serum and intestinal fluid was noted in these patients together with a normal histological appearance and negative immunofluorescent studies. It should be emphasized that in one of these patients (Rogé et al. 1970) the complete remission had lasted for six years after withdrawal of the antibiotic therapy. It is also noteworthy that, in the three published cases, the initial serum level of α-CD protein was relatively low.

The overt malignant tumours which arise in the late course of α-CD were first classified as reticulum cell sarcoma or Hodgkin's disease. According to the present views of the pathologists, they should be considered as large cell 'immunoblastic' lymphomas. Several lines of evidence suggest that, if we assume that the plasmacytic proliferation of α-CD is monoclonal in nature, these large lymphomatous cells may be derived from the same B cell clone as the initial plasma cell proliferation. The two types of proliferation can be seen intermingled in the lymph nodes and in the gut (Bognel et al. 1972). Rough endoplasmic reticulum may be found by electron microscopy in the apparently poorly differentiated malignant cells (Doe 1975). All transitional forms between the large undifferentiated malignant cells and the mature plasma cells may be found in some patients. Intracytoplasmic α-CD protein may be undetectable by immunofluorescence in the most malignant and undifferentiated cells (Bognel et al. 1972). However, α-CD protein has been identified in one patient in the perinuclear cisternae of the large lymphomatous cells found in the bone marrow (F. Reyes, personal communication). Furthermore, the study of membrane-bound immunoglobulins has provided conclusive evidence that the sarcomatous cells of morphologically similar lymphomas arising in two other immunoproliferative disorders, namely chronic lymphocytic leukaemia and Waldenström's macroglobulinaemia, originate from the same clone as the previous lymphoid proliferation (Brouet et al. 1975). Alpha chains were recently found in our laboratory on the surface of large lymphoma cells in one patient with α-CD.

The typical clinicopathological pattern of the intestinal form of α-CD may be associated with unusual immunoglobulin findings. In two patients, an entire IgA myeloma globulin was found in the serum and Bence-Jones protein was present in the urine of one of these cases (Chantar et al. 1974; Tangun et al. 1975). In another young girl who was under the care of Dr Stephen Bender in Frankfurt and who presented with the typical clinicopathological features of intestinal α-CD, we demonstrated a γ-heavy chain disease protein in the serum and in the intestinal biopsy. In a few patients with the usual clinicopathological pattern, we have been unable to detect the α-CD protein in the serum. Such a failure may reflect the insensitivity of the techniques used or the advanced undifferentiated stage of the malignancy. Careful prospective studies should include a systematic search for the abnormal protein in jejunal fluid and, in negative cases, at the intracellular level by immunofluorescence and biosynthetic studies, since non-secretory forms of α-CD may exist and immediate degradation of the incomplete α chain may occur. Such a study is necessary in order to establish whether the majority, if not all, cases of so-called 'Mediterranean lymphoma' represent the late malignant phase of α-CD. These Mediterranean lymphomas—that is, diffuse primary intestinal lymphoma associated with malabsorption and occurring in underprivileged young patients—were first reported in Israel (Ramot et al. 1965; Eidelman et al. 1966). These initial reports did not include immunoglobulin studies. A retrospective pathological study (Rappaport et al. 1972) revealed that the majority of these lymphomas begin as an apparently benign infiltration of the small intestine by plasma cells. Our hypothesis (Seligmann & Rambaud 1969) that many of these lymphomas are in fact α-CD, provided their definition is restricted to cases showing a diffuse plasma cell proliferation with or without superimposed sarcoma, has been confirmed by the study of serum immunoglobulins in numerous such patients.

PATHOGENESIS

TABLE 1

Geographic origin of 100 patients with alpha chain disease

Africa		South America	
Tunisia	20	Columbia	1
Algeria	18	North Argentina	1
South Africa	2	Mexico	1
Morocco	1	Europe	
Middle East		Spain	9
Iran	10	South Italy	5
Israel	8	Turkey	6
Lebanon	2	Yugoslavia	2
Syria	1	Greece	2
Libya	1	Portugal	1
Iraq	1	Finland	1
Far East		Netherlands	1*
Pakistan	2	Great Britain	1*
Cambodia	1	North America	
India	1	USA	1*

* Respiratory forms of the disease.

The geographic distribution of α-CD patients is very peculiar (Table 1). There now appears to be a wide spectrum of racial or ethnic origins and cases have been found in many parts of the world. It should be emphasized that the patients from the Netherlands, Great Britain and United States were those with the respiratory form of the disease and without detectable intestinal involvement. The digestive form of the disease appears to be extremely rare in western 'developed' nations and there is a clear predilection for underprivileged populations. These findings suggest that environmental factors providing a local and protracted antigenic stimulation may play an important role in its pathogenesis (Seligmann et al. 1971). One common factor among susceptible populations of various ethnic origins is their exposure to an environment of poor hygiene in areas with a high degree of infestation by intestinal pathogens. Studies conducted in affected populations have shown that chronic gastrointestinal infection and diarrhoea are common and serial intestinal biopsies in healthy people have shown an increased lymphocytic and plasma cell infiltration within the lamina propria of the small bowel. Since orally ingested microorganisms are known to be a powerful proliferative stimulus to the secretory IgA system, the early phase of α-CD could represent an aberrant humoral immune response following sustained topical antigenic stimulation of the intestinal mucosa. The specific or non-specific nature of the postulated stimulating microorganisms is open to question. Limited bacteriological, parasitological and virological studies have not revealed evidence for a specific agent associated with α-CD. However, the postulated antigenic stimulation may have occurred many years before α-CD became clinically manifest. The clinical onset of the disease has occurred in some patients more than ten years after withdrawal from the environmental factors. Microorganisms involved in the pathogenesis of α-CD may be present only during infancy or childhood and absent in identifiable form years later at the time of diagnosis. Unfortunately, the absence of Fab in α-CD protein precludes its use for identifying putative antigenic stimuli. These environmental factors could trigger the clonal proliferation directly. Alternatively, they may only be predisposing factors causing a non-specific stimulation of immunocytes which could potentiate the oncogenic effect of a virus interfering with genes controlling IgA synthesis (Rambaud & Matuchansky 1973).

The postulated environmental antigenic stimulus might be associated with an underlying immunodeficiency. This could be a defect rendering the host more susceptible to infection with oncogenic organisms or a basic defect of the feedback mechanisms controlling the cellular proliferative response to stimulation. Immunodeficiency could be due to malnutrition, especially in early infancy, or to genetic factors. In fact, the role of environmental factors does not exclude the possibility of predisposing genetic factors. Although limited family studies have failed to reveal consistent Ig abnormalities, a search for genetic markers may help to identify predisposed subjects. Raised serum levels of the intestinal iso-enzyme of alkaline phosphatase were reported in patients with α-CD and Mediterranean lymphoma and in their healthy relatives (Ramot & Streifler 1966; Doe et al. 1972; Lewin et al. 1976).

It is remarkable that the plasma cell proliferation resulting from the postulated antigen stimulation appears to lead to α-CD rather than to myeloma. This fact suggests the following hypotheses (WHO Meeting Report 1976). An abnormal B cell clone synthesizing the α-CD protein could be produced in the gut through a series of recombinant events during embryogenesis. Another possibility is that a somatic mutational event gives rise to a cell producing the α-CD protein, permitting it to enter the gut-associated lymphoid system and to home into the lamina propria. In either case, the abnormal clone would overgrow in abnormal microenvironmental situations and could for instance be susceptible to the proliferative stimulus of bacterial lipopolysaccharide in the intestinal lumen. In addition, the abnormal clone could have a selective advantage for proliferation because of the lack of antibody activity of its immunoglobulin product, possibly resulting in the suppression of a feedback mechanism.

Alpha chain disease is characterized by a continuous sequence of events ranging from an apparently benign hyperplastic process reversible by the administration of antibiotics to an overt neoplastic proliferation. The elucidation of this sequence of events, as well as continued structural and cellular studies, may offer a revealing insight into the development of lymphomas in the gut-associated lymphoid system.

ACKNOWLEDGEMENTS

I am grateful to Mrs Edith Mihaesco and Drs Françoise Danon and Jean-Louis Preud'-homme for their important contribution to the study of alpha chain disease in our laboratory and to Drs Jean-Claude Rambaud, Michael Potter and Blas Frangione for helpful discussions.

References

BOGNEL, J. C., RAMBAUD, J. C., MODIGLIANI, R., MATUCHANSKY, C., BOGNEL, C., BERNIER, J. J., SCOTTO, J., HAUTEFEUILLE, P., MIHAESCO, E., HUREZ, D., PREUD'HOMME, J. L. & SELIGMANN, M. (1972) Etude clinique, anatomo-pathologique et immunochimique d'un nouveau cas de maladie des chaines alpha suivi depuis cinq ans. *Rev. Eur. Etud. Clin. Biol.* 17, 362-374

BROUET, J. C., LABAUME, S. & SELIGMANN, M. (1975) Evaluation of T and B lymphocyte membrane markers in human non-Hodgkin malignant lymphomas. *Br. J. Cancer 31*, Suppl. II, 121-127

BUXBAUM, J. N. & PREUD'HOMME, J. L. (1972) Alpha and gamma heavy chain diseases in man: intracellular origin of the aberrant polypeptides. *J. Immunol. 109*, 1131-1137

CHANTAR, C., ESCARTIN, P., PLAZA, A. G., CORUGEDO, A. F., ARENAS, J. I., SANZ, E., ANAYA, A., BOOTELLO, A. & SEGOVIA, J. M. (1974) Diffuse plasma cell infiltration of the small intestine with malabsorption associated to IgA monoclonal gammapathy. *Cancer 34*, 1620-1630

COWAN, N. J., SECHER, D. S. & MILSTEIN, C. (1974) Intracellular immunoglobulin chain synthesis in non-secreting variants of a mouse myeloma: detection of inactive light-chain messenger RNA. *J. Mol. Biol. 90*, 691-701

DOE, W. F. (1975) Alpha chain disease. Clinicopathological features and relationship to so-called Mediterranean lymphoma. *Br. J. Cancer 31*, Suppl. II, 350-355

DOE, W. F., HENRY, K., HOBBS, J. R., AVERY JONES, F., DENT, C. E. & BOOTH, C. C. (1972) Five cases of alpha-chain disease. *Gut 13*, 947-957

EIDELMAN, S., PARKINS, A. & RUBIN, C. (1966) Abdominal lymphoma presenting as malabsorption. A clinicopathologic study of 9 cases in Israel and a review of the literature. *Medicine 45*, 111-137

FAUX, J. A., CRAIN, J. D., ROSEN, F. S. & MERLER, E. (1973) An alpha heavy chain abnormality in a child with hypogammaglobulinemia. *Clin. Immunol. Immunopathol. 1*, 282-290

FLORIN-CHRISTENSEN, A., DONIACH, D. & NEWCOMB, P. B. (1974) Alpha chain disease with pulmonary manifestations. *Br. Med. J. 2*, 413-415

FRANGIONE, B. & FRANKLIN, E. C. (1973) Heavy chain diseases: clinical features and molecular significance of the disordered immunoglobulin structure. *Seminars Hematol. 10*, 53-64

FRANGIONE, B. & MILSTEIN, C. (1969) Partial deletion in the heavy chain disease protein ZUC. *Nature (Lond.) 224*, 597-599

FRANKLIN, E. C. & FRANGIONE, B. (1975) Structural variants of human and murine immunoglobulins. *Contemp. Top. Mol. Immunol. 4*, 89-126

GALIAN, A., LECESTRE, M. J., SCOTTO, J., BOGNEL, C., MATUCHANSKY, C. & RAMBAUD, J. C. (1977) Pathological study on alpha chain disease with, special emphasis on evolution. *Cancer*, in press

GREY, H. M., ABEL, C. A., YOUNT, W. J. & KUNKEL, H. G. (1968) A subclass of human γA-globulins (γA2) which lacks the disulfide bonds linking heavy and light chains. *J. Exp. Med. 128*, 1223-1236

LEWIN, K. J., KAHN, L. B. & NOVIS, B. H. (1976) Primary intestinal lymphoma of 'Western' and 'Mediterranean' type, alpha chain disease and massive plasma cell infiltration. A comparative study of 37 cases. *Cancer*, in press

MONGES, H., AUBERT, L., CHAMLIAN, A., REMACLE, J. P., MATHIEU, B., COUGARD, A. & ARROYO, H. (1975) Maladie des chaines alpha à forme intestinale. Présentation d'un cas traité par antibiothérapie avec rémission clinique, histologique et immunologique. *Arch. Fr. Mal. App. Dig. 64*, 223-231

NATORI, S. & GAREN, A. (1970) Molecular heterogeneity in the amino-terminal region of alkaline-phosphatase. *J. Mol. Biol. 49*, 577-588

RAMBAUD, J. C. & MATUCHANSKY, C. (1973) Alpha-chain disease. Pathogenesis and relation to Mediterranean lymphoma. *Lancet 1*, 1430-1432

RAMBAUD, J. C., BOGNEL, C., PROST, A., BERNIER, J. J., LE QUINTREC, Y., LAMBLING, A., DANON, F., HUREZ, D. & SELIGMANN, M. (1968) Clinico-pathological study of a patient with 'Mediterranean' type of abdominal lymphoma and a new type of IgA abnormality ('alpha chain disease'). *Digestion 1*, 321-336

RAMBAUD, J. C., MODIGLIANI, R., GALIAN, A., DANON, F. & BERNIER, J. J. (1976) Rémission complète clinique, histologique et immunologique d'un cas de maladie des chaines alpha traité pendant deux mois par antibiothérapie orale. *Arch. Fr. Mal. App. Dig.*, in press

RAMOT, B. & STREIFLER, C. (1966) Raised serum-alkaline phosphatase. *Lancet 2*, 587

RAMOT, B., SHANIN, N. & BUBIS, J. J. (1965) Malabsorption syndrome in lymphoma of small intestine. *Israel J. Med. Sci. 1*, 221-226

RAPPAPORT, H., RAMOT, B., HULU, N. & PARK, J. K. (1972) The pathology of so-called Mediterranean abdominal lymphoma with malabsorption. *Cancer 29*, 1502-1511

ROGÉ, J., DRUET, P. & MARCHE, C. (1970) Lymphome méditerranéen avec maladie des chaines alpha. Triple rémission clinique, anatomique et immunologique. *Pathol. Biol. 18*, 851-858

SELIGMANN, M. & RAMBAUD, J. C. (1969) IgA abnormalities in abdominal lymphoma (α-chain disease). *Israel J. Med. Sci. 5*, 151-157

SELIGMANN, M., DANON, F., HUREZ, D., MIHAESCO, E. & PREUD'HOMME, J. L. (1968) Alpha chain disease: a new immunoglobulin abnormality. *Science (Wash.) 162*, 1396-1397

SELIGMANN, M., MIHAESCO, E., HUREZ, D., MIHAESCO, C., PREUD'HOMME, J. L. & RAMBAUD, J. C. (1969) Immunochemical studies in four cases of alpha chain disease. *J. Clin. Invest. 48*, 2374-2389

SELIGMANN, M., MIHAESCO, E. & FRANGIONE, B. (1971) Studies on alpha chain disease. *Ann. N.Y. Acad. Sci. 190*, 487-500

STOOP, J. W., BALLIEUX, R. E., HIJMANS, W. & ZEGERS, B. J. M. (1971) Alpha chain disease with involvement of the respiratory tract in a Dutch child. *Clin. Exp. Immunol. 9*, 625-635

TANGUN, Y., SARACBASI, Z., INCEMAN, S., DANON, F. & SELIGMANN, M. (1975) IgA myeloma globulin and Bence-Jones proteinuria in a diffuse plasmacytoma of small intestine. *Ann. Intern. Med. 83*, 673

WHO Meeting Report (1976) Alpha chain disease and small intestinal lymphoma. *Bull. W.H.O.*, in press

WOLFENSTEIN-TODEL, C., MIHAESCO, E. & FRANGIONE, B. (1974) 'Alpha-chain disease' protein Def: internal deletion of a human immunoglobulin A_1 heavy chain. *Proc. Natl Acad. Sci. U.S.A. 71*, 974-978

WOLFENSTEIN-TODEL, C., MIHAESCO, E. & FRANGIONE, B. (1975) Variant of a human immunoglobulin: α chain disease protein AIT. *Biochem. Biophys. Res. Commun. 65*, 47-53

Discussion

Davies: Your Table 1 (p. 271) showing the geographical origin of the cases recorded a number in Algeria. Were they diagnosed in France or in Algeria?

Seligmann: A number were diagnosed in France; subsequently some were diagnosed in Algiers. I went there soon after we found the first cases and retrospectively we found a number of cases there. Interestingly enough, some of these patients were thought to have peritoneal tuberculosis, which is not surprising from the clinical pattern of the disease. Many of the 20 or so cases in Tunis were diagnosed there. When the local clinicians know how to detect the disease, the percentage of cases in which we find the alpha chain disease protein in the sera sent to us becomes very high.

Booth: The geographical distribution is interesting, because the question is whether it is in fact geographical or racial. The vast majority of the cases are from that Mediterranean area in which the Arabs lived at some stage in their history. That applies to Southern Italy, Greece and all the countries you mentioned. The only one that does not fit is Finland. Among the Israeli cases, no case has been recorded in the Ashkenazim. Going further East, I don't know of any case recorded in China, and there is no case yet from Black Africa. If it is an infection or a question of reaction to a recurrent infection, the obvious place to look is Australia among the aborigines, because the incidence of gut infection in children particularly is very high. I have corresponded with Australian friends and no case has yet been found there. So it could be genetic rather than environmental in causation.

In Africa, the cases in Cape Town described by Novis and his colleagues (1971) are interesting. I have seen some of them, and they call them Cape Coloured people. There was a lot of slave trading down that area by the Arabs for a long period and one wonders if Mediterranean blood didn't get mixed in at some stage.

Seligmann: This reminds me of letters I have had from Spain where they say that the patient is pure Spanish without a drop of Arabic blood, which is totally impossible! My guess would be that this disease is probably frequent in Central and South America, which would probably solve the problem of a genetic or geographic correlation. The disease has not been looked for there very much, but in Mexico City when they began to look one case was found very quickly. A similar case has been published from Texas. I should add that one of the cases recently studied in Paris by Rambaud was a French person who was born in Algeria and had lived there for a number of years.

As you say, there is no case from Black Africa, although we asked friends to look carefully for it in Dakar and the Ivory Coast. We hypothesized that if our views on the pathogenesis of alpha chain disease were right, one might expect that in these Black African countries, in view of the kind of parasites common there, you would find μ-chain disease. In fact, two cases of μ-chain disease were found in the Ivory Coast, once I had asked people to look for it (Bonhomme *et al.* 1974; Danon *et al.* 1975). So this is possibly something similar in pathogenesis.

Davies: Your suggestion that because there is a lack of the appropriate Fab fragment, you are failing to get a feedback mechanism operating, is very interesting. It perhaps indicates that if you took normal serum IgA from people in the same area and gave it to the patients, you would get this feedback operating. That is to say, you are presumably missing a particular kind of antibody. Presumably the disease is a rare manifestation of a fairly common infection. If so, you might be able to treat it by simply giving IgA.

Seligmann: This is possible. I agree that treatment in the first stage of the disease in addition to the administration of oral antibiotics may be the proper immunoglobulins, some of them having the right antibody activity. In fact Dr Rosen has told me that in his case of the respiratory form of alpha chain disease in a young boy, the patient is doing well with progressively decreased levels of the alpha chain disease protein. He gave some antibiotics but the main treatment was gammaglobulins.

Rosen: The child no longer has his abnormal α-chain but remains very hypogammaglobulinaemic. He is doing well on replacement therapy.

Booth: On the question of tumours in the gut, one can get intestinal obstruction with big lumps of tissue. The lesson of this meeting has been that these IgA cells must be turning over rapidly. If the half-time of an IgA cell is normally 4.7 days, what is the doubling time or half-time of these cells or tumours in the intestine? Is there a normal circulation going on? I presume there is, because our first case was a patient in whom we found primitive-looking plasma cells in the blood (Doe *et al.* 1972). So presumably there is an enormous circulation. How one maintains that circulation and at the same time develops a tumour big enough to block the intestine baffles me completely.

Gowans: It might be the reverse: perhaps the cells are abnormal and have a long life and that's why accumulations develop.

Seligmann: I have no answer to this question about the lifespan of these cells. In the circulation, in the first stage you don't usually see plasma cells in the blood; in the second malignant stage they may be found. Even in the first stage you may see a few α-chain-containing plasma cells in the marrow (Seligmann *et al.* 1969).

Booth: In myeloma how long do plasma cells survive?

Gowans: Mattioli & Tomasi (1973) studied the lifespan of IgA-secreting cells by giving continuous thymidine infusions to mice. They found a half-life of 4.7 days, although some labelled cells persisted for 7-8 weeks.

White: If you produce plasma cell proliferation in a rabbit by hyperimmunization, three weeks later it's completely back to normal. The plasma cells cannot therefore have a half-life of more than a few days.

Evans: Are the plasma cells that you see in the first stage capable of division, or do they originate from lymphoid precursors which are not obviously plasma cells?

Seligmann: Mitotic figures are rare in the first stage of plasmacytic infiltration in this disease. Divisions are seen more often in the second stage with the tumours. I cannot answer the question more precisely.

Evans: Are the peripheral blood leucocytes normal, in terms of their surface cell markers?

Seligmann: In the few cases where this has been studied they were normal, but I should add that in the few cases where membrane-bound immunoglobulins have been studied in alpha chain disease, no heavy chain was usually detected on the surface of the proliferating cells.

Booth: It is sometimes difficult to demonstrate immunofluorescent staining on the gut containing all these plasma cells.

Seligmann: We often had faint staining for intracytoplasmic α chains (Seligmann *et al.* 1969), but our technique was not as good as that of Dr Brandtzaeg! He tells me that in the case he studied he found bright staining.

Brandtzaeg: We also checked for the J chain, and this is relevant to the secretory IgA system origin of this disease. The J chain is present in the cells although its synthesis seems to be defective.

Booth: Do you find the alpha chain?

Brandtzaeg: Yes, but in the Finnish boy Dr E. Savilahti and I studied the cells seemed to be very immature.

Booth: The Finnish case was predominantly ileal as opposed to jejunal disease, as well as in the large intestine, so this case was somewhat different from those described by Dr Seligmann.

Seligmann: It is interesting that this is the only digestive case recorded in Northern Europe. Earlier (p. 38) it was suggested that the IgA system in the large intestine may be different from that in the small intestine. The Finnish case could be more like the respiratory forms.

Beeson: Would you expand on the antibiotic therapy? Were you aiming at anaerobes or aerobes; what drugs did you use; and did you have any failures?

Seligmann: Treatment is purely empirical. The antibiotics given in cases where remission was complete were usually tetracyclines. In no case so far have antibiotics been given according to the sensitivity to antibiotics of the intestinal flora, if something abnormal was found. The shortest delay between the beginning of treatment and complete remission was 2–3 months and the longest delay to complete remission was one year. As far as I know, the number of patients with well-documented complete remission, including serum studies, biopsies and so on, is four or five so far.

There were some failures. One problem is that many of these patients did not have systematic laparotomy and in my opinion and that of my gastro-enterological colleague, J. C. Rambaud, the first thing you should do in alpha chain disease without overt malignant tumours is a laparotomy and multiple biopsies to ascertain whether the patient is at the stage of purely plasmacytic infiltration or whether there are lymphomatous tumours and immunoblastic proliferation. It is difficult to say that antibiotics have failed in patients who have not undergone systematic laparotomy, because at the sarcomatous stage one would expect antibiotics to fail. The patients with a good follow-up are rare. Many have been studied in countries where a good follow-up is difficult and there are only a few cases, but the data are enough to say that in some patients, who are presumably at the first stage, you can get a complete remission.

Booth: J. C. Rambaud's and your practice of staging seems logical when you compare it with lymphomas.

Brandtzaeg: I don't think we can presume that the cells are different, even though the site of the lesion is. On Dr Davies' suggestion of treating these patients with IgA, I think it must be colostral IgA from the mothers in the geographical region, because this is a defect of the secretory IgA system.

Rosen: Dr Seligmann, is it possible that you haven't detected an IgA2 heavy chain because the chain isn't covalently held together and you may be getting degradation because of the structural anomaly?

Seligmann: This is a possibility which we have suggested, but we have no way to prove or disprove it at present. In fact, cellular studies with antisera specific for subclasses should be done in cases without detectable α-chain protein in the serum.

Cebra: Do any of the structural studies suggest that any part of the V gene message is being translated to give rise to any of your proteins? Since you don't find any surface product representing part of the α chain, and yet you suggest a compartmentalization of these cells, presumably the lodging properties shown by these cells and probably by normal IgA immunoblasts are not attributable to surface IgA? One possibility to explain lodging of IgA cells is that glycosyltransferases that build oligosaccharides onto IgA might be involved in changes in membrane glycoproteins or glycolipids of B cells. Have any of your structural studies concerned the oligosaccharides of these heavy chain proteins?

Seligmann: We have very few data on the variable part of these proteins, since the only sequences we have are eight residues in one case and two residues in the other! These eight residues don't resemble much of what is known in V regions. For this reason, one hypothesis is that it could be something else than the variable region, which could be still more exciting. It could be a precursor or a viral genome or something else. We can't be sure that it is the V region that is defective.

The absence of membrane-bound chains on these cells is not a constant finding. Recently we had a patient in whom α-chains were detected on the surface of large sarcomatous cells for the first time. In our experience, the absence of heavy chains on the membrane of the cells in many but not all cases is common in all kinds of heavy chain diseases. We found the same in some cases of γ- and μ-chain disease. The carbohydrate content of α-chain disease protein is high (Seligmann *et al.* 1971) but the oligosaccharide moiety has not been studied.

Rosen: There must be several of them, to get PAS-positive staining.

Gowans: Are the Peyer's patches hypertrophic in the early stages of the disease, on the assumption that the cells would be originating there?

Seligmann: I have no personal experience here, as very few patients have been studied *post mortem*.

Gowans: At laparotomy, are the patches grossly hypertrophic?

Seligmann: No.

White: When one produces myeloma experimentally by giving a stimulus like paraffin oil, does one ever see this two-stage process? In other words, do you see a stage of diffuse plasma cell infiltration without obvious malignancy, or is it a kind of tumour right from the start?

Seligmann: I have discussed this many times with Mike Potter. The answer is that there is not a long-term 'pre-malignant' phase.

White: The question is whether there is diffuse plasma cell infiltration. It seems you do get this and at one focus you get a neoplasm. That isn't the picture that I have derived from descriptions of experimental myeloma production.

Evans: Human myeloma cases sometimes show diffuse infiltration of marrow; after melphalan treatment such cases may develop soft tissue tumours of morphologically undifferentiated but immunoglobulin-producing cells. This may be comparable with the observations in alpha chain disease.

Seligmann: The situation where you have chronic proliferation of B cells followed by an acute exacerbation with a B cell sarcoma is well known. We know this in chronic lymphocytic leukaemia, with or without treatment, and in macroglobulinaemia. It can also happen in myeloma and heavy chain diseases. So this is usual in the natural history of chronic B cell malignancies. We were able to prove in some such instances that the blastic or sarcoma cells derive from the same clone as the previous chronic malignancy (Brouet *et al.* 1973, 1975), since we found the same Ig chains on both types of cells and the same antibody activity in the membrane-bound immunoglobulins in one case, which is proof of the same variable region. The special point about alpha chain disease is that the first stage may not be truly malignant, as opposed to macroglobulinaemia or chronic lymphatic leukaemia, which are usually viewed as chronic malignant processes.

Lachmann: How does this differ from the so-called benign monoclonal gammopathy which becomes myeloma after a variable period of years?

Seligmann: It differs in any case in the frequency in which malignancy occurs, because in alpha chain disease malignancy would probably occur in most patients after a few years, and this kind of evolution of benign monoclonal gammopathy is documented in very few patients and after a very long time.

Lachmann: In other words, the first stage may be longer than the life of the patient!

Mayrhofer: How does this pattern of events compare to that in those patients with coeliac disease whose illness takes a deteriorating course, eventually leading to development of an IgA-secreting lymphoma?

Seligmann: Our alpha chain disease patients have no past history of anything looking like coeliac disease.

Booth: It is really quite different. The lymphoma in coeliac disease is usually patchy and not a diffuse involvement of the intestine. It can also involve areas other than the gut.

Mayrhofer: Is it often associated with increased IgA levels?

Booth: In some cases but not all.

Mayrhofer: Does the tumour produce the IgA?

Booth: I don't think that's known.

André: Are there any modifications of the intestinal flora in patients with non-malignant alpha chain disease?

Seligmann: This has not been looked for carefully in many patients, but where it has, there has been no important abnormality. The anaerobic flora has not been well studied in many patients.

André: After tetracycline therapy, are there any obvious changes?

Seligmann: This has not been studied systematically yet.

References

BONHOMME, J., SELIGMANN, M., MIHAESCO, C., CLAUVEL, J. P., DANON, F., BROUET, J. C., BOUVRY, P., MARTINE, J. & CLERC, M. (1974) Mu chain disease in an African patient. *Blood* 43, 485-492

BROUET, J. C., PREUD'HOMME, J. L., SELIGMANN, M. & BERNARD, J. (1973) Blast cells with monoclonal surface immunoglobulin in two cases of acute blast crisis supervening on chronic lymphocytic leukaemia. *Br. Med. J. 4*, 23-24

BROUET, J. C., LABAUME, S. & SELIGMANN, M. (1975) Evaluation of T and B lymphocyte membrane markers in human non Hodgkin malignant lymphomas. *Br. J. Cancer 31*, Suppl. II, 121-127

DANON, F., MIHAESCO, C., BOUVRY, M., CLERC, M. & SELIGMANN, M. (1975) A new case of heavy Mu chain disease. *Scand. J. Haematol. 15*, 5-9

DOE, W. F., HENRY, K., HOBBS, J. R., AVERY JONES, F., DENT, C. E. & BOOTH, C. C. (1972) Five cases of alpha-chain disease. *Gut 13*, 947-957

MATTIOLI, C. A. & TOMASI, T. B. (1973) The life span of IgA plasma cells from the mouse intestine. *J. Exp. Med. 138*, 452

NOVIS, B. H., BANKS, S., MARKS, I. N., SELZER, A., KAHN, L. & SEALY, R. (1971) Abdominal lymphoma presenting with malabsorption. *Q. J. Med. 40*, 521-540

SELIGMANN, M., MIHAESCO, E., HUREZ, D., MIHAESCO, C., PREUD'HOMME, J. L. & RAMBAUD, J. C. (1969) Immunochemical studies in four cases of alpha-chain disease. *J. Clin. Invest. 48*, 2374

SELIGMANN, M., MIHAESCO, E. & FRANGIONE, B. (1971) Studies on alpha chain disease. *Ann. N.Y. Acad. Sci. 190*, 487

Immunological studies in inflammatory bowel disease

M. B. PEPYS*, M. DRUGUET, H. J. KLASS, A. C. DASH, D. D. MIRJAH and AVIVA PETRIE

Department of Medicine, Royal Postgraduate Medical School, London

Abstract Three aspects of immunological function were studied in patients with Crohn's disease and ulcerative colitis (inflammatory bowel disease): atopic status and serum IgE levels; serum concentration of C-reactive protein; and C3 activation. The incidence of atopy, assessed by prick testing with common allergens, did not differ in patients with inflammatory bowel disease from healthy controls. 12 of 39 patients with Crohn's disease and 5 of 20 with ulcerative colitis, among whom were some non-atopic subjects, had elevated serum levels of IgE. Serum levels of C-reactive protein in patients were significantly greater than normal, even in those in whom the disease was clinically quiescent. Symptomatic patients with Crohn's disease had significantly higher levels than similar patients with ulcerative colitis and in Crohn's disease the levels correlated well with an overall assessment of severity and disease activity. Although conversion of C3 was detected in fresh serum samples from inflammatory bowel disease patients and not controls, only minimal traces were present in just 7 of 89 samples of EDTA-plasma from 47 patients; this finding did not correlate with disease activity. However, there were low titres of immunoconglutinin in the sera of some patients, but not in controls, suggesting that complement activation may be occurring *in vivo*.

Ulcerative colitis and Crohn's disease are severe, chronic inflammatory conditions of the intestine, the aetiology and pathogenesis of which are unknown. They cause appreciable morbidity and may be fatal, and the incidence of Crohn's disease in England has tripled in the past decade or so (Miller *et al.* 1974). In both conditions the pathology of the lesions includes mononuclear lymphoid cells as well as other features which suggest that immunological mechanisms may be operative. A variety of immunological abnormalities have been described in these patients, but although certain phenomena are generally accepted

---

* *Present address:* Department of Immunology, Royal Free Hospital, Pond Street, London

there remains controversy about others (reviewed in Jewell & Hodgson 1976). It is not possible to formulate a generally acceptable hypothesis of aetiopathogenesis on the basis of existing observations, and all of the immunological findings could be secondary or epiphenomena. Even so, immunological mechanisms might be important in some of the manifestations of disease, and might also help to differentiate between these two conditions in which, despite a considerable clinical overlap, the prognosis and management may be quite different.

We report here the results of studies of three different aspects of immunological function in patients with inflammatory bowel disease.

ATOPIC STATUS AND SERUM IgE LEVELS

Atopy may be considered in immunological terms as a predisposition to respond to common normal environmental antigens by the production of IgE antibodies (Pepys 1975). Abnormal environmental exposure can induce IgE antibody formation in non-atopic individuals (Pepys 1975). Atopic individuals and their atopic status may be identified by prick testing of the skin with extracts of the common, chiefly inhaled, allergens (Pepys 1975). Prick testing is a precise procedure which, if it elicits the characteristic weal and flare reaction, indicates the presence of reaginic antibodies which are generally of IgE class, although short-term mast cell-sensitizing IgG antibodies have also been demonstrated in man (Parish 1970).

There is a strong correlation between atopic status, defined by prick testing, and the occurrence of certain diseases, particularly extrinsic asthma, 'hay-fever' and infantile eczema. IgE antibodies are clearly implicated in the pathogenesis of the first two conditions. Quite apart from these diseases the atopic status of an individual, in terms of this propensity to produce IgE antibody, can modify profoundly the immunological and pathological consequences of abnormal exposure to antigens in the environment (Pepys 1969). Knowledge of the atopic status of patients with diseases of unknown but possibly immunological pathogenesis, such as inflammatory bowel disease, is therefore clearly of interest.

In the present study the atopic status of patients with Crohn's disease and ulcerative colitis was assessed using the following information: past and present history of asthma, 'hay-fever' or non-seasonal rhinitis clearly provoked by an extrinsic agent, and eczema; history of these conditions among first degree relatives; and the results of prick testing with a batch of common allergens (Bencard Ltd, Worthing) (Table 1). The food extracts were included though they are not as a rule helpful in identifying food allergens; no reactions

TABLE 1

Allergens used for prick testing

Grass pollens	Cat fur
Tree pollens	Dog fur
Shrub pollens	
	Milk
Dermatophagoides pteronyssinus	Whole egg
	Fish
Moulds	Wheat
Aspergillus fumigatus	

Allergen extracts were obtained from Bencard Ltd, Worthing.

to them were observed in any patients. Controls who were similarly assessed were matched approximately for age and sex with the patients but were otherwise randomly selected, and were members of the medical, nursing and technical staff of the RPMS. The results are shown in Tables 2 and 3.

Analysis of the results in Table 3 by the χ^2 test demonstrated no significant differences between the three groups. The most meaningful observation is the incidence of one or more positive prick tests, namely about 26% in both disease groups. In large-scale testing of healthy subjects screened pre-employment for evidence of atopy the incidence is of the order of 30% (J. Pepys, personal communication 1976). Our control group had a higher than expected incidence of reactions, 50% giving one or more positive prick test reactions.

The incidence of asthma, 'hay-fever'/rhinitis and eczema was comparable to that reported by Jewell & Truelove (1972), and greater than that observed by Hammer et al. (1968). However, they both found a very low incidence among

TABLE 2

Atopic status in inflammatory bowel disease

Group	Prick tests negative[a]		Prick tests positive[a]					
	No family history of atopy	Family history of atopy	No atopic symptoms[b]			Atopic symptoms[b]		
			1	1-3	>3	1	1-3	>3
Crohn's disease	17	14	2	2	0	1	2	4
Ulcerative colitis	12	7	1	2	0	0	3	1
Controls	9	6	0	3	1	4	2	5

[a] Subjects were prick tested with the allergens shown in Table 1. No individuals with negative prick tests had a history or suffered from asthma, 'hay-fever' or eczema.
[b] Asthma, 'hay-fever' or eczema.

TABLE 3

Atopic status in inflammatory bowel disease

Group (No.)	Positive prick test(s)[a]: atopic symptoms[b]		Positive prick test(s)[a]: total		First degree relatives with history of atopic symptoms[b]		
	No.	%	No.	%	No.	No. at risk	%
Crohn's disease (42)	7	16.7	11	26.2	23	184	12.5
Ulcerative colitis (26)	4	15.4	7	26.9	12	120	10.0
Controls (30)	10	33.3	15	50.0	15	109	13.8

[a] Subjects giving one or more positive prick test reactions with the allergens shown in Table 1.
[b] Asthma, 'hay-fever' or eczema.

controls, including normals and patients with other diseases. It is difficult to ascertain the true incidence of these atopy-associated or allergic diseases in the general population, owing to problems of definition and recognition. There are also differences in methods used in previous surveys and variations in incidence and manifestations with age, social and other factors. Perhaps the best survey is that of Blair (1974), who examined in detail 9145 members of a single general practice and found the incidence of asthma, 'hay-fever' and infantile eczema alone or in any combination to be 7.2%. This would suggest that the incidence in our patients and our controls may be high but the numbers of individuals are relatively small, and for the reasons stated interpretation of this sort of result should be most cautious. The firmest evidence remains the result of prick testing, an objective and well-validated procedure which, contrary to the essentially historical data in other studies of this question, does not support an association between atopy and inflammatory bowel disease.

IgE antibodies are induced under ordinary circumstances by mucosal exposure to antigens, and there is evidence that even transient deficiency of IgA can predispose to reaginic antibody formation (Soothill 1974). One possible mechanism is that impaired IgA responses may modify the mucosal barrier to antigen penetration and permit IgE production to be stimulated. Patients with inflammatory bowel disease have mucosal ulceration which may be expected to allow enhanced penetration of luminal antigens, and it is therefore of some interest to examine their IgE responses. Knowledge of patients' atopic status is essential in these studies for, although total serum IgE levels do not correlate particularly well with severity of clinical allergy in atopic subjects, they do nonetheless tend to be elevated above the very low levels (mean 36.3 units/ml, Nye et al. 1975) found in a strictly non-atopic population.

We measured total serum IgE by the relatively insensitive modified radial

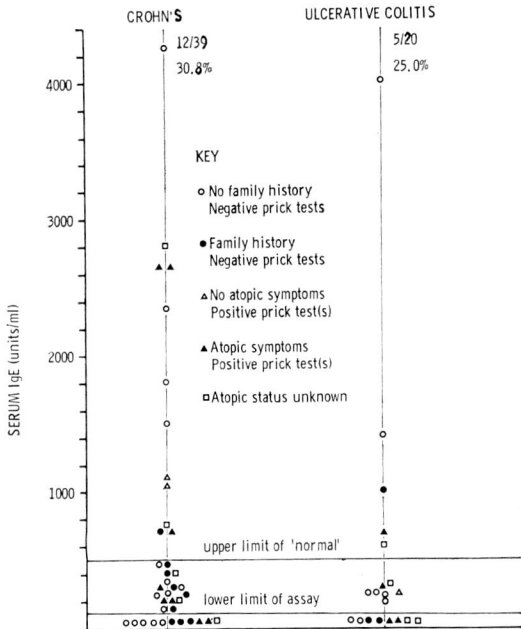

FIG. 1. Serum IgE levels in patients with inflammatory bowel disease. Family history and atopic symptoms refer to asthma, 'hay-fever' and infantile eczema. Prick tests were made with the allergens listed in Table 1. The proportions shown for each group are the patients with IgE levels above normal.

immunodiffusion method (Rowe 1969) which does not detect less than 100 units/ml. The levels among 'normal' individuals, who do not suffer from any clinical allergic symptoms, do not exceed 500 units/ml, shown in Fig. 1 as the upper limit of 'normal'. The present technique was not sufficiently sensitive to provide information about the lower range of IgE values; furthermore, the significance of the values recorded between 100 and 500 units/ml is not clear. These might be more frequent than would be found among healthy strictly non-atopic subjects, but a more discriminating assay is required to elucidate this. However, a proportion of patients with Crohn's disease or ulcerative colitis have definite elevation of total serum IgE, and some of these patients are non-atopic by all criteria.

There have been two previous studies of serum IgE in inflammatory bowel disease (Bergman *et al.* 1973; Brown *et al.* 1973), in neither of which were raised levels found, but IgE antibodies have a high affinity for the surface of mast cells and basophils, and it is these cell-bound molecules which are biologically important rather than the material free in the blood. The significance of the present findings is not clear, though they do suggest that there may be enhanced stimulation of IgE formation in at least some patients with inflammatory bowel disease in the absence of any evidence of atopy. It would be of interest to know the antigen specificity of their IgE, and studies of this point are under way.

It is conceivable that IgE antibody directed against dietary or microbial antigens in the lumen could play a role in perpetuating damage caused by an initial insult which weakened the mucosal barrier to antigen. Also IgE-mediated immediate hypersensitivity reactions are known to play a permissive role in the development of IgG-mediated Arthus type reactions (Cochrane 1971). The lesions of both Crohn's disease and ulcerative colitis contain greatly increased numbers of IgG plasma cells (Baklien & Brandtzaeg 1975), and it has been suggested (Brandtzaeg 1974) that breakdown in the normal secretory IgA barrier at the mucosa can permit penetration of antigen and induction of local IgG antibody responses with an enhanced capacity for the mediation of tissue-damaging hypersensitivity reactions. It is of interest that a beneficial effect has recently been observed in ulcerative colitis of sodium cromoglycate, a drug which blocks IgE-dependent hypersensitivity reactions (Mani et al. 1976).

C-REACTIVE PROTEIN

C-reactive protein (CRP) is a normal plasma protein which occurs in trace amounts, usually less than 2 μg/ml, in normal healthy individuals but which increases dramatically in a wide variety of pathological processes including trauma, infection, collagen disease and malignancy. It was initially detected by its interaction with pneumococcal C-substance, but in recent years it has been found to have a calcium-dependent binding capacity for a large number of different substances which are present in the body (Siegel et al. 1975) (Table 4), many of which may be expected to be more 'exposed' in damaged than in healthy tissue. Interaction between CRP and some of its substrates efficiently activates the classical pathway of complement (Siegel et al. 1974, 1975), and furthermore CRP has been reported to bind selectively to T lymphocytes and to inhibit some of their functions (Mortensen et al. 1975). CRP could therefore be an important modulator of inflammatory and immunological responses.

We have studied CRP in patients with inflammatory bowel disease in an attempt to correlate serum levels with diagnosis and disease activity, and in order to initiate an assessment of whether CRP might play a part in pathogenesis of the lesions or of other associated abnormalities. CRP was isolated from pathological plasma by absorption onto agar (Ganrot & Kindmark 1969), elution with EDTA, absorption with insolubilized anti-normal human serum

TABLE 4

Properties of C-reactive protein

Normal plasma protein	Mol.wt. $\sim$ 120 000

Acute-phase reactant

Calcium-mediated binding to:
  Pneumococcal C-substance, lecithin
  Polycations: histones, leucocyte cationic protein, myelin basic protein, protamine
  Polyanions: heparin, nucleic acid, dextran sulphate

Reacts with low molecular weight substances: phosphoryl choline, mononucleotides, SO_4^{2-}

Fixes complement by classical pathway

Binds to T cells *in vitro*; inhibits some of their properties

antibodies, and finally precipitation of residual impurities with 20% sodium sulphate. Anti-CRP serum was raised by immunization of a rabbit with the purified protein and used to measure the serum concentration of CRP by electroimmunodiffusion. The assay was calibrated using purified CRP as standard and it could detect 2 μg/ml with an error of $\pm$ 7% in replicate samples.

The patients studied were: 41 with Crohn's disease involving small, small and large or large bowel alone, diagnosed by clinical, radiological and where possible histological criteria; 43 with ulcerative colitis or proctititis diagnosed by clinical and radiological features and in whom Crohn's disease had been excluded as far as possible. The controls were 70 healthy members of the medical, nursing and technical staff of the RPMS whose age and sex distribution approximated to that of the patient populations. Venous blood samples were allowed to clot for 1–4 hours at room temperature before separation of serum and storage at -20 °C. One sample was tested for each control subject, whilst a total of 500 samples taken at different times from patients were examined.

There are considerable difficulties in assessing the severity and disease activity in inflammatory bowel disease, and there have been several attempts to quantitate clinical observations so that patients can be allocated to various categories. For the presentation of results here we tried to obtain groups suffering from ulcerative colitis and Crohn's disease of comparable overall clinical severity and we have therefore separated them only into the three broad categories, severe, moderate and quiescent, which are defined in Table 5. If an individual remained within a given category for more than one CRP measurement, the mean of all the levels (which were normally distributed) was used in plotting the results shown in Fig. 2. The statistical significance of differences between the various groups is shown in Table 6.

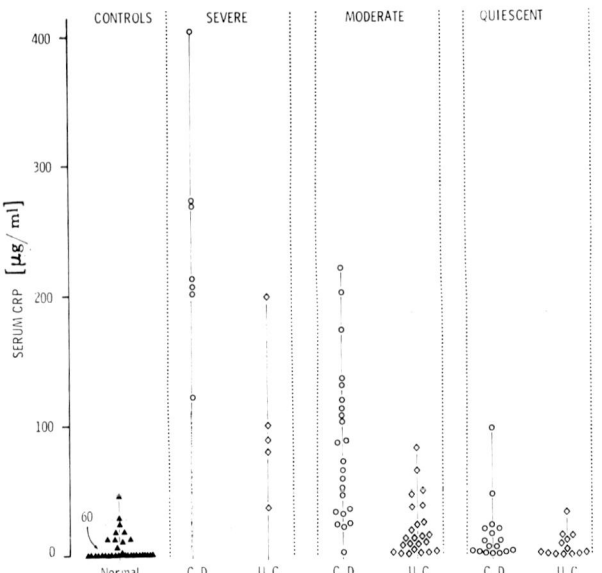

FIG. 2. Serum C-reactive protein levels in patients with inflammatory bowel disease. Each point represents a single individual. C.D., Crohn's disease; U.C., ulcerative colitis. For full details see text.

TABLE 5

Categories of disease activity in inflammatory bowel disease

Severe
Acute symptoms and signs necessitating immediate hospital admission
Abnormalities of ESR, Hb, WBC, serum albumin, rectal histology

Moderate
Variable symptoms, marked or mild, treatable as out-patients or by elective admission
Abnormalities among ESR, Hb, WBC, serum albumin, rectal histology

Quiescent
No clinical symptoms. Occasional abnormalities of ESR, rectal histology

On the basis of this analysis and the longitudinal study of many patients during the course of illness and therapy three main interpretations are possible:

1. Among symptomatic patients those with Crohn's disease had significantly higher CRP levels than those with ulcerative colitis, and in pairs of individuals closely matched for disease activity the level was always greater in Crohn's disease. This measurement may therefore be useful in distinguishing between

TABLE 6

Statistical analysis of serum levels of C-reactive protein in inflammatory bowel disease
(1) Kruskal-Wallis one way non-parametric analysis of variance $P<0.001$
(2) Wilcoxon tests for differences between pairs of groups[a]

	Normal	Severe C.D.	Severe U.C.	Moderate C.D.	Moderate U.C.	Quiescent C.D.	Quiescent U.C.
Normal	–						
Severe C.D.	$P<0.01$	–					
Severe U.C.	$P<0.01$	$P<0.01$	–				
Moderate C.D.	$P<0.01$	$P<0.01$	N.S.	–			
Moderate U.C.	$P<0.01$	$P<0.01$	$P<0.01$	$P<0.01$	–		
Quiescent C.D.	$P<0.01$	$P<0.01$	$P<0.01$	$P<0.01$	N.S.		
Quiescent U.C.	$P<0.01$	$P<0.01$	$P<0.01$	$P<0.01$	N.S.	N.S.	–

[a] Statistical tables do not indicate significance greater than 1% level.
U.C., ulcerative colitis; C.D., Crohn's disease.

the two diseases in cases where the diagnosis is in doubt. Even life-threatening colitis did not produce very high CRP levels. For example two patients, whose levels on admission to hospital and before treatment are shown in Fig. 2 in the severe ulcerative colitis group, underwent emergency colectomy because of failure to respond to medical therapy within days. Comparable CRP values were frequent in moderately symptomatic out-patients with Crohn's disease.

2. In Crohn's disease the CRP levels correlated well with disease activity, whereas in ulcerative colitis the levels were appreciably greater in symptomatic than in asymptomatic patients only when the disease was extemely severe. In most individuals with either disease the CRP level tended to fall towards normal with remissions, either spontaneous or induced by therapy.

3. Even in the clinically quiescent state the CRP levels of the group as a whole differed significantly from normal, and a few patients with Crohn's disease in whom there were few or no symptoms had appreciably elevated levels. We have insufficient evidence to know whether measurement of serum CRP concentration can predict a clinical relapse, but it nonetheless seems to be a clinically useful aid in the assessment of activity as a basis for management.

Precise correlation of CRP concentration with other laboratory indices of disease activity is currently under way, but it is already clear that the CRP level does not just reflect the erythrocyte sedimentation rate, and is a much more sensitive indicator than serum albumin concentration or white blood cell count. Other aspects of the results of CRP measurement which are of interest are that it is elevated even in cases of Crohn's disease in which the colon is grossly spared, and that none of the treatments used, including salazopyrine, corticosteroids, ACTH, azathioprine or metronidazole, seem to affect it unless there is remission of disease activity by both clinical and laboratory criteria.

Elevation of serum CRP is a non-specific response to tissue injury, but is probably fundamental as it appears early in both ontogeny (Felix et al. 1966) and phylogeny (Baldo & Fletcher 1973). The stimulus to CRP production and the determinants of the serum level attained are not known. The higher values we have observed in Crohn's disease may just reflect the more extensive tissue damage than occurs in ulcerative colitis. It is, however, also conceivable that the raised concentration of plasma CRP might influence inflammatory reactions in a number of ways resulting from its capacity for binding to phospholipids ubiquitous in cell membranes, for complement fixation and for adhering to T cells and inhibiting some of their functions. In contrast to the reported binding of CRP to T cells during in vitro culture (Mortensen et al. 1975) we, using a fluorescent rabbit F(ab)$_2$ anti-human CRP reagent, have not detected any lymphocytes bearing CRP in the peripheral blood of patients with high serum CRP levels. This raises the possibility that interaction between lymphocytes and CRP might affect their recirculatory behaviour, for example by acting as a trapping mechanism in damaged tissue. Many of the infiltrating lymphocytes in Crohn's disease are T cells (Strickland et al. 1975; Meuwissen et al. 1976).

COMPLEMENT ACTIVATION

Complement is an important mediator of inflammation both at the humoral and at the cellular level. It also participates in cellular aspects of induction of the allergic response, probably as a consequence of the interaction between fixed C3 and the C3 receptors of B cells and macrophages (Pepys 1976). We have detected mononuclear cells with C3 receptors in cryostat sections of biopsies of lesions and resected tissue from all of four patients with Crohn's disease who were studied (M. B. Pepys & A. C. Dash, unpublished observations). There have been reports of immune complexes in the serum of patients with both Crohn's disease and ulcerative colitis (Doe et al. 1973; Jewell & Mac-Lennan 1973), and for all these reasons it was of interest to see whether there is any evidence of in vivo complement activation in inflammatory bowel disease. We have used two approaches, first, examination of plasma for C3 conversion products and, second, assay of serum immunoconglutinins, which are autoantibodies against fixed complement, chiefly C3 (Lachmann 1967).

Initially, using a modified Laurell technique (Laurell 1965) of two-dimensional immunoelectrophoresis to study EDTA–plasma freshly separated in the cold, we found only very occasional traces of C3 conversion (Table 7). Subsequently

TABLE 7

Plasma C3 conversion in inflammatory bowel disease

Method[a]	Group	No. of patients	No. of samples	No. with C3 conversion[d]	
				Patients	Samples
'Insensitive'[b]	Crohn's disease	37	134	3	4
	Ulcerative colitis	20	50	2	2
'Sensitive'[c]	Crohn's disease	34	68	6	1+5 (trace)
	Ulcerative colitis	13	21	1	1 (trace)

[a] Two-dimensional immunoelectrophoresis.
[b] Well origin, 1:5 dilution of sample, 5-10V/cm.
[c] Slot origin, neat sample, 10-20 V/cm.
[d] No sample showed more than 5% conversion; most much less.

Teisberg & Gjone (1975) reported that C3 conversion was often to be found in sera of patients with inflammatory bowel disease, but not in controls, and that the degree of conversion correlated with the extent and activity of disease. We therefore repeated our study comparing serum and plasma samples taken at the same time from each patient, and in addition using a Laurell technique which was capable of detecting minimal traces of C3 conversion and was more sensitive than that used in our first study. Fresh serum was separated one hour after venesection into plain glass tubes kept at 21 °C, whilst plasma was obtained by taking blood into EDTA on ice and centrifuging at 4° C; both sorts of samples were then stored in liquid nitrogen before testing.

We confirmed that there was some C3 conversion in all the sera from patients but in none of the healthy controls (Table 8). However, the degree of conversion did not correlate with the extent or activity of disease, and there was no conversion in any of the plasma samples.

TABLE 8

Plasma and serum C3 conversion in inflammatory bowel disease

Group	No.	C3 conversion in:[a]	
		Plasma/EDTA	Fresh serum
Crohn's disease	8	0	8
Ulcerative colitis	5	0	5
Controls	10	0	10

[a] Detected by sensitive two-dimensional immunoelectrophoresis.
No sample showed more than 5% conversion.

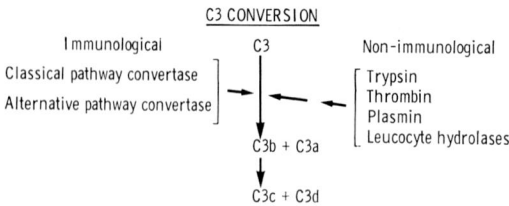

FIG. 3. C3 convertase enzymes.

C3 is known to be labile in serum as a result of its susceptibility to a variety of proteolytic enzymes (Fig. 3), and we had used EDTA–plasma freshly separated in the cold expressly to minimize this problem and to examine the *in vivo* C3 profile. It is difficult to ascribe C3 conversion in serum to *in vivo* complement activation, and we suggest that these findings may reflect acceleration of the normal *in vitro* conversion which occurs with clotting (Krøll 1970). This might result from a variety of factors which are absent in healthy controls, for example: polymorphonuclear leucocytosis, elevated CRP levels or alterations in other plasma proteins with biological activity in this respect. The conversion of factor B observed by Teisberg & Gjone (1975) in their patients can also be attributed to *in vitro* C3 conversion stimulating the C3b feedback loop of the alternative pathway (Lachmann & Nicol 1973).

We retested a number of EDTA–plasma samples by the more sensitive technique and found traces of C3 conversion in a small proportion (Table 7, p. 293). We conclude that this method does not provide very much evidence for *in vivo* C3 activation in the circulation in inflammatory bowel disease.

Immunoconglutinins in serum which had been heat-inactivated and absorbed with sheep erythrocytes were detected by agglutination of sheep erythrocytes sensitized with human complement. The sera of some of the patients contained low titres of immunoconglutinins, none greater than 1:4 (Table 9). The results on this small number of sera suggest that the occurrence of immunoconglutinin may be significant. Preliminary study of the levels of anti-C3 activity in parotid saliva did not reveal any difference between patients and controls.

The presence of immunoconglutinins in serum supports the idea that *in vivo* complement activation is taking place in inflammatory bowel disease, and accords with the finding of Potter *et al.* (1975) that there is an accelerated fractional catabolic rate of C3 in these patients with evidence for C3 consump-

TABLE 9

Serum immunoconglutinin in inflammatory bowel disease

Group	Number of individuals			Significance[b]
	Positive[a]	Negative	Total	
Crohn's disease	10	13	23	$P=0.0135$
Ulcerative colitis	6	10	16	$P=0.0536$
Control	0	11	11	

[a] Agglutination of complement-coated erythrocytes by inactivated absorbed serum. No serum titre was $> 1:4$.
[b] Fisher's exact test for difference from the controls.

tion at an extravascular site. There is thus some evidence suggesting that complement activation may be a feature of inflammatory bowel disease. More critical studies are required and, for example, a more sensitive assay for immunoconglutinin, which we are currently developing, might provide a clearer distinction between the levels in patients, with disease of varying extent and severity, and controls.

CONCLUSIONS

The present studies shed some light on different aspects of immunological function in inflammatory bowel disease, although they do not favour any particular aetiopathogenetic hypothesis. From the practical point of view the results suggest that the measurement of serum CRP concentration may help to distinguish Crohn's disease from ulcerative colitis, and to assess disease activity in Crohn's disease.

ACKNOWLEDGEMENTS

We wish to thank Professor C. C. Booth and Professor G. Neale for their help and encouragement and permission to study their patients; Dr J. E. Lennard-Jones, Dr N. J. Buckell, Dr H. J. F. Hodgson and Dr D. P. Jewell for providing sera from their patients with acute ulcerative colitis; and Miss Julie Mitchell, Department of Clinical Immunology, Cardiothoracic Institute, London SW3 for the IgE measurements.

References

BAKLIEN, K. & BRANDTZAEG, P. (1975) Comparative mapping of the local distribution of immunoglobulin-containing cells in ulcerative colitis and Crohn's disease of the colon. Clin. Exp. Immunol. 22, 197-209.

BALDO, B. A. & FLETCHER, T. C. (1973) C-reactive protein-like precipitins in plaice. *Nature (Lond.) 246*, 145-146

BERGMAN, L., JOHANSSON, S. G. O. & KRAUSE, U. (1973) Immunoglobulin concentrations in serum and bowel secretions in Crohn's disease. *Scand. J. Gastroenterol. 8*, 401-406

BLAIR, H. (1974) The incidence of asthma, hay-fever and infantile eczema in an East London Group Practice of 9145 patients. *Clin. Allergy 4*, 389-399

BRANDTZAEG, P. (1974) Mucosal and glandular distribution of immunoglobulin components. Immunohistochemistry with a cold ethanol fixation technique. *Immunology 26*, 1101-1113

BROWN, W. R., LANSFORD, C. L. & HORNBROOK, M. (1973) Serum IgE concentrations in patients with gastrointestinal disorders. *Digestive Diseases 18*, 641-645

COCHRANE, C. G. (1971) Mechanisms involved in the deposition of immune complexes in tissues. *J. Exp. Med. 134*, Suppl., 75-89

DOE, W. F., BOOTH, C. C. & BROWN, D. L. (1973) Evidence for complement-binding immune complexes in adult coeliac disease, Crohn's disease and ulcerative colitis. *Lancet 1*, 402-403

FELIX, N. S., NAKAJIMA, H. & KAGAN, B. M. (1966) Serum C-reactive protein in infections during the first six months of life. *Pediatrics 37*, 270-277

GANROT, P. O. & KINDMARK, C. O. (1969) A simple two-step procedure for isolation of C-reactive protein. *Biochim. Biophys. Acta 194*, 443-448

HAMMER, B., ASHURST, P. & NAISH, J. (1968) Diseases associated with ulcerative colitis and Crohn's disease. *Gut 9*, 17-21

JEWELL, D. P. & HODGSON, H. J. F. (1976) Autoimmune and inflammatory diseases of the gastrointestinal tract, in *Immunological Aspects of the Liver and Gastrointestinal Tract* (Ferguson, A. & MacSween, R. N. M., eds.), pp. 203-250, Medical and Technical Publishing Co. Ltd, Lancaster

JEWELL, D. P. & MACLENNAN, I. C. M. (1973) Circulating immune complexes in inflammatory bowel disease. *Clin. Exp. Immunol. 14*, 219-226

JEWELL, D. P. & TRUELOVE, S. C. (1972) Reaginic hypersensitivity in ulcerative colitis. *Gut 13*, 903-906

KRØLL, J. (1970) Changes in the β_{1C}-β_{1A}-globulin during the coagulation process demonstrated by means of a quantitative immunoelectrophoresis method, in *Protides of the Biological Fluids*, vol. 17 (Peeters, H., ed.), pp. 529-532, Pergamon Press, Oxford

LACHMANN, P. J. (1967) Conglutinin and immunoconglutinins. *Adv. Immunol. 6*, 480-527

LACHMANN, P. J. & NICOL, P. (1973) Reaction mechanism of the alternative pathway of complement fixation. *Lancet 1*, 465-467

LAURELL, C.-B. (1965) Antigen-antibody crossed electrophoresis. *Anal. Biochem. 10*, 358-361

MANI, V., LLOYD, G., GREEN, F. H. Y., FOX, H. & TURNBERG, L. A. (1976) Treatment of ulcerative colitis with oral disodium cromoglycate. *Lancet 1*, 439-441

MEUWISSEN, S. G. M., FELTKAMP-VROOM, T. M., BRUTEL DE LA RIVIÈRE, A., VON DEM BORNE, A. E. G. Kr. & TYTGAT, G. N. (1976) Analysis of the lympho-plasmacytic infiltrate in Crohn's disease with special reference to identification of lymphocyte subpopulations. *Gut, 17*, 770-780

MILLER, D. S., KEIGHLEY, A. C. & LANGMAN, M. J. S. (1974) Changing pattern in epidemiology of Crohn's disease. *Lancet 2*, 691-693

MORTENSEN, R. F., OSMAN, A. P. & GEWURZ, H. (1975) Effects of C-reactive protein on the lymphoid system. I. Binding to thymus-dependent lymphocytes and alteration of their function. *J. Exp. Med. 141*, 821-839

NYE, L., MERRETT, T. G., LANDON, J. T. & WHITE, R. J. (1975) A detailed investigation of circulating IgE levels in a normal population. *Clin. Allergy 5*, 13-24

PARISH, W. E. (1970) Short term anaphylactic IgG antibodies in human sera. *Lancet 2*, 591-592

PEPYS, J. (1969) *Hypersensitivity Diseases of the Lung due to Fungi and Organic Dusts*, Karger, Basle

PEPYS, J. (1975) Atopy, in *Clinical Aspects of Immunology*, 3rd edn (Gell, P. G. H., Coombs, R. R. A. & Lachmann, P. J., eds.), p. 877, Blackwell Scientific Publications, Oxford

Pepys, M. B. (1976) Role of complement in the induction of immunological responses. *Transplant. Rev. 32*, 93-120

Potter, B. J., Hodgson, H. J. F. & Jewell, D. P. (1975) C3 metabolism in inflammatory bowel disease. *Gut 16*, 833

Rowe, D. S. (1969) Radioactive single radial immunodiffusion: a method for increasing the sensitivity of immunochemical quantification of proteins in agar gel. *Bull. W.H.O. 40*, 613-616

Siegel, J., Rent, R. & Gewurz, H. (1974) Interactions of C-reactive protein with the complement system. I. Protamine-induced consumption of complement in acute phase sera. *J. Exp. Med. 140*, 631-647

Siegel, J., Osmand, A. P., Wilson, M. F. & Gewurz, H. (1975) Interactions of C-reactive protein with the complement system. II. C-reactive protein-mediated consumption of complement by poly-L-lysine polymers and other polycations. *J. Exp. Med. 142*, 709-721

Soothill, J. F. (1974) Immunodeficiency and allergy, in *Progress in Immunology II* (Brent, L. & Holborow, J., eds.), vol. 5, pp. 183-191, North-Holland, Amsterdam & Oxford

Strickland, R. G., Husby, G., Black, W. C. & Williams, R. C. (1975) Peripheral blood and intestinal lymphocyte sub-populations in Crohn's disease. *Gut 16*, 847-853

Teisberg, P. & Gjone, E. (1975) Humoral immune system activity in inflammatory bowel disease. *Scand. J. Gastroenterol. 10*, 545-549

Discussion

Gowans: I gather that these two diseases, ulcerative colitis and Crohn's disease, are very similar in certain respects. Can you elaborate on the similarities and the differences?

Pepys: Ulcerative colitis is a disease with acute and chronic inflammation in the colon; that is, with respect to the gut, it is restricted to the large bowel. It starts at the anus and may progress proximally to affect the whole colon. The lesions are always in contiguity. It presents a fairly homogeneous clinical picture. Crohn's disease may affect the bowel from the mouth to the anus and perianal skin. It is characterized by gross lesions in discontinuity. The histological marker present in many cases but not all is a granuloma which is not seen in ulcerative colitis.

Gowans: Are there any grounds for supposing that they have a common aetiology?

Pepys: When they affect the large bowel they may be clinically indistinguishable. There are some cases in which a diagnosis is never made, or is made only at operation or post mortem. There is a lot of overlap.

Booth: The fundamental pathological difference is that the pathology in the colon in ulcerative colitis is a mucosal ulceration that seems to involve the surface enterocytes as the primary lesion, whereas in Crohn's disease the lesion is a submucosal granuloma. Those are the extremes: in between are a whole range of changes.

Evans: I would not describe it as a *submucosal* granuloma; the mucosa is involved as well.

What concerned me, Dr Pepys, is the comparability of your groups. If you had compared cases of Crohn's disease with no obvious small bowel lesion, with cases of total colitis in ulcerative colitis, you might have a more valid comparison in terms of the volume of tissue involved. If you have included patients with ulcerative proctitis who may not have total colitis and compared them with patients with Crohn's disease who may have involvement of small intestine and the large intestine as well, it does not surprise me that there is a significant difference in an acute-phase reaction.

Pepys: As I said, the classification of patients with inflammatory bowel disease is difficult. It is often not possible to assess the overall extent of tissue damage even when all the clinical data are available. We tried to make the groups as comparable as possible in terms of overall clinical severity. For example, the 'severe' group contained patients with acute total ulcerative colitis and patients with acute total Crohn's colitis. Some of the ulcerative colitis patients went on to emergency colectomy because medical therapy failed. There were nonetheless significant differences in the C-reactive protein (CRP) levels between the two diseases, and this was the case even in less severely ill patients. On the question of small or large bowel involvement, our experience has been that patients with Crohn's disease affecting only the small intestine have CRP levels comparable to those seen in colonic disease.

Lachmann: On the whole, the measurement of acute-phase reactants has always turned out to be somewhat non-specific. Have you any evidence that if you regress the erythrocyte sedimentation rate (ESR) and the C-reactive protein levels in these two diseases, there are significant differences?

Pepys: The correlation coefficients (r) between serum CRP level and other clinical laboratory indices are shown in Table 1. No significant correlations were found among the ulcerative colitis patients for whom full data were

TABLE 1 (Pepys)

Relationship between serum concentration of C-reactive protein and other clinical laboratory tests

	ESR	WBC	Hb	Albumin
Crohn's disease (44 patients)				
Correlation coefficient (r)	0.669	0.403	−0.141	−0.465
Significance (p)	<0.001	<0.01	N.S.	<0.01
$(1-r^2)\%$	55.2	83.8	98.0	78.4
Ulcerative colitis (20 patients)				
Correlation coefficient (r)	0.435	0.274	−0.122	−0.247
Significance (p)	N.S.	N.S.	N.S.	N.S.
$(1-r^2)\%$	81.1	92.5	98.5	93.9

available. Since r^2 represents the proportion of the variance of y (CRP level) which can be attributed to its linear regression on x (the other variables), the value of $1-r^2$ indicates the proportion of the variance of CRP which is independent of each of the other variables. Our results therefore suggest that measurement of serum CRP in Crohn's disease provides appreciably different information from that obtained by measuring ESR, WBC or serum albumin. This is borne out by sequential observations in individual patients.

Lachmann: Are you saying that the patients with Crohn's disease have discordantly high C-reactive protein levels compared to other parameters of the acute phase of inflammation, whereas ulcerative colitis patients have low C-reactive protein levels compared with the other parameters?

Pepys: All we can say is that for comparable abnormalities of ESR, WBC, etc., patients with Crohn's disease tend to have higher levels of serum CRP than patients with ulcerative colitis.

Jones: It is important to recognize that C-reactive protein may interfere with some of the tests used to detect immune complexes. Nevertheless, we have evidence in patients with coeliac disease, Crohn's disease and ulcerative colitis that a whole battery of tests are positive for immune complexes. For instance, we measure C3 and C4 levels, haemolytic complement, anti-complementary activity, C1q binding, and cryoprecipitability. Many of these tests may be affected by C-reactive protein, although I think that not all are. The question is of whether the levels of C-reactive protein are high enough to react with C1q.

We can confirm Bill Doe's evidence that coeliac disease patients when challenged with gluten develop immune complexes which aggregate platelets and that this activity subsequently fades (see Booth *et al.*, this volume, pp. 329–346). Perhaps the strongest evidence that at least some of this is due to immune complexes is that several of our patients with particularly high levels of anti-complementary activity and platelet aggregation have cryoglobulins, and it would be difficult to explain this phenomenon, which may be transient, in terms of C-reactive protein.

Pepys: The interaction of CRP with a variety of substrates activates the classical complement pathway via C1q very efficiently (Kaplan & Volanakis 1974; Siegel *et al.* 1975) and the concentration of CRP required is often exceeded in the sera of patients with inflammatory bowel disease. Some of the lipoprotein substrates with which CRP reacts are ubiquitous, and this may be a mechanism for the C3 conversion which we see in serum but not in plasma. I do not know whether the presence of CRP in serum can lead to C1q binding in your test system.

Lachmann: I imagine, Dr Jones, that you do your C1q precipitation in the presence of EDTA. The reaction of C-reactive protein is calcium-dependent and should therefore not interfere.

Jones: That is possible. Do you know how C-reactive protein reacts with platelets in the platelet aggregation test for immune complexes? We find this test positive in some of our cases of Crohn's disease.

Pepys: CRP does not aggregate platelets on its own, but it inhibits the aggregation of platelets by either aggregated IgG or thrombin, and also the activation but not the activity of platelet factor 3 (Fiedel & Gewurz 1976). I do not know how this might affect your use of a platelet aggregation test for 'immune' complexes. With regard to the interaction between CRP and C1q it is worth noting that, although the binding of CRP to its substrates requires calcium ions, this may not be the case for CRP-C1q binding. Aggregated CRP might bind C1q just as aggregated IgG does.

Jones: The other point is that immune complexes are found most frequently in patients with colitis who have peripheral manifestations, such as joint involvement, vasculitis and pyoderma gangrenosa. Although C-reactive protein may be an important trap, there is sufficient evidence to suggest that immune complexes account for at least some of the peripheral phenomena in these conditions.

Lachmann: Would you agree that immune complexes in diseases where there may be breaches of the mucosal barrier allowing increased absorption of macromolecular material may not be of *primary* aetiological significance, even if they may help to cause the distant effects? The fact that immune complexes occur is not very surprising, in situations where abnormal amounts of food and bacterial antigens are absorbed.

Jones: Yes, I agree that they may account for epiphenomena. We have another observation on macromolecular antigens which may relate to that. We have been interested in circulating antibodies to bacteriophage ϕX174 (a phage of a non-pathogenic *E. coli* which is found in the stools of about one in five normal healthy individuals). We have only ever found circulating antibodies to this phage in three out of the 200 subjects that we studied. We have never found antibodies in patients with severe coeliac disease, where a leaky gut with access to intestinal antigens would be expected. We have found three subjects in whom an intravenous injection of ϕX174 produced a secondary response instead of the normal primary response. One had Crohn's disease, one had rheumatoid arthritis and one had chronic liver disease. This phage is a common gut antigen and it is therefore interesting and puzzling that antigens seem to be able to leak from the gut into the blood and produce circulating immune complexes, yet we don't find many people sensitized to this very immunogenic bacteriophage.

White: Have you proof that the IgA form of the antibody would work in your tests for phage neutralization?

Jones: Our bacteriophage neutralization test is extremely sensitive. We do have some evidence that circulating IgA neutralizes the bacteriophage.

Lehner: We have measured C-reactive protein in recurrent aphthous ulcers and in Behçet's syndrome (a condition in which patients suffer with oral and genital ulcers, skin lesions, often with iritis, arthrosis and thrombophlebitis). We find high levels of CRP, particularly in Behçet's syndrome, by the single radial immunodiffusion method (Adinolfi & Lehner 1976). Elevated CRP levels, however, are found in many conditions and it is unwise to attach too great a significance to this.

As CRP is one of the acute-phase proteins, have you assayed the others? We have found that while concentrations of CRP and C9 may be considerably increased, particularly in Behçet's syndrome, this does not apply to α1 antitrypsin. I wonder which acute-phase proteins you are referring to, as there may be only a selective increase in some of them.

Pepys: We have not measured other acute-phase reactants in our patients although this has been done in inflammatory bowel disease (Weeke & Jarnum 1971). Our experience with C3 and C4 levels is that they tend to correlate with severity of disease, but in very severe or protracted illness they may remain low. This is not so with CRP, which remains elevated even terminally. I agree that the elevation of CRP concentrations is very non-specific and is a feature of almost any febrile or tissue-damaging illness irrespective of its aetiology. In the present context it is clinically valuable because it helps to distinguish between two overlapping diseases, and because it provides an index of disease activity in Crohn's disease. At a more fundamental level CRP is an interesting protein to study because of its rapid production, its dramatic increases in serum concentration, and its capacity to fix complement and to bind to and modify the activities of T lymphocytes.

Soothill: I find the absence of C3 conversion *in vivo* very pleasing and perhaps surprising. When we (Matthews & Soothill 1970) demonstrated this after feeding milk to milk-allergic patients I was worried that possibly it was not a direct effect of the milk, but an effect of other antigens getting in because of milk allergic damage to the bowel. Your patients had very damaged large intestines and some of your cases of Crohn's disease will have damaged small intestines too, so I was glad that you did not find C3 conversion.

Secondly, Ezer & Hayward (1974) showed that the serum of patients with Crohn's disease inhibited the C3-binding sites of normal B lymphocytes. We interpreted this as evidence of C3 activation *in vivo*, and possibly of immune complex. This appears to be slightly incompatible with your essentially negative information.

Pepys: There are several problems in the interpretation of those observations. Firstly, since serum from patients with Crohn's disease was used the inhibition may have been due to *in vitro* phenomena following clotting rather than to changes occurring *in vivo*. It would be interesting to repeat the experiments with fresh EDTA-plasma. Secondly, substantial concentrations of fluid phase C3 conversion products are required to inhibit C3-dependent rosette formation on lymphocytes (Pepys & Butterworth 1974), so unless the major part of the serum C3 was converted and the serum was used neat, I am surprised at the extent of inhibition described.

Thayer has demonstrated reduced numbers of C3 receptor lymphocytes in patients with Crohn's disease and ulcerative colitis (Thayer *et al*. 1975). In more limited studies we have not seen this. I do not know whether CRP can block lymphocyte C3 receptors. According to Gewurz's group, CRP does not stick to B cells (Mortensen *et al*. 1975).

Lachmann: I am very interested to see your data on C3 conversion. Two patterns of C3 conversion products have been found *in vivo* under rather different conditions. Occasionally C3c (or possibly C3b) is found in freshly taken, warm plasma from patients with severe, presumably intravascular, complement activation; for example, in diseases like systemic lupus erythematosus. This is uncommon. C3c (and even more so, C3b) have a short half-life in plasma *in vivo* and one would not expect to find them unless they were being generated quite fast. A different C3 conversion product, C3d, is detected quite commonly in certain patients with renal disease. C3d is a long half-life fragment of C3 which appears to be generated extravascularly and to come back into the circulation (Charlesworth *et al*. 1974). There seems no reason to doubt that this C3d is really made *in vivo*. In the case of small amounts of C3c (or C3b) in fresh plasma, as have been reported by Versey *et al*. (1973), the possibility that this has been formed *in vitro* is, on the other hand, very real. It is known that in the acute phase of inflammation C3 levels, and levels of factor B of the alternative pathway, can be markedly raised. The high levels of these components potentiate the feedback mechanisms which give rise to C3 conversion. In 'acute-phase' patients even more than in others one can picture any one of a number of factors including for example the presence of slightly raised levels of cold autoantibodies to the patient's own red cells giving rise to minor C3 conversion. Do you take blood and clot it while warm in these tests, to make sure that this does not happen?

Pepys: The tests in which serum and plasma were studied in parallel were all done at room temperature, because we wanted to replicate Teisberg & Gjone's (1975) experiment.

Brandtzaeg: Teisberg found that C3 conversion products disappear after a gluten-free diet is given and reappear after the introduction of gluten into the diet of coeliac disease patients. Does this not indicate that the technique is valid in showing *in vivo* complement activation?

Pepys: I have seen those data, but they were obtained on serum. Before ascribing C3 conversion to *in vivo* complement activation it is necessary to prevent the processes which are known to activate C3 during coagulation.

Brandtzaeg: Do you think the argument about an increased enzymic level in serum also applies to coeliac disease?

Pepys: I don't know. I would like to see the same study done on EDTA-plasma collected and separated in the cold.

Brandtzaeg: I understand that Dr Teisberg has had some technical problems using plasma instead of serum.

Rosen: I just wonder if these patients' lymphocytes can be infected with EB virus, since the C3 receptor may be identical or adjacent to the EB virus receptor of the B lymphocyte?

Pepys: I don't know. We have measured the concentration of C3 receptor lymphocytes in the peripheral blood of patients with inflammatory bowel disease and we do not find it to be low, as reported by Thayer *et al.* (1975). We have not studied it systematically because the isolation of mononuclear cells from the blood invariably distorts the proportions of the different lymphocyte populations (Brown & Greaves 1974), making it impossible to calculate their true circulating ratios and absolute concentrations. In addition monocytes also have C3 receptors. In an attempt to overcome these problems and to quantify precisely the absolute concentrations of circulating lymphocyte populations we are developing techniques for studying various markers in whole blood (Pepys 1976). In Crohn's disease and colitis we find some lymphocytes in the affected tissues which bear C3 receptors (M. B. Pepys & A. C. Dash, unpublished work).

References

ADINOLFI, M. & LEHNER, T. (1976) Acute phase proteins and C9 in patients with Behçet's syndrome and aphthous ulcers. *Clin. Exp. Immunol.* 25, 36-39

BOOTH, C. C., PETERS, T. J. & DOE, W. F. (1977) Immunopathology of coeliac disease, this volume, pp. 329-346

BROWN, G. & GREAVES, M. F. (1974) Enumeration of absolute numbers of T and B lymphocytes in human blood. *Scand. J. Immunol.* 3, 161-172

CHARLESWORTH, J. A., WILLIAMS, D. G., SHERINGTON, E., LACHMANN, P. J. & PETERS, D. K. (1974) Metabolic studies of the third component of complement and the glycine-rich beta glycoprotein in patients with hypocomplementaemia. *J. Clin. Invest. 53*, 1578-1587

EZER, G. & HAYWARD, A. R. (1974) Inhibition of complement dependent lymphocyte rosette formation: a possible test for activated complement products. *Eur. J. Immunol. 4*, 148

FIEDEL, B. A. & GEWURZ, H. (1976) Effects of C-reactive protein on platelet function. I. Inhibition of platelet aggregation and release reactions. *J. Immunol. 116*, 1209-1294

KAPLAN, M. K. & VOLANAKIS, J. E. (1974) Interaction of C-reactive protein complexes with the complement system. I. Consumption of human complement associated with the reaction of C-reactive protein with pneumococcal C-polysaccharide and with the choline phosphatides, lecithin and sphingomyelin. *J. Immunol. 112*, 2135-2147

MATTHEWS, T. S. & SOOTHILL, J. F. (1970) Complement activation after milk feeding in children with cow's milk allergy. *Lancet 2*, 893

MORTENSEN, R. F., OSMAND, A. P. & GEWURZ, H. (1975) Effects of C-reactive protein on the lymphoid system. I. Binding to thymus-dependent lymphocytes and alteration of their functions. *J. Exp. Med. 141*, 821-839

PEPYS, M. B. (1976) Characterization and enumeration of lymphocyte populations in whole human peripheral blood, in *In Vitro Methods in Cell-Mediated and Tumour Immunity* (Bloom, B. R. & David, J., eds.), pp. 172-202, Academic Press, New York

PEPYS, M. B. & BUTTERWORTH, A. E. (1974) Inhibition by C3 fragments of C3-dependent rosette formation and antigen-induced lymphocyte transformation. *Clin. Exp. Immunol. 18*, 273-282

SIEGEL, J., OSMAND, A. P., WILSON, M. F. & GEWURZ, H. (1975) Interactions of C-reactive protein with the complement system. II. C-reactive protein-mediated consumption of complement by poly-L-lysine polymers and other polycations. *J. Exp. Med. 142*, 709-721

TEISBERG, P. & GJONE, E. (1975) Humoral immune system activity in inflammatory bowel disease. *Scand. J. Gastroenterol. 10*, 545-549

THAYER, W. R., CHARLAND, C. & FIELD, C. (1975) Complement bearing and other lymphocytes in inflammatory bowel disease. *Gastroenterology 68*, 997

VERSEY, J. M., HOBBS, J. R. & HOLT, P. J. L. (1973) Complement metabolism in rheumatoid arthritis. 1. Longitudinal studies. *Ann. Rheum. Dis. 32*, 557

WEEKE, B. & JARNUM, S. (1971) Serum concentration of nineteen serum proteins in Crohn's disease and ulcerative colitis. *Gut 12*, 297-302

Effects of local delayed hypersensitivity on the small intestine

ANNE FERGUSON and T. T. MACDONALD

Gastro-Intestinal Unit, University of Edinburgh and Western General Hospital, Edinburgh and University Department of Bacteriology and Immunology, Western Infirmary, Glasgow

Abstract There are many T and B cells in the small intestinal mucosa and local T cell immunity could have a role both in protective immunity and as a cause of disease (i.e. hypersensitivity). This latter aspect has been investigated by using several animal models to assess the effects of local delayed hypersensitivity on the structure and function of the small intestine.

Heterotopically transplanted grafts of fetal small intestine in mice (isografts and allografts) have been examined by conventional histology, scanning and transmission electron microscopy, by making direct measurements of villi, crypts, and lymphoid cell infiltrate, and by counting the number of mitoses per crypt. This cell-mediated immune reaction causes lymphocyte infiltration which is most marked in the lamina propria, hyperplasia of the crypts of Lieberkühn, increased cell loss with villous atrophy and a flat surface, but the individual enterocytes appear fairly normal.

Graft-versus-host disease causes exactly the same changes in structure and in cell kinetics as does rejection. However, crypt hyperplasia has been found to precede villous atrophy by several days. Preliminary experiments on local contact hypersensitivity suggest that intraluminal injection of oxazolone in the gut of sensitized mice also produces villous atrophy and crypt hyperplasia.

It is postulated that these effects are likely to be produced via lymphokines: by an 'enteropathic' factor which damages the lamina propria and basement membrane, and a factor which is mitogenic for crypt stem cells.

In mice infected with *Giardia lamblia*, crypt hyperplasia and lymphocyte infiltration of the epithelium are present and there is accelerated epithelial cell turnover. In rats infected with *Nippostrongylus brasiliensis*, the flat mucosa has been shown to be due to the thymus-dependent immune response and not directly to the damage produced by the parasite itself.

A common factor in the variety of conditions associated with villous atrophy and crypt hyperplasia may well be a local cell-mediated immune reaction to food, microbial, parasite or other antigens which causes changes in enterocyte turnover rate and malabsorption.

The small intestine has the unique and essential function of nutrient absorption, a function which resides in the sheet of enterocytes—columnar epithelial cells which cover the villi. However, large numbers of cells of the immune system are also to be found in the intestinal mucosa. These are dispersed singly or in small groups among the epithelial and connective tissue components of the intestine and they comprise T, B and null cells, together with mononuclear phagocytes, mast cells and eosinophils. Thus the gut has the cellular capacity for truly protective local immunity (e.g. antibody to enteric pathogens) and for entirely pathological, hypersensitivity reactions (e.g. food allergy). The situation can also be envisaged where a protective immune reaction will, of necessity, be accompanied by some tissue damage and in this paper we describe and discuss the harmful effects which may be produced by local delayed hypersensitivity reactions in the small intestine.

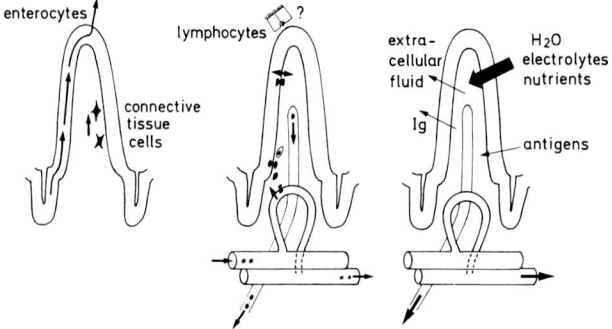

FIG. 1. Some of the components of the small intestine which are continually renewed or replaced.

The apparently regular arrangement of its crypts and villi is misleading when one considers the small intestinal mucosa as the backcloth for an immune reaction lasting several days. The epithelial, stromal and lymphoid cells are continually renewed or replaced, and the absorbed and exuded fluids will dilute, dissolve and wash away any soluble antigen in the vicinity (Fig. 1). Despite this, it is evident that some living and non-living antigens will persist for sufficient time to allow the evolution of a cell-mediated immune (CMI) reaction in the intestinal mucosa; these include parasites and viruses, particulate antigens and cellular or subcellular components of the tissue itself (Table 1).

ALLOGRAFT REJECTION AS A MODEL OF DELAYED HYPERSENSITIVITY

When grafts of fetal mouse intestine are implanted heterotopically into adult mice of the same inbred strain, they take, grow and retain their normal morpho-

TABLE 1

Antigens which persist in the small intestinal mucosa for sufficient time to allow evolution of a cell-mediated immune reaction

Microorganisms and parasites:
  Lumen-dwelling
  Adherent
  In mucosa

Non-living:
  Attached to cells or stroma
  Precipitated
  Large particles

Small intestinal tissue:
  Histocompatibility antigens
  Autoantigens
  Organ-specific antigens

? Foods taken three or four times daily

logical appearances for several months (Ferguson & Parrott 1972). If donor and host are from different strains, grafts grow for a few days, then are infiltrated with lymphocytes and rejected (Ferguson & Parrott 1973). Such allografts of small intestine, implanted under the kidney capsule, provide a useful and inexpensive model of a local delayed hypersensitivity reaction. They have the additional advantage that, since the implanted tissue is fetal, there are no antigens within the lumen of the graft, no local immune reactions to foods or microorganisms, and any pathological features observed can be attributed directly to the rejection process. Rejection of allografts in this system is a thymus-dependent phenomenon (Table 2) (Ferguson & Parrott

TABLE 2

Thymus-dependence of small intestinal allograft rejection

Experimental design		*Number of grafts implanted (> 10 days previously)*	*Number of grafts with complete mucosal destruction*
Donor	Host		
CBA →	BALB/c	46	45
BALB/c →	CBA	26	24
BALB/c →	Thymus-deprived CBA	32	5

Grafts of fetal small intestine were implanted under the kidney capsules of adult mice and subsequently examined histologically.

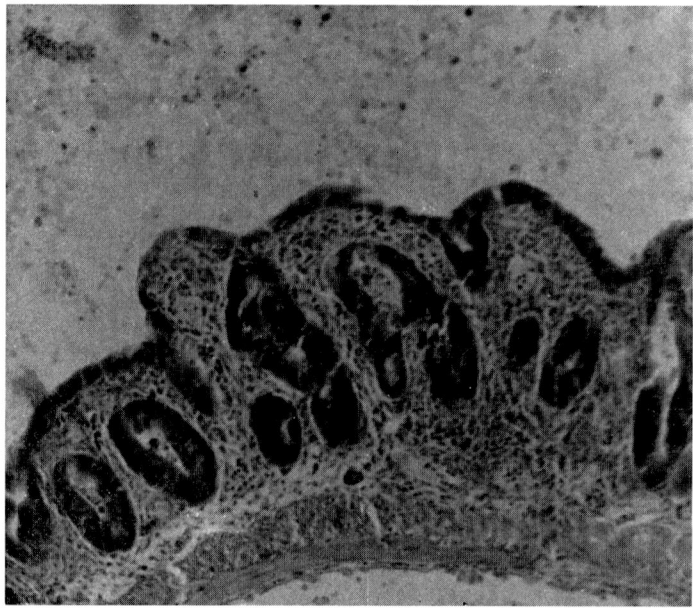

Fig. 2. Typical histology of rejection of a mouse small intestinal allograft.

1973) and, since destruction of the mucosa precedes the appearance of serum antibody by several days (Table 3) (Elves & Ferguson 1975), it is the cellular component of the thymus-dependent reaction which is implicated.

We have concentrated mainly on histopathological studies of the effects of rejection on the small intestine, and some of our findings have already been published (Ferguson & Parrott 1973; MacDonald & Ferguson 1976a) or are in press (Ferguson et al. 1976a; MacDonald & Ferguson 1976b). In all experiments, isografts (between animals of the same strain) have been compared with allografts (host and donor of different strains). Tissues have been examined by using conventional histology, scanning and transmission electron microscopy, direct measurements of villi, crypts and enterocytes, counts of intestinal lymphoid cells and studies of mitotic activity in crypt cells.

The most striking histological effect of rejection is seen before the mucosa is completely destroyed (Fig. 2). Grafts are infiltrated with lymphocytes, villi are short or absent and crypts of Lieberkühn appear abnormally long. This appearance is not unique to rejection of intestine in the mouse. Similar findings have been reported in dog intestinal allografts (Holmes et al. 1971) and in mice with graft-versus-host disease (Reilly & Kirsner 1965) where the histological lesion is accompanied by malabsorption (Hedberg et al. 1968; Palmer & Reilly

TABLE 3

Time-course and thymus-dependence of the humoral immune response to small intestinal allografts

Experimental design		Proportion of host mice with serum antibody to graft strain antigens, at different times after graft implantation:			
Donor	Host	5 days	9 days	12 days	15 days
CBA ⇄ BALB/c		0/12	0/12	12/12	12/12
BALB/c →Thymus-deprived CBA		–	0/2	–	0/5

1971). These animal experiments produce changes very similar to those seen in intestinal biopsies in human coeliac disease and parasite infection (Ferguson 1975, 1976). Thus elucidation of the mechanisms whereby the local CMI reaction of rejection changes intestinal architecture may allow more rational interpretation of the significance of villous atrophy in clinical disease.

VILLI IN ALLOGRAFTS OF SMALL INTESTINE

The enterocytes are formed by cell division in the crypts of Lieberkühn. They move up on to the villi and are shed from villous tips some 2–3 days later. It has become generally accepted that the shapes and height of villi are determined by the size of the population of enterocytes at any one time—if there are fewer mature enterocytes the villi change from finger-like or deltoid shapes to become ridges, then low convolutions. For a few days after implantation, the villi of allografts resemble those of normal intestine and of isografts. Once rejection is established the villi become shorter and the surface is ridged or flat; this feature is best seen by using scanning electron microscopy (Fig. 3). Yet despite the striking changes in the shapes of the villi, individual enterocytes appear remarkably normal during rejection, to both light and electron microscopic evaluation. Sheets of virtually intact columnar enterocytes can be seen in the lumen of many grafts (illustrated as Fig. 3 in Ferguson & Parrott 1973). We have found that the epithelium of allografts tends to separate very readily from the underlying basement membrane during fixation and cutting of sections, and in transmission electron micrographs abnormally wide spaces have been seen between the enterocytes lining the surface of the gut. One further point draws attention from the enterocytes themselves to the other tissue components. Large numbers of lymphocytes are found in the mucosa of rejecting grafts. These tend to be concentrated in the lamina propria, there are relatively few within the epithelium, and indeed intraepithelial lymphocytes

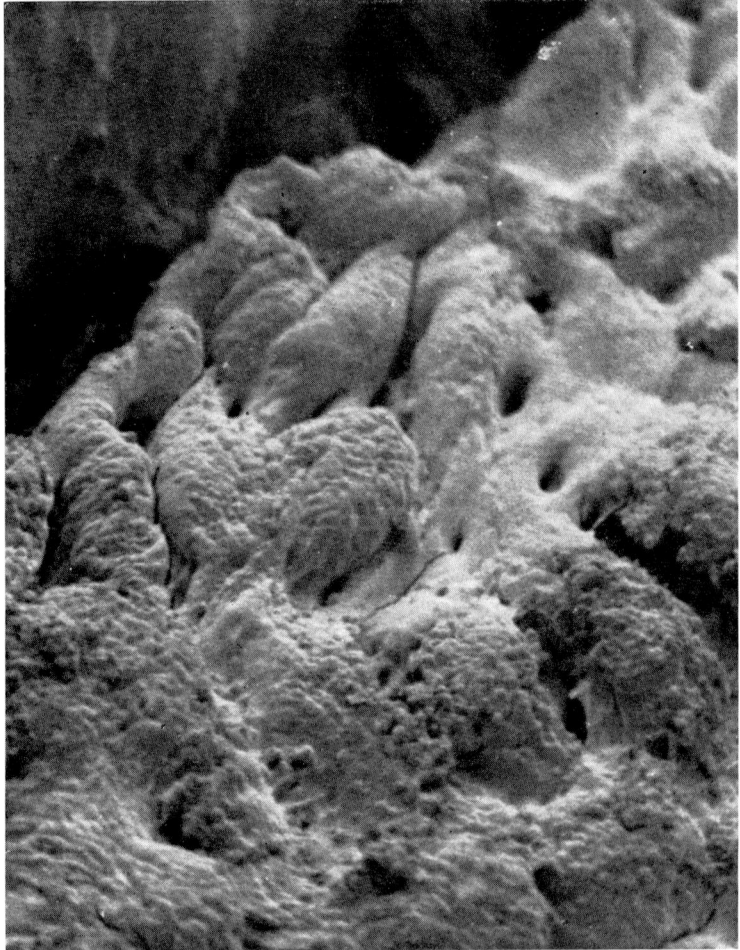

Fig. 3. Scanning electron micrograph of the luminal surface of a small intestinal allograft. (Supplied by Dr K. E. Carr, Department of Anatomy, University of Glasgow.)

were found in only 38 of 50 grafts with flat surface appearance (MacDonald & Ferguson 1976a). Thus the 'villous atrophy' and increased cell loss in rejection do not seem to be due to a direct result of early enterocyte death. We suggest that damage to or destruction of the underlying stroma—lamina propria and basement membrane—is a more likely mechanism (Fig. 4).

CRYPTS IN ALLOGRAFTS OF SMALL INTESTINE

On subjective evaluation of rejecting allografts it appeared that the crypts of

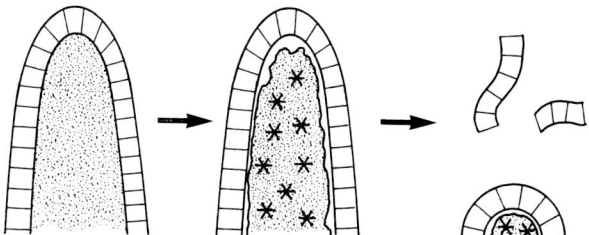

FIG. 4. A mechanism whereby the cell-mediated immune reaction of rejection, mainly confined to the lamina propria, produces villous atrophy.

Lieberkühn were longer than in isografts, and this was borne out by formal measurements of histological sections (MacDonald & Ferguson 1976a). Further to examine the significance of crypt hyperplasia, we used microdissection and metaphase arrest to examine the properties of single crypts. Mice bearing grafts were given colchicine two hours before they were killed (colchicine blocks mitosis in metaphase). Grafts were fixed in Clarke's fixative and Feulgen stained in bulk; groups of crypts were dissected out, squashed under a cover slip (Fig. 5), and the numbers of metaphases per crypt were counted. The results of this experiment are summarized in Fig. 6. In the crypts of normal small intestine and in isografts, there were some 2–4 mitoses per crypt per hour, whereas in allografts five days after implantation, 12.5 crypt cells entered mitosis hourly—crypt hyperplasia which had been considerably underestimated in direct measurements of crypt length. Between days 7 and 9, the cell production rate per crypt dropped significantly and this may be evidence of a late cytotoxic or ischaemic effect of the immune reaction on these rapidly dividing cells.

TIME COURSE OF CHANGES IN CRYPTS AND VILLI IN GRAFT-VERSUS-HOST DISEASE

Allografts provide only small pieces of tissue for examination, so we have used graft-versus-host (GVH) disease in order to examine more closely the time-course of changes in crypts and villi. GVH disease was induced in CBA × BALB/c F1 hybrid neonatal mice by injecting 25×10^6 parental spleen cells intraperitoneally, five days after birth. Mice were killed at intervals up to age 19 days and were given colchicine two hours before death. A detailed analysis of mucosal cytokinetics was obtained by measuring the various aspects listed in Table 4. The results of this study are published elsewhere (Ferguson & MacDonald 1976b) but the comparisons between villi, crypts and crypt

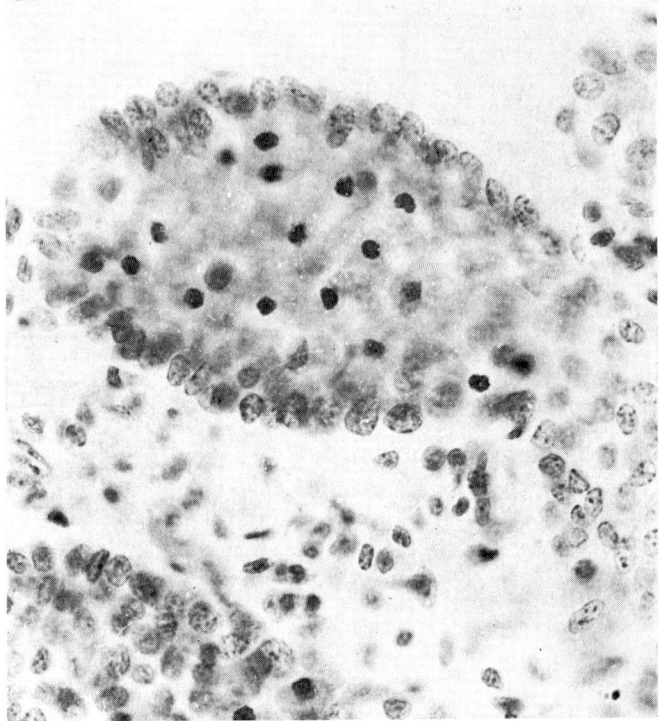

FIG. 5. Single crypts of Lieberkühn, dissected from a small intestinal allograft. The animal had been given colchicine 2 hours before death, so that mitoses are blocked in metaphase.

TABLE 4

Measurements of small intestinal architecture and cytokinetics

Length of villi
Shapes of villi (finger-like in mouse)
Length of crypts
Number of duplicating crypts
Cell production per crypt per hour
Number of crypts associated with each villus (i.e. ratio crypts: villi)
Cell loss per villus per hour (calculated)

mitosis in GVH animals and in their littermates are summarized in Fig 7. Striking crypt hyperplasia was found in the GVH mice aged 10 days when compared with their littermates, although the villi were the same height in both groups. Thus although crypt hyperplasia may in some conditions be a com-

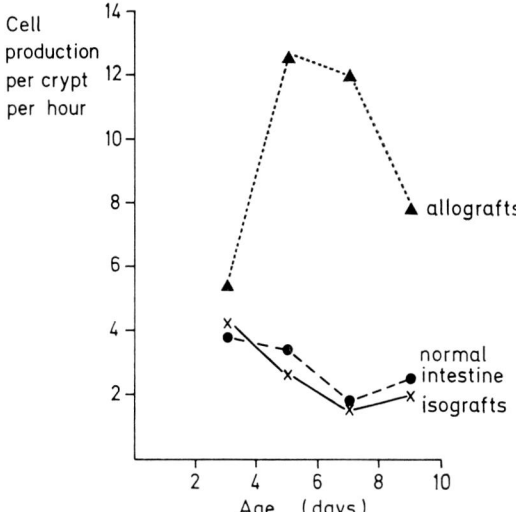

FIG. 6. The rate of cell production per hour (as assessed by metaphase arrest) in allografts (CBA → BALB/c) and isografts (CBA → CBA; BALB/c → BALB/c) of mouse jejunum, and in normal jejunum of the same age.

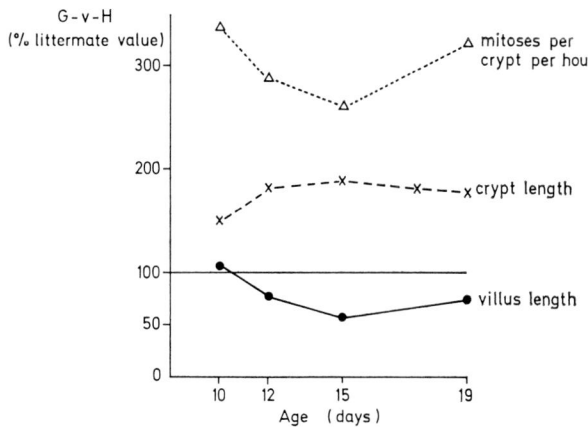

FIG. 7. Values for villous height, crypt length and mitoses per crypt per hour, in neonatal mice with graft-versus-host disease. Results are expressed as a % of the values for normal littermates of the same age.

pensatory response to loss of part of the mature enterocyte population, this cannot be the case in these experiments, since the 3–4-fold increase in crypt mitosis preceded villous atrophy by several days. We have therefore concluded that one of the direct effects of a local CMI reaction is stimulation of mitosis of crypt stem cells.

CONTACT HYPERSENSITIVITY IN THE SMALL INTESTINE

Contact hypersensitivity (e.g. to tuberculin, dinitrochlorobenzene, oxazolone) is another experimental model of a local CMI reaction. There is a single report in the literature of dinitrochlorobenzene challenge, by feeding, of sensitized pigs (Bicks et al. 1967). This produced malabsorption, as assessed by xylose absorption, lymphocyte infiltration of the intestine, oedema and necrosis.

We have used a number of regimes in attempts to produce local hypersensitivity to oxazolone in sensitized mice. Five different schedules for oxazolone feeding were unsuccessful, but villous atrophy and crypt hyperplasia have been found in two groups of experiments—where oxazolone in olive oil was injected into a Thiry-Vella loop at laparotomy, and when oxazolone, dissolved in 50% alcohol, was injected into the lumen of the jejunum at laparotomy.

These preliminary findings indicate that crypt hyperplasia and villous atrophy occur even when a CMI reaction is directed against antigens other than those of the intestine itself. They support the theory that the tissue damage is mediated via lymphokines rather than by a direct toxic effect of T cells on the enterocytes.

ENTEROPATHIC LYMPHOKINES?

A local CMI reaction may damage adjacent tissue by at least two mechanisms—direct T cell cytotoxicity, and via the action of the soluble factors, lymphokines. Light and electron microscopy have not yet provided evidence of a cytotoxic effect of the lymphocytes within allografts, but it seems likely that the two striking effects of local CMI—villous atrophy and crypt hyperplasia—are produced by 'enteropathic' lymphokines or factors. Two actions are postulated:

(1) destruction or distortion of the stroma of the lamina propria so that enterocyte adhesion is impaired—a truly enteropathic factor,

(2) stimulation of mitosis in the stem cells of the crypts of Lieberkühn—a crypt mitogenic factor.

These factors are as yet only theoretical. But as a first stage in their detection we have used several conventional assays in attempts to demonstrate secretion

TABLE 5

Secretion of lymphokines by isografts and allografts of mouse small intestine

Lymphokine	Assay system		Isografts	Allografts
Macrophage migration inhibition factor (MIF)	Migration of mouse spleen cells into planchettes filled with organ culture fluid		12% inhibition	18% inhibition
Skin reactive factor (SRF)	Intradermal injection of organ culture fluid; sequential measurements of double skin thickness		0.12 mm peak increment	0.11 mm peak increment
Chemotactic factor for macrophages (CF)	Distance migrated into Millipore filter by mouse peritoneal exudate cells % chemotaxis	*Gey's fluid alone* 39 ± 5 μm (mean $\pm$ S.E.)	40 ± 3 μm 6%	41 ± 6 μm 13%
Inhibition of macrophage chemotaxis (CIF)	As above; casein added to stimulate chemotaxis % inhibition of chemotaxis	54 ± 6 μm	55 ± 7 μm −2%	45 ± 6 μm 60%

of lymphokines by the T cells in allografts. (This work has been done in collaboration with Mr R. Russell.)

Isografts and allografts (6–8 days after implantation) were dissected from the kidney capsules of host mice, and were either cultured on the grids of disposable organ culture dishes for six hours (the culture fluid then being used for assay of macrophage migration inhibition factor, MIF, and skin reactive factor, SRF) or were placed directly in Boyden chemotaxis chambers. Results of the experiments are summarized in Table 5. There was no evidence of secretion by grafts of MIF or of SRF into organ culture fluids; however, allografts were found to secrete an inhibitor of macrophage chemotaxis.

CMI AND THE 'ENTEROPATHY' OF PARASITE INFECTIONS

Immunity to parasites involves a range of immune reactions, and these affect the parasites at different stages of their life cycle. IgE and T lymphocytes are clearly important and probably in both cases effective protective immunity will of necessity produce some tissue damage. The nature of the immune response to *Giardia lamblia* is unknown. However, in children (Ferguson

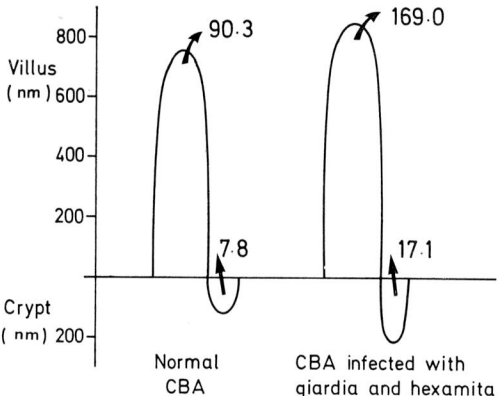

FIG. 8. Small intestinal architecture and cytokinetics in healthy CBA mice and in CBA mice infected with the parasites *Giardia* and *Hexamita*. The numbers indicate cell production per crypt per hour (measured directly) and cell loss per villus per hour (calculated).

et al. 1976b) and in mice (Table 6) infected with *Giardia* there are increased numbers of intraepithelial lymphocytes and several pieces of work suggest that the intraepithelial lymphocytes are T cells. Also in patients with hypogammaglobulinaemia but normal T cell immunity, *Giardia* infection is usually accompanied by partial villous atrophy and malabsorption (Ochs & Ament 1976), findings which we would interpret as probably due to intense CMI reactions unmodulated by local antibody. Accordingly, we have made detailed studies of intestinal architecture in *Giardia*-infected mice, and have found that although there is no villous atrophy and no obvious crypt enlargement on conventional histological examination, crypt mitosis is doubled by *Giardia* infection (Fig. 8) and there is a more rapid transit of enterocytes up the sides of villi (Table 7). We have not had the opportunity to examine the effects of *Giardia* infection on the cell kinetics of the small intestine in congenitally athymic mice. On the basis of our work described in this paper it is likely that a lymphokine causes

TABLE 6

Influence of thymus and of *Giardia lamblia* infection on intraepithelial lymphocytes

Experimental group	No. of animals	Intraepithelial lymphocyte count (per 100 epithelial cells)	
		Mean	S.E.
CBA mice (6 wk)	5	13.6	1.8
Nu nu mice (6 wk)	6	2.0	0.4
Sha sha mice (6 wk), *Giardia*-infected	7	21.8	3.0

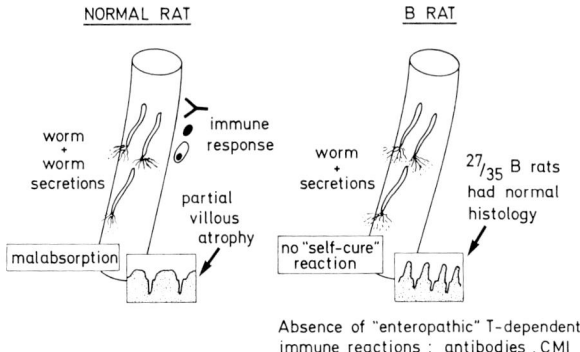

FIG. 9. An explanation for the lack of morphological damage to the small intestinal mucosa in thymus-deprived rats infected with the parasite *Nippostrongylus brasiliensis*.

crypt hyperplasia in this parasitic infection, so we would predict that thymus-dependent crypt hyperplasia would not be found in athymic mice infected with this or other parasites.

When rats are infected with *Nippostrongylus brasiliensis*, oedema, villous atrophy and crypt hyperplasia are found in those areas of the small intestine where the parasites are localized. We used T cell-depleted, B rats (thymectomy, 850 R irradiation, repopulated with autologous bone marrow) to determine whether these tissue changes are produced directly by parasites or are side-effects of the anti-parasite immune response (Ferguson & Jarrett 1975). The results are illustrated in Fig. 9. With the infective dose used (4000 larvae), changes in the appearance of the small intestinal mucosa were found in virtually all immunologically intact infected animals. However, villous atrophy and crypt hyperplasia were absent in 27 of 35 parasitized B rats. Thymus dependence of the worm-associated tissue damage has also been found by E. J. Ruitenberg

TABLE 7

Rate of transit of enterocytes in CBA and *sha sha* mice

Experimental group	*No. of mice*	Height of leading labelled cell (number of nuclei from villus–crypt junction)	
		Mean	S.E.
CBA mice	6	23.8	3.0
Sha sha mice	6	44.3	3.9

Each mouse had been given 25 μCi[^{3}H]thymidine i.p., 25 hours before death. Autoradiographs of sections of jejunum were exposed for 18 days.

(personal communication) in his work on the immune response to *Trichinella* in normal and *nu nu* mice.

HYPOTHESIS

Our experiments have shown that local CMI reactions, probably acting via lymphokines, can produce crypt hyperplasia and villous atrophy with ready separation of enterocytes from the basement membrane. However, CMI does not seem to damage the individual epithelial cells and does not correlate with the presence or absence of increased numbers of intraepithelial lymphocytes. Factors other than a local delayed hypersensitivity reaction are likely to be the cause of enterocyte changes and to influence the distribution of intestinal lymphocytes in diseases such as coeliac disease and acute gastroenteritis. However, although a variety of changes in small intestinal architecture can be produced experimentally, the flat mucosa with crypt hyperplasia and malabsorption is by far the most frequently encountered lesion in human and animal diseases. We suggest that a common factor in all of these conditions is probably a local CMI reaction to food, microbial, parasite or other antigens. This local hypersensitivity reaction results in crypt hyperplasia, fast epithelial cell turnover, reduced epithelial cell adhesion and villous atrophy, with the clinical end result of a malabsorption syndrome.

IMPLICATIONS: LOCAL CMI REACTIONS AND MALNUTRITION

Areas of the world where nutrition is borderline or insufficient are also those areas where enteric infections and parasite infestation are endemic. It is to be hoped that effective bacterial, viral and parasite vaccines will be developed and used in the populations concerned, but if further work confirms that local CMI reactions can indeed cause malabsorption, then the nature of such vaccines and immunization schedules must be tailored to promote local immunity with a minimum of local delayed hypersensitivity.

ACKNOWLEDGEMENTS

This work has been supported by grants from the National Fund for Research into Crippling Diseases and the Camilla Samuel fund.

References

BICKS, R. O., AZAR, M. M. & ROSENBERG, E. W. (1967) Delayed hypersensitivity reactions in the intestinal tract. II. Small intestinal lesions associated with xylose malabsorption. *Gastroenterology* 53, 437-443

FERGUSON, A., MACDONALD, T. T., WATT, C. & CARR, K. E. (1976a) Hypersensitivity reactions in the small intestine. 4. Effects of allograft rejection on intestinal architecture; transmission and scanning electron microscopic studies. *Gut*, in press

ELVES, M. W. & FERGUSON, A. (1975) The humoral immune response to allografts of foetal small intestine in mice. *Br. J. Exp. Pathol. 56*, 454-458

FERGUSON, A. (1975) Lymphocytes in coeliac disease, in *Coeliac Disease* (Hekkens, W. T. J. M. & Peña, A. S., eds.), pp. 265-276, Stenfert Kroese, Leiden

FERGUSON, A. (1976) Models of intestinal hypersensitivity. *Clin. Gastroenterol. 5*, 271-288

FERGUSON, A. & JARRETT, E. E. E. (1975) Hypersensitivity reactions in the small intestine. 1. Thymus dependence of experimental partial villous atrophy. *Gut 16*, 114-117

FERGUSON, A., MCCLURE, J. P. & TOWNLEY, R. R. W. (1976b) Intraepithelial lymphocyte counts in jejunal biopsies of children with diarrhoea. *Acta Paediatr. Scand. 65*, 541-546

FERGUSON, A. & PARROTT, D. M. V. (1972) Growth and development of 'antigen-free' grafts of foetal mouse intestine. *J. Pathol. 106*, 95-101

FERGUSON, A. & PARROTT, D. M. V. (1973) Histopathology and time course of rejection of allografts of mouse small intestine. *Transplantation 15*, 546-554

HEDBERG, C. A., REISER, S. C. & REILLY, R. W. (1968) Intestinal phase of the runting syndrome in mice. 2. Observations on nutrient absorption and certain disaccharidase abnormalities. *Transplantation 6*, 104-110

HOLMES, J. T., KLEIN, M. S., WINAWER, S. J. & FORTNER, J. G. (1971) Morphological studies of rejection in canine jejunal allografts. *Gastroenterology 61*, 693-706

MACDONALD, T. T. & FERGUSON, A. (1976a) Hypersensitivity reactions in the small intestine. 2. Effects of allograft rejection on mucosal architecture and lymphoid cell infiltrate. *Gut 17*, 81-91

MACDONALD, T. T. & FERGUSON, A. (1976b) Hypersensitivity reactions in the small intestine. 3. The effects of allograft rejection and of graft-versus-host disease on epithelial cell kinetics. *Cell Tissue Kinet.*, in press

OCHS, H. D. & AMENT, M. E. (1976) Gastrointestinal tract and immunodeficiency, in *Immunological Aspects of the Liver and Gastrointestinal Tract* (Ferguson, A. & MacSween, R. N. M., eds.), pp. 83-120, Medical & Technical Publishing Co. Ltd, Lancaster

PALMER, R. H. & REILLY, R. W. (1971) Bile salt depletion in the runting syndrome. *Transplantation 12*, 479-483

REILLY, R. W. & KIRSNER, J. B. (1965) Runt intestinal disease. *Lab. Invest. 14*, 102-107

Discussion

Bienenstock: Functional MIF activity can apparently be found in high quantities in normal human intestinal secretions, according to Waldman (Gadol *et al.* 1976).

Ferguson: We have shown that a MIF can be secreted by small bowel biopsies from coeliac patients when cultured with gliadin, but we did not find MIF activity when biopsies from normal persons or from coeliac disease patients were cultured in the absence of antigen. Frederick & Bohl (1976) have found MIF secretion by suspensions of lamina propria cells of guinea pigs, but only when these cells were cultured in the presence of specific antigen (transmissible gastroenteritis virus in their experiments). We have not looked in normal human intestinal secretions but I would expect that many substances such as enterotoxin and trypsin would interfere with migration, so that it would be difficult to show that the effect in question was indeed due to the presence of a lymphokine.

Bienenstock: Waldman has shown that this activity is compatible with the published molecular size of MIF. That does not prove that it is MIF. But if MIF *is* present normally, perhaps other lymphokines are there normally too? If so, this goes against your thesis that a lymphokine is responsible for villous flattening.

Ferguson: There are of course many T and B lymphocytes in normal gut. Their functions are still uncertain. We feel it is unlikely that, in normal animals which are not infected by parasites, local cell-mediated immune reactions influence the shapes of villi and crypts. The histology of the small intestinal mucosa in CBA, BALB/c and nude mice is very similar although there are substantial numbers of mucosal lymphocytes in the CBA and BALB/c strains but very few in the nude mice. I could not predict the source of MIF as secreted by normal uninfected gut, but I doubt if it would be from the T cells in transit through the tissue.

Gowans: On the point of the mechanism of destruction of the allografts, I was interested in your description of a gap developing under the epithelium and of the enterocytes falling away from the stump underneath. A gap suggests the development of oedema. I suspect that the lymphatic drainage of your grafts may be poor so that damage due to the allograft reaction may lead rapidly to an accumulation of fluid. Have you considered a simple mechanical shearing due to oedema? A second question: how quickly does blood supply fail in the allografts? Is this the crucial event determining graft destruction?

Ferguson: These grafts are attached to the capsule of the kidney and not to the underlying tissue, and in established grafts one sees apparently normal, although small, blood vessels. There are large lymphatic-like spaces at the edges of the grafts, but neither in isografts or allografts has oedema of the mucosa appeared to be a feature, and this point has been examined both by light and by electron microscopy. One reason why we think there is lymphoid cell traffic into and out of these grafts is that large lymphocytes can be seen in the lymphatic spaces draining allografts.

Gowans: That is why I thought they might be obstructed. I was recalling your own comment that the accumulations of lymphocytes in and around the grafts might have been due 'to obstruction of lymphatic drainage of the grafts' (Ferguson & Parrott 1972).

Ferguson: In the normal small bowel a considerable amount of water is absorbed across the epithelium. Some of this leaves the mucosa as lymph and I think it's likely that lymphocytes are passively propelled along in this stream of fluid, rather than that lymphocytes actively migrate along the lymphatics from the gut to the lymph nodes. Certainly it's my experience of Thiry-Vella loops that the lymphatics within the villus cores often contain many lymphocytes, many more than one would expect in a segment of normal intestine that is actively absorbing jejunal fluids.

We have not examined the blood vessels by electron microscopy, but by light microscopy there does not seem to be any obvious capillaritis or arteritis. On rejection the grafts do not become black, as do rejecting skin grafts; they just slowly disappear, although fragments of the smooth muscle layer are recognizable for a long time. Nevertheless I would not be surprised if the final ulceration of the mucosa prior to complete rejection was partly due to a local anoxia.

Gowans: You mentioned that there may be a big traffic of lymphoid cells through the lamina propria of the normal gut. I am sure you will agree that histological studies will not tell us the answer. You have to go back over 40 years to find someone who has taken the trouble to cannulate individual lacteals in order to examine this point. Baker (1933) found in cats that prenodal lymph draining Peyer's patches contained many cells while that draining the intestine between patches contained many fewer cells. This should be an easy experiment to repeat employing modern methods of micromanipulation and until it is repeated the matter will remain unresolved.

Booth: It would be interesting to know whether one sees, in the electron microscope, endothelial cell swelling in the capillaries beneath the basement membrane. Do you get macrophages moving in? Are polymorphs seen? What sort of activity goes on in that subepithelial layer?

Ferguson: Polymorphs have not been seen in rejecting allografts. We have seen rows of cells with the appearance of lymphocytes, sitting under the basement membrane. With regard to the fine structure of the basement membrane, the electron microscopist, Dr K. E. Carr, has concentrated on the surface morphology and the enterocyte appearances up to now. In view of our present hypothesis on the significance of the basement membrane, she is now examining the lamina propria closely.

André: Is there a difference in graft-versus-host reaction if one grafts a piece of gut with or without Peyer's patches?

Ferguson: A baby mouse has tiny Peyer's patches which contain mainly T cells, and are presumably areas of T cell traffic. As far as I know the workers who have examined the small bowel in graft-versus-host disease have not looked to see whether the reaction is worse, or whether ulceration occurs more rapidly, around the Peyer's patches. Most of the grafts in our experiments will not contain a Peyer's patch, because the transplanted intestine is a length of only 5 mm, but we have noted that in areas where there is an obvious nodule of lymphoid tissue in a rejecting graft, that area is crammed with blast cells. It does look as if this is a route of entry of T cells into the grafts. However, in other parts of the same graft a millimetre or two away from the presumed Peyer's patch but in the same section, the histological stage of rejection, and the nature of the lymphoid cell infiltrate, are identical to the appearances we find in other allografts at the same stage of rejection, in which no Peyer's patch has been present.

Evans: I want to ask a general question about the acceptability in immunological terms of a truly localized delayed hypersensitivity reaction in the gut which is not demonstrable anywhere else. Your models have been developed with coeliac disease in mind, and a major problem in coeliac disease is that you cannot demonstrate by skin testing any significant difference in terms of delayed hypersensitivity between coeliac patients and other patients, with wheat proteins. You can get skin reactions on biopsy but there is no real evidence that this is a delayed hypersensitivity reaction. Are you developing the thesis here that you get a truly localized delayed hypersensitivity reaction with no spillover into the other systems?

Ferguson: It was purely fortuitous that our early studies of the morphology of rejection showed a similarity to the small bowel in coeliac disease. If I had not worked as a clinical gastroenterologist before my period in laboratory immunology, I would probably have failed to appreciate the significance of this chance finding. At the moment I see no reason to postulate that the cells which can mediate a delayed hypersensitivity reaction to gluten are confined to the mucosal surfaces. In a disease like tuberculosis there are sensitized T cells throughout the body and a local reaction will occur at any site where an appropriate amount of antigen has been concentrated. Indeed this latter aspect is a great problem in trying to suggest that coeliac disease is due only to a delayed hypersensitivity reaction. I do not think that molecules of gluten will stay in the small intestine for a sufficient length of time to allow the evolution of a cell-mediated immune reaction. However, if gluten is precipitated in immune complexes, or if it has stuck to reticulin or to the surface of enterocytes, or if for some other reason coeliac patients retain gluten antigen in their gut, then I can envisage the evolution of a cell-mediated immune reaction.

If one does skin tests with soluble antigens, these diffuse into the tissue fluids and are no longer present at the site 12–24 hours later. Thus in order to demonstrate delayed hypersensitivity to gluten in coeliac disease it will be necessary to do skin tests by using particulate preparations of a range of gluten antigens, both in normal people and in coeliac patients.

Evans: Are you saying that the methods of skin testing for delayed hypersensitivity need an immobilized antigen in order to be valid?

Ferguson: Yes.

Pepys: It has been known for a long time that the antigens which produce delayed hypersensitivity reactions in the skin of man need to be antigens which fix, like tuberculin, and remain in the tissue for a long time. The tuberculin reaction can be modulated by agents which affect vasomotor tone and vascular permeability. Addition of histamine to the tuberculin causes the tuberculin to diffuse away and prevents the appearance of a positive reaction. Alternatively, the introduction of adrenaline together with a high dilution of tuberculin makes the antigen fix in a more localized area and may bring out a positive reaction which is not seen with that dilution of tuberculin in the absence of adrenaline (Pepys 1955).

Another reason for the failure to demonstrate delayed hypersensitivity reactions to gluten in the skin in coeliac patients may be that they have Arthus reactions which could act like histamine in 'diluting out' the antigen. Coeliac patients were found to have clear Arthus reactions on skin testing with gluten antigens which correlated with their serum titres of anti-gluten antibodies (P. Baker & A. E. Read, personal communication); on a gluten-free diet, the reactions went away as the levels of anti-gluten antibody fell.

Pierce: I am not certain how long an antigen has to remain in tissue to induce a delayed hypersensitivity reaction. Some of our studies of the response of rats to cholera toxoid suggest that soluble protein antigens may remain in the gut mucosa for several days after a single exposure (Pierce & Gowans 1975). This is suggested by the observation that a single gut booster induces a systemic traffic of IgA immunoblasts which home selectively to the lamina propria of the boosted portion of the gut 4–5 days after boosting. Since this homing is antigen-specific I presume it is due to antigen trapped in the mucosa at the time of boosting and persisting there for at least 4–5 days, though I realize other explanations are possible. My point is that there is no evidence in these circumstances of anything looking like a local delayed hypersensitivity reaction, and the rats do not sicken or die from apparent systemic delayed hypersensitivity reactions. Perhaps persistence of antigen for 4–5 days is not long enough.

Ferguson: Surely for antigen to persist for several days it would need to be intracellular. The macrophage is a suitable candidate which has been completely ignored in our discussions so far.

Cebra: Has the cholera toxoid lost all its tissue-fixing properties at the time you use it?

Pierce: Yes. It no longer binds to cell membrane as cholera *toxin* does.

Lachmann: These tests are also used the other way round. The retention of antigen can be used as a test for cellular immunity to it. If you inject radio-labelled tuberculin into the skin of a tuberculin-sensitive guinea pig and of a normal guinea pig the rates of clearance are very different, the antigen being retained in the skin of the immunized animal.

Bienenstock: On this question of local cellular immunity, O'Neill in my laboratory has shown that in guinea pigs fed with BCG he can demonstrate MIF production specific for PPD from cells derived from Peyer's patches and to a lesser extent from the lamina propria, in the absence of skin-test positivity and in the absence of the turning on of splenic lymphocytes (M. O'Neill & J. Bienenstock, unpublished). So local feeding of antigen can give rise to the local production of MIF; whether it is B or T cell-derived is another issue.

Cebra: Since undifferentiated crypt cells have been implicated in the transport of secretory IgA out into the gut lumen, I wonder if an involvement of more of these cells in cell division to generate enterocytes, as you indicate occurs in certain situations, interferes with the secretory process. In your *Giardia*-infected mice have you measured the overall concentration of secretory IgA in the gut fluid to see whether there is a sharp fall in the level?

Secondly, it is difficult to disperse the cells in the lamina propria and recover intact and reasonably viable plasma cells. As Dr Bienenstock mentioned, you can get a fair number of small round cells out, and these could be looked at to determine the proportion of T cells. It would be even more interesting to use antisera against Ly1 or Ly2,3 to determine the proportion of suppressor T cells present in animals in which you suspect delayed hypersensitivity.

Ferguson: There is little information on the nature of protective immunity to *Giardia*, and I am unaware of any work on IgA or secretory IgA responses in this infection. With regard to the nature of the lymphocytes in the gut, Dr Bienenstock's department has reported that there are T cells, null cells and B cells in preparations of intestinal lymphocytes.

Bienenstock: There are very few B cells. In fact our methods are questionable, in the sense of whether they represent the cell population in the lamina propria (Rudzik & Bienenstock 1974).

Pierce: If one is drawing a parallel between host-versus-graft reaction and what takes place in parasitization with the introduction of foreign antigens, it is not clear to me why, during *Nippostrongylus* infection or other parasitic infections, the individual does not go on to reject the bowel completely, though obviously he doesn't.

Ferguson: In patients with coeliac disease there are many tiny areas of ulceration in the affected areas of the small bowel. In addition large deep benign ulcers have been reported in a small proportion of such patients. We have suggested that an established cell-mediated immune reaction will speed up the rate of cell turnover—a potentially protective although non-specific mechanism for the exfoliation of parasite-infected or virus- or bacteria-infected epithelial cells. Perhaps it is only when there is an intense cell-mediated immune reaction, as is seen in rejection, that one finds changes in the general architecture, malabsorption and, in extreme cases, ulceration.

Lehner: You suggested two lymphokines as explaining some of your findings and I particularly wonder about the mitogenic factor, which has only been shown to cause mitosis in lymphoid cells and not in epithelial cells. Have you looked for evidence of the latter?

Ferguson: Assays of mitogenic factor are usually done with lymphocytes or lymphoid cell lines. However, in their work on leishmaniasis in the guinea pig, Bryceson *et al.* (1972) found that the thickening of the skin in leishmaniasis was a thymus-dependent reaction.

Lehner: You have shown chemotactic inhibition by means of casein attraction of cells. What is the mechanism?

Ferguson: Casein is used as a standard chemotactic agent. If one wishes to assay a factor which will inhibit chemotaxis, the cells are attracted through a filter by using casein in the lower chamber, and it is possible to see whether the substance under consideration inhibits the casein-induced chemotaxis.

Lehner: Casein has been shown to be a good B cell mitogen. I wondered if this would affect your results.

Parrott: I doubt whether the fact that casein is mitogenic would make any difference to its chemotactic effect. The concentrations at which mitogens such as Con A are chemotactic are much lower than those at which they are mitogenic (Wilkinson *et al.* 1976).

Cebra: How much physical association is there between the basal part of the plasma membrane of the epithelial cells and the basement membrane? It would seem that as cells are dividing out, they must slide over the basement membrane; that is probably not being constantly regenerated at the same rate as overlying enterocytes.

Ferguson: The region of the basement membrane and basal lamina is indeed formed continuously, but it is not known how much is produced by the epithelial cells and how much is a liquid or solid component of the ground substance of the lamina propria. In specimens of small intestine which have been allowed to autolyse overnight, the epithelium strips off and scanning electron microscopy can be used to examine the underlying basement membrane. There are holes in this basement membrane (Toner *et al.* 1970) and the numbers seem to correspond to the numbers of lymphocytes crossing the basement membrane in conventional sections. However, I think the epithelial cells move at a different rate from the basement membrane.

Booth: Marsh & Trier (1974) labelled the fibroblasts in the basement membrane, in fact, and showed that they moved up the villus in the same way that the enterocytes do.

Ferguson: They also (Marsh & Trier 1974) showed that the fibroblasts moved more rapidly up the side of the villi than did labelled enterocytes.

Cebra: I am wondering whether the supposed T lymphocytes may have only one kind of lymphokine, the mitogenic factor, and the other effect is produced by a breaking of the tight junctions that join the epithelial cells together, so that in order to get a sheet cells off, all that is needed is to break it in a few places. It could be done mechanically by the lymphocytes forcing their way between the epithelial cells and breaking open junctions, rather than by an effect on adhesion to the basement membrane.

Ferguson: In coeliac disease a high number of intraepithelial lymphocytes is a constant finding in untreated patients (Ferguson 1974). This is not so for other conditions where the mucosa is flattened, for example *Nippostrongylus* infection. In fact there are fewer lymphocytes than normal between the epithelial cells in the flattened mucosa in worm infections (T. T. MacDonald & A. Ferguson, unpublished 1975). Neither are there increased numbers in acute gastroenteritis or in graft rejection (Ferguson *et al.* 1976; MacDonald & Ferguson 1976). Thus damage by intraepithelial lymphocytes cannot explain the villus atrophy.

References

BAKER, R. D. (1933) The cellular content of chyle in relation to lymphoid tissue and fat transportation. *Anat. Rec. 55,* 207

BRYCESON, A. D. M., PRESTON, P. M., BRAY, R. S. & DUMONDE, D. C. (1972) Experimental cutaneous leishmaniasis. II. Effect of immunosuppression and antigenic competition on the course of infection with *Leishmania enriettii* in the guinea-pig. *Clin. Exp. Immunol. 10,* 305-335

FERGUSON, A. (1974) Lymphocytes in coeliac disease, in *Coeliac Disease* (Hekkens, W. T. J. M. & Peña, A. S., eds.), pp. 265-276, Stenfert Kroese, Leiden

FERGUSON, A. & PARROTT, D. M. V. (1972) The effect of antigen deprivation on thymus-dependent and thymus-independent lymphocytes in the small intestine of the mouse. *Clin. Exp. Immunol. 12,* 477-488

FERGUSON, A., MCCLURE, J. P. & TOWNLEY, R. R. W. (1976) Intraepithelial lymphocyte counts in small intestinal biopsies from children with diarrhoea. *Acta Paediatr. Scand. 65,* 541-546,

FREDERICK, G. T. & BOHL, E. H. (1976) Local and systemic cell-mediated immunity against transmissible gastroenteritis, an intestinal viral infection of swine. *J. Immunol. 116,* 1000-1004

GADOL, N., WALDMAN, R. H. & CLEM, L. W. (1976) Inhibition of macrophage migration by normal guinea pig intestinal secretions. *Proc. Soc. Exp. Biol. Med. 15,* 654-658

PEPYS, J. (1955) Specific and non-specific factors in the tuberculin reaction. *Am. Rev. Tubercul. 71,* 49-73

MACDONALD, T. T. & FERGUSON, A. (1976) Hypersensitivity reactions in the small intestine.

2. The effects of allograft rejection on mucosal architecture and lymphoid cell infiltrate. *Gut*, *17*, 81-91

MARSH, M. N. & TRIER, J. S. (1974) Morphology and cell proliferation of subepithelial fibroblasts in adult mouse jejunum. II. Radioautographic studies. *Gastroenterology* *67*, 636-645

PIERCE, N. F. & GOWANS, J. L. (1975) Cellular kinetics of the intestinal immune response to cholera toxoid in rats. *J. Exp. Med. 142*, 1550-1563

RUDZIK, O. & BIENENSTOCK, J. (1974) Isolation and characteristics of gut mucosal lymphocytes. *Lab. Invest. 30*, 260-266

TONER, P. G., CARR, K. E., FERGUSON, A. & MACKAY, C. (1970) Scanning and transmission electron microscopic studies of human intestinal mucosa. *Gut 11*, 471-481

WILKINSON, P. B., ROBERTS, J. A., RUSSELL, R. J. & MCLOUGHLIN, M. (1976) Chemotaxis of mitogen-activated human lymphocytes and the effects of membrane active enzymes. *Clin. Exp. Immunol. 25*, 280-287

Immunopathology of coeliac disease

C. C. BOOTH, T. J. PETERS and W. F. DOE

Department of Medicine, Royal Postgraduate Medical School, London

Abstract Coeliac disease may be defined as a condition in which there is an abnormal jejunal mucosa with loss of villi, which improves morphologically after treatment with a gluten-free diet. Pathologically, there is damage to the jejunal enterocytes, with hyperplasia of crypt cells so that overall enteropoiesis is increased. On conventional or scanning electron microscopy the enterocytes are markedly abnormal. Histochemically, the normal punctate appearance of the lysosomes is lost and sensitive lysosomal enzyme assays on mucosal biopsy samples using isopycnic centrifugation techniques show that there is an increase in total lysosomal activity with reduction in lysosomal latency.

Studies following gluten feeding in patients whose mucosa has returned to normal after treatment with a gluten-free diet show that pathological abnormalities appear within 4–8 hours of gluten challenge. Complement together with extracellular IgM can be demonstrated in the lamina propria, suggesting the formation of immune complexes. In untreated coeliac disease there is a significant reduction in serum levels of C3 and C4. There is also evidence indicating the presence of immune complexes in the serum. Coeliac disease may therefore be an intestinal model of an immune complex disease, in which an antigen derived from gluten reacts with an antibody formed locally in the gut, fixing complement and causing damage to the enterocyte by activation of lysosomes.

Dicke (1950) was the first to show that coeliac disease is produced in some way by a normal dietary constituent, gluten, which is present in wheat and rye flour. Subsequent studies have repeatedly shown that there is a toxic factor present in gluten which damages the absorbing cells of the jejunal mucosa in subjects with the disorder, whether the condition presents in childhood or in adult life. The mechanism by which this toxicity occurs is not yet established with certainty but there is increasing evidence that coeliac disease can be considered as an immunological disorder in which there is a reaction between an antigen present in gluten and an antibody secreted by the immunocytes of the intestinal mucosa. This is associated with complement fixation and subsequent cell damage. The purpose of this paper is to review the evidence which suggests that coeliac disease is at least in part an immune complex disease.

DEFINITION

The term 'coeliac disease' is often used to describe a variety of conditions in which an abnormal jejunal mucosa is associated with malabsorption. For the purpose of this paper coeliac disease will be defined as an abnormality of the jejunal mucosa which improves morphologically after treatment with a gluten-free diet.

MORPHOLOGY

In coeliac disease the appearances of the intestinal mucosa are strikingly abnormal. There are variations in the severity of the lesion in different patients (Stewart et al. 1967) but at low power under the dissecting microscope the mucosa is usually flat and devoid of villi. At higher power the mucosa can be seen to be divided by grooves into a mosaic pattern. The crypts of Lieberkühn, not being hidden by villi, open directly on to the surface of the mucosa and their orifices can be clearly seen. The histology of the flat mucosa reveals three main features. The enterocytes are no longer columnar but are flat, cuboidal, and reduced in number. The enteroblasts (or crypt cells) are increased, the crypt layer being markedly thickened compared with the normal, and there is an infiltration of the lamina propria with abundant lymphocytes and plasma cells. There is clear evidence that there is damage to the enterocytes, the hyperplasia of the enteroblasts being compensatory in an attempt to make up for damage to the surface cells, a situation analogous to haemolytic anaemia (Booth 1970). The appearances of the abnormal jejunal enterocyte improve dramatically when a gluten-free diet is given, the response being more rapid and more striking in children than in adults. These observations refer to the jejunal enterocyte, for the ileum in this condition is either normal or less severely involved than the jejunum (Rubin et al. 1960; Booth et al. 1962; Stewart et al. 1967), which would be expected if the intestine were being damaged by an orally ingested toxin.

HISTOCHEMISTRY

The anatomical changes already described are associated with abnormalities in the histochemistry of the intestinal cell. Brush border enzymes are usually abnormal and frequently reveal a reduction of alkaline phosphatase as well as diminished staining of other brush border enzymes (Riecken et al. 1966). Lysosomal enzymes can also be shown to be abnormal. In the untreated jejunal mucosa the lysosomal enzymes, for example acid phosphatase and esterase, are not present as discrete organelles as they should be in the normal situation, but are diffusely scattered throughout the disorganized enterocyte. As Wattiaux & de Duve (1956) have suggested, it is possible that this diffusion of intensely hydrolytic enzymes into the cytoplasm may contribute to cell damage. The changes shown are not specific to coeliac disease and probably simply reflect the gross damage that gluten causes to the susceptible enterocyte.

CYTOCHEMICAL STUDIES

The cytochemistry of jejunal biopsies in untreated coeliac disease has been compared with the results in control subjects and in patients who have been treated satisfactorily with a gluten-free diet (Peters et al. 1975). As others have shown, there are gross reductions in the activities of the major brush border enzymes, but the results for the lysosomal enzymes have been shown to be quite different. Table 1 shows the specific activities of six acid hydrolases and of lactate dehydrogenase, a cytosol enzyme, in homogenates of biopsies from control subjects and from patients with coeliac disease. Mean activities of all acid hydrolases were found to be significantly higher in untreated patients than in control subjects. The increase in activity differed for each enzyme, with acid phosphatase showing the smallest rise. Enzyme activities in patients treated with a gluten-free diet decreased towards normal values. For acid phosphatase

TABLE 1

Activities of acid hydrolases and of lactate dehydrogenase in jejunal biopsies from control subjects and patients with adult coeliac disease

Enzyme	Control subjects	Untreated coeliac disease	Treated coeliac disease
N-Acetyl-β-glucosaminidase	2.12 ± 0.15 (20)	3.28 ± 0.31 (9)$P<0.001$	2.71 ± 0.25 (5)$P<0.05$
α-Galactosidase	0.185 ± 0.012 (20)	0.402 ± 0.021(7)$P<0.001$	0.301 ± 0.063(7)$P<0.01$
Acid phosphatase	16.2 ± 2.1 (21)	22.5 ± 2.1 (9)$P<0.05$	14.9 ± 3.2 (6)N.S.
Acid β-galactosidase	1.15 ± 0.31 (19)	2.20 ± 0.23 (7)$P<0.001$	1.65 ± 0.39 (7)$P<0.05$
β-Glucuronidase	2.01 ± 0.19 (19)	4.41 ± 0.24 (7)$P<0.001$	3.02 ± 0.42(11)$P<0.05$
Acid diesterase	0.74 ± 0.21 (8)	1.74 ± 0.31 (4)$P<0.01$	0.82 ± 0.31 (4)N.S.
Lactate dehydrogenase	4120 ± 850 (16)	1400 ± 210 (7)$P \pm 0.05$	3680 ± 940 (7)N.S.

Activities are expressed as mean values ± S.E.M. (munits/mg of protein) with the number of samples assayed in duplicate shown in parentheses. P is probability that the difference from values in control subjects is due to chance alone. N.S., not significant.
(From Peters et al. 1975.)

and acid diesterase there was no significant difference between control values and values in treated patients. The other acid hydrolases showed significantly elevated activities in the treated patients compared with controls but the values were lower than in the untreated patients. The cytosol enzyme, lactate dehydrogenase, in contrast to the acid hydrolases, showed a significant decrease in untreated coeliac mucosa with a return to normal activity after treatment.

Fractionation experiments

Using fractionation techniques, it was possible to demonstrate the latent, sedimentable, recovered and released acid hydrolase activities in the fractionated mucosal biopsies obtained both from normal subjects and from the patients with coeliac disease before and after treatment. These results are set out in Table 2. The latent N-acetyl -β-glucosaminidase activity was strikingly reduced

TABLE 2

Latent, sedimentable, recovered, and released acid hydrolase activities in jejunal biopsies from control subjects and patients with adult coeliac disease

Enzyme	*Control subjects*	*Untreated coeliac disease*	*Treated coeliac disease*
N-Acetyl-β-glucosaminidase:			
Latent	73.6±1.19(13)	59.7±1.99(7)$P<0.001$	68.2±1.56(6)$P<0.05$
Sedimentable	69.0±2.0 (10)	56.9±1.5 (6)$P<0.001$	62.6±1.5 (5)N.S.
Recovered	91.2±2.9 (13)	82.2±4.3 (6)N.S.	92.6±5.2 (5)N.S.
Released	62.3±2.2 (11)	69.4±5.1 (6)N.S.	69.9±5.1 (5)N.S.
β-Glucuronidase:			
Sedimentable	76.9±1.8 (12)	68.8±2.8 (5)$P<0.05$	77.6±1.34(5)N.S.
Recovered	92.1±4.6 (12)	85.5±2.6 (5)N.S.	87.0±9.2 (5)N.S.
Released	56.5±3.6 (12)	63.4±6.2 (5)N.S.	59.5±6.1 (5)N.S.
Acid phosphatase:			
Sedimentable	72.4±4.6 (5)	60.4±1.3 (6)$P<0.05$	68.8±2.1 (5)N.S.
Recovered	87.7±7.4 (5)	72.6±2.8 (6)N.S.	80.3±5.5 (5)N.S.
Released	51.6±4.9 (5)	72.9±4.9 (6)$P<0.05$	69.2±7.1 (5)N.S.
Acid β-galactosidase:			
Sedimentable	69.3±2.8 (8)	59.3±1.2 (4)$P<0.05$	68.3±4.2 (5)N.S.
Recovered	82.3±2.6 (8)	85.0±1.4 (4)N.S.	86.8±3.5 (5)N.S.
Released	52.2±2.8 (8)	70.8±6.3 (4)$P<0.05$	50.9±3.5 (5)N.S.

Latent, sedimentable, recovered and released activities, expressed as percentage, are defined in the text. Results are shown as mean values ± S.E.M. with the number of samples estimated in duplicate in parentheses. P is probability that the difference from values in control subjects was due to chance alone.
(From Peters *et al.* 1975.)

in untreated patients but biopsies from treated patients showed activities nearer to those of control subjects. The patterns of change of the sedimentable, recovered, and released activities of the four acid hydrolases were very similar. Biopsies from patients with untreated coeliac disease showed decreased sedimentable acid hydrolases. This was most marked for N-acetyl -β-glucosaminidase but the other enzymes also showed a significant decrease. The sedimentable acid hydrolase activities (%) in the biopsies from treated patients were all within the normal range. No significant change in recovered enzyme activity was found for any of the four enzymes in the three groups of patients studied. The released enzyme activity (%) showed higher values for the biopsies from untreated coeliac disease than for the control subjects, but only for acid β-galactosidase and acid phosphatase were the differences statistically significant. For these two enzymes the activities returned to the normal range after treatment.

The interpretation of the increased fragility of lysosomes in the mucosa in coeliac disease is uncertain. First, it may indicate an increased permeability of the lysosomal membrane. Secondly, the changes in latent activity may reflect an increase in the size of lysosomes in the coeliac mucosa such as has been shown by electron microscopy (Padykula *et al.* 1961; Riecken *et al.* 1966; Rubin *et al.* 1966; Shiner 1967). The role of the lysosome in the pathogenesis of enterocyte damage is not completely established by these experiments but would be compatible with an immunological mechanism of cytolysis.

IMMUNOLOGICAL ABNORMALITIES IN COELIAC DISEASE

There appears to be an overall reduction in lymphoreticular tissue throughout the body in untreated adult coeliac patients. This is indicated by the small spleen that may be found in adult coeliac disease and by the signs of splenic atrophy which are recognized in the blood, the presence of Howell-Jolly bodies being particularly striking. McCarthy *et al.* (1966) have shown that there is a reduction in peripheral lymphoid tissue and it has also been found that the lymphocytes in coeliac patients may show impaired transformation, whether they be circulating lymphocytes (Blecher *et al.* 1969) or lymphocytes teased out from mesenteric lymph nodes (Housley *et al.* 1969). All these findings suggest lymphoreticular dysfunction and this is supported by studies of the immunoglobulins in coeliac disease (Hobbs & Hepner 1968) which have shown reduced levels of IgM in 60% of untreated patients. This is a secondary phenomenon, since the levels return to normal after treatment with a gluten-free diet. The reduced level of IgM is not due to increased loss of IgM into the gut from damaged mucosa, because the overall rate of synthesis of IgM in coeliac disease is reduced (Brown et al. 1969), probably reflecting the general depression of lymphoreticular function in this disease. It is tempting to speculate that this may be an important factor in untreated patients, in whom there is a greatly increased incidence of lymphoma and intestinal neoplasia (Gough et al. 1962; Austad et al. 1967; Harris et al. 1967).

The immunological response to gluten in coeliac disease is not mediated through reaginic sensitivity since, as Hobbs et al. (1969) and Asquith et al. (1969) have shown, serum IgE levels are normal unless coeliac patients also have atopic manifestations such as asthma or allergic rhinitis. Furthermore, immunofluorescent studies do not implicate IgE-containing cells in the gut mucosa and the concentration of IgE in the jejunal fluid is not apparently increased. Circulating antibodies to gluten fractions and other food substances, especially milk proteins, are often found in untreated coeliac patients, both in childhood and in adult life (Heiner et al. 1961; Alarcøn-Segovia et al. 1964; Kivel et al. 1964; Taylor et al. 1964; Bayless et al. 1967). The techniques used in these studies have varied considerably and it is therefore difficult to make comparisons between the work of different groups but it seems unlikely that any of these serum antibodies are specifically correlated with the mucosal damage of coeliac disease, since they can be found in other disorders, such as ulcerative colitis.

Histological studies of the jejunal mucosa show that there is a dense infiltration of the lamina propria with lymphocytes and plasma cells in coeliac disease. There is also an increase in the inter-epithelial lymphocyte (theliolymphocyte) population in the intestinal mucosa. The immunoglobulin classes of the plasma cells of the lamina propria have been studied by immunofluorescence by a number of workers. It is clear that the normal preponderance of IgA cells in the gut is also found in the mucosa of coeliac patients (Rubin et al. 1965). Crabbé (1967), in a single patient, however, reported an excess of IgM-producing cells in the untreated coeliac mucosa and subsequent studies on larger numbers of patients have confirmed this finding (Douglas et al. 1969; Søltoft 1970). In seven untreated coeliac patients Douglas and his colleagues (1969) showed that there was an excess of IgM-producing cells, an abnormality which persisted in all but two of fifteen patients treated with a gluten-free diet. The excess of these cells was localized to the jejunum, since examination of the rectum and bone marrow showed a normal distribution of immunocytes.

COMPLEMENT IN COELIAC DISEASE

Studies of the complement system in coeliac disease suggest that activation of complement may play an important role in the pathogenesis of the mucosal

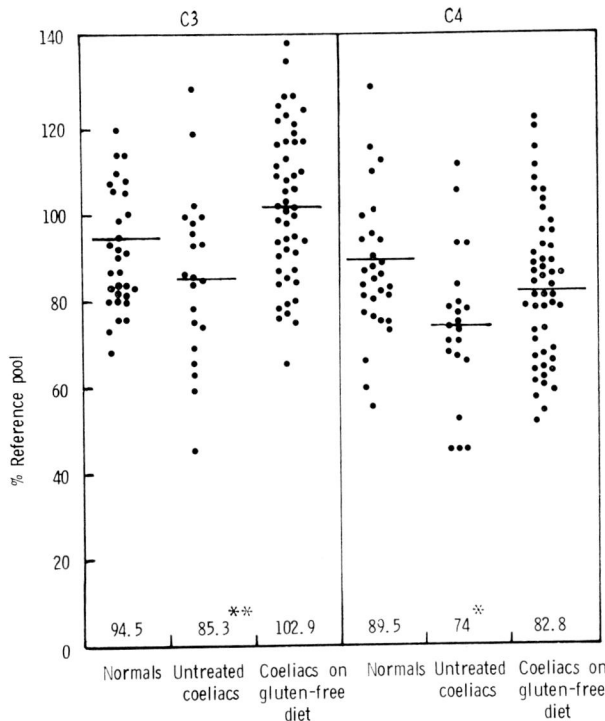

FIG. 1. Levels of C3 and C4 in plasma from normal subjects, coeliac patients taking a normal diet, and those who had been taking a gluten-free diet for over six months. Means are represented by horizontal bars. (From Doe et al. 1975.)

lesion. Deposits of the third component of complement have been detected in the jejunal mucosa of childhood and adult coeliac patients after they have received a single gluten challenge (Shiner & Ballard 1972; Doe et al. 1972b). Furthermore Rossipal (1972) has shown significant reductions in serum C3 after sustained gluten challenge in childhood coeliacs who have been successfully treated with a gluten-free diet. Studies of the levels of various complement components in the serum have been made by Doe et al. (1975). The results of studies of plasma levels of C3 and C4 in 30 normal subjects, 20 coeliac patients taking a normal diet and 53 coeliac patients taking a gluten-free diet for at least six months, are shown in Fig. 1. Mean plasma C3 was lower in untreated coeliac patients than in normal controls, but this difference was not statistically significant. A significantly higher mean C3 level was found in coeliac patients taking a gluten-free diet than in the untreated group ($P<0.001$). Mean C4 levels were significantly lower in untreated coeliacs than in controls ($P<0.01$), but while

TABLE 3

Relationship between gluten-free diet and presence of C1q precipitation in sera from adult coeliac disease patients

Adult coeliac disease patients	No. of patients	C1q positive	
		No.	%
Normal diet	50	20	40
Gluten-free diet for > 6 months	77	8*	10*

*$P<0.001$ ($\chi_1^2 = 13.79$).
(From Doe et al. 1973).

the treated coeliac group had a higher mean C4 level, this difference did not achieve significance.

Further studies have utilized the C1q precipitation test for detecting complement-binding soluble antigen–antibody complexes in the sera of patients with coeliac disease (Doe et al. 1973). The techniques used were those described by Agnello et al. (1970). Studies were done in 50 patients with adult coeliac disease who were receiving a normal diet and in 77 who had had a gluten-free diet for longer than six months. The results are set out in Table 3. Of the 50 patients with adult coeliac disease on a normal diet, 20 (40%) showed a positive C1q precipitation test. Results after a gluten-free diet, however, were significantly different. In this group only 10% had a persistently positive C1q precipitation test. These studies, together with the observations previously referred to, suggest the possibility that there may be circulating immune complexes involving the binding of complement in the serum of patients with coeliac disease, and it is therefore important to know whether complement fixation occurs at the level of the intestine.

IMMUNOLOGICAL ABNORMALITIES AFTER GLUTEN CHALLENGE

The possibility that gluten challenge might induce an antigen–antibody reaction in the jejunal mucosa in coeliac disease has been previously studied in children by Shiner & Ballard (1972) and ultrastructural changes have been documented by Shiner (1973). When gluten is given in a dose of 30 g to an adult patient whose mucosa has recovered after treatment with a gluten-free diet, the morphological changes can be sequentially studied by repeated jejunal biopsies. The data obtained in our laboratory from such studies in five adult patients with coeliac disease in the 48 hours after they had received a gluten challenge can be summarized as follows. Four hours after gluten had been ingested remarkably little change was found in the intestinal mucosa. There was slight oedema in some biopsies and an occasional eosinophil could be seen but it was not until eight to twelve hours after gluten challenge that significant abnormalities occurred. As Shiner & Ballard (1972) and Shiner (1973) have pointed out, the earliest changes occur in the sub-epithelial region, endothelial cell swelling being noted in blood vessels in the lamina propria. By 12 hours, however, there is a diffuse cellular infiltration which in our studies was at this time due to infiltration with polymorphonuclear leucocytes, and was associated on immunofluorescent study with the deposition of complement and extra-cellular IgM. At 24 hours the mucosa had become frankly abnormal with stunted villi and grossly abnormal enterocytes. At this time, however, the infiltration of the lamina propria was predominantly due to mononuclear cells, active macrophages, and plasma cells. By 48 hours most of the abnormality had disappeared and the villi were showing signs of recovery. A similar sequence of pathological events can be demonstrated when gluten is directly instilled into the ileum (Rubin et al. 1962).

There were at the same time important changes in the inter-epithelial lymphocytes (Fig. 2, p. 338). These began to increase at four hours after gluten challenge in some patients and reached a peak level at 12 or 24 hours after the gluten was given (Ferguson 1975). The precise significance of these lymphocyte changes is not known but it is clear that even though there may be a reaction between antigen and antibody, with complement fixation occurring at the level of the lamina propria, there are at the same time important changes occurring in the lymphocytes. Since the majority of the inter-epithelial lymphocytes are in fact T lymphocytes, this observation may indicate an important contribution of cell-mediated immunity in addition to humoral immunity in the pathogenesis of cell damage.

ASSOCIATION OF COELIAC DISEASE WITH CRYOGLOBULINAEMIA

There is additional evidence to suggest that immune complexes are concerned with coeliac disease, at least in some cases. Doe et al. (1972a) described four patients with coeliac disease, all of whom had cryoglobulinaemia. It has been suggested that mixed cryoglobulins represent circulating antigen–antibody complexes (Lospalluto et al. 1962; Meltzer & Franklin 1967) which may result in the deposition of immune complexes in vessels, causing arteritis and other features of immune complex disease. The four patients described by Doe et al. (1972a) all had vasculitis and cryoglobulinaemia. Three patients had extensive skin rashes and in the first patient the dermatological appearances were suggestive of cryoglobulinaemia. Two of these patients showed a morphological improvement in the jejunal mucosa when a gluten-free diet was given; one

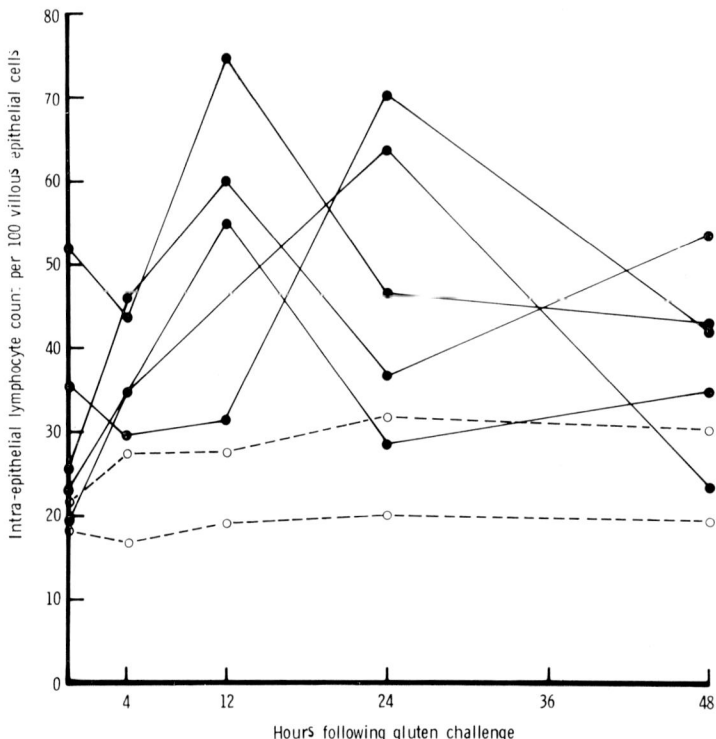

FIG. 2. Serial inter-epithelial lymphocyte counts in five adult coeliac disease patients who received an oral challenge of 30 g gluten after a prolonged period of gluten withdrawal. (From Ferguson 1975.)

patient had a history suggesting malabsorption which dated from childhood, and the other patient had originally presented with malabsorption which had responded satisfactorily to treatment with a gluten-free diet some years earlier. He had, however, then become unresponsive to gluten, and had developed a severe mucosal abnormality with dense collagen deposited under the basement membrane of the enterocytes. It is curious that this relationship between coeliac disease and cryoglobulinaemia has until now only been reported in one laboratory.

CONCLUSION

The evidence presented in this paper suggests that coeliac disease may be due to a reaction between antigen and antibody occurring at gut level. If this is so, the question has to be asked whether there is an *abnormal* entry of large amounts of antigen which then produces a *normal* immunological response of the immunocytes of the intestine. Alternatively, there might be a *normal* entry of whatever amounts of antigen can normally penetrate the small intestinal mucosa, with an *abnormal* immune response. Studies of the relationship between coeliac disease and HLA antigens have repeatedly indicated a close relationship between coeliac disease and HLA-B8 (Falchuk *et al.* 1972; Stokes *et al.* 1972) and more recently with HLA-DW3 (Keuning *et al.* 1976). Coeliac disease is known to be genetically determined, although the precise nature of its genetic background is not completely clear. The present evidence suggests that it is inherited as a dominant with incomplete penetrance (MacDonald *et al.* 1965). These two pieces of evidence would be in keeping with the idea that coeliac disease is due to an abnormal immune response gene, the basic abnormality being a genetically determined failure to clear antigens which enter the lamina propria of the gut.

ACKNOWLEDGEMENT

We thank the many colleagues at the Royal Postgraduate Medical School who have been associated with us in these studies during the past ten years. We also gratefully acknowledge the generous support of the Medical Research Council and the Wellcome Trust.

References

AGNELLO, V., WINCHESTER, R. J. & KUNKEL, H. G. (1970) Precipitin reactions of the Clq component of complement with aggregated γ-globulin and immune complexes in gel diffusion. *Immunology* 19, 909-919

ALARCØN-SEGOVIA, D., HERSKOVIC, T., WAKIM, K. G., GREEN, P. A. & SCUDAMORE, H. H. (1964) Presence of circulating antibodies to gluten and milk fractions in patients with nontropical sprue. *Am. J. Med.* 36, 485-499

ASQUITH, P., THOMPSON, R. A. & COOKE, W. T. (1969) Serum-immunoglobulins in adult coeliac disease. *Lancet* 2, 129

AUSTAD, W. I., CORNES, J. S., GOUGH, K. R., MCCARTHY, C. F. & READ, A. E. (1967) Steatorrhea and malignant lymphoma. The relationship of malignant tumors of lymphoid tissue and celiac disease. *Am. J. Dig. Dis.* 12, 475-490

BAYLESS, T. M., PARTIN, J. S. & PARTIN, J. C. (1967) Serum precipitins to milk, gluten and rice in tropical sprue. *Johns Hopkins Med. J.* 120, 310-316

BLECHER, T. E., BRZECHWA-AJDUKIEWICZ, A., MCCARTHY, C. F. & READ, A. E. (1969) Serum immunoglobulins and lymphocyte transformation studies in coeliac disease. *Gut* 10, 57-62

BOOTH C. C. (1970) The enterocyte in coeliac disease. *Br. Med. J.* 3, 725-731 and 4, 14-17

BOOTH, C. C., STEWART, J. S., HOLMES, R. & BRACKENBURY, W. (1962) Dissecting microscope appearances of intestinal mucosa, in *Intestinal Biopsy (Ciba Found. Study Group. 14)*, pp. 2-19, London, Churchill

BROWN, D. L., COOPER, A. G. & HEPNER, G. W. (1969) IgM metabolism in coeliac disease. *Lancet* 1, 858-861

CRABBÉ, P. A. (1967) *Signification du Tissu Lymphoïde des Muqueuses Digestives*, pp. 118, 119, Editions Arscia, Bruxelles

DICKE, W. K. (1950) Coeliakie. Een onderzoek naar de nadelige invloed van sommige graansoorten op de lijder aan coeliakie. [Coeliac disease. A study of the harmful effect of some wheat species on the coeliac disease patient] Thesis, University of Utrecht

DOE, W. F., EVANS, D., HOBBS, J. R. & BOOTH, C. C. (1972a) Coeliac disease, vasculitis, and cryoglobulinaemia. *Gut 13*, 112-123

DOE, W. F., HENRY, K., HOLT, L. & BOOTH, C. C. (1972b) An immunological study of adult coeliac disease. *Gut 13*, 324-325

DOE, W. F., BOOTH, C. C. & BROWN, D. L. (1973) Evidence for complement binding immune complexes in adult coeliac disease, Crohn's disease and ulcerative colitis. *Lancet 1*, 402-403

DOE, W. F., HENRY, K. & BOOTH, C. C. (1975) in *Coeliac Disease* (Hekkens, W. T. J. M. & Peña, A. S., eds.), p. 189, Stenfert Kroese, Leiden

DOUGLAS, A. P., CRABBÉ, P. A. & HOBBS, J. R (1969) An immunochemical study of plasma cells in the intestinal mucosa in adult coeliac disease. *Gut 10*, 413

FALCHUK, Z. M., ROGENTINE, G. N. & STROBER, W. J. (1972) Predominance of histocompatibility antigen HL-A8 in patients with gluten-sensitive enteropathy. *J. Clin. Invest. 51*, 1602-1605

FERGUSON, A. (1975) Lymphocytes in coeliac disease, in *Coeliac Disease* (Hekkens, W. T. J. M. & Peña, A. S., eds.), p. 265, Stenfert Kroese, Leiden

GOUGH, K. R., READ, A. E. & NAISH, J. M. (1962) Intestinal reticulosis as a complication of idiopathic steatorrhoea. *Gut 3*, 232-239

HARRIS, O. D., COOKE, W. T., THOMPSON, H. & WATERHOUSE, J. A. H. (1967) Malignancy in adult coeliac disease and idiopathic steatorrhoea. *Am. J. Med. 42*, 899-912

HEINER, D. C., LAHEY, M. E., WILSON, J. R. & PECK, G. A. (1961) *Am. J. Dis. Child. 102*, 446

HOBBS, J. R. & HEPNER, G. W. (1968) Deficiency of gamma-M-globulin in coeliac disease. *Lancet 1*, 217-220

HOBBS, J. R., HEPNER, G. W., DOUGLAS, A. P., CRABBÉ, P. A. & JOHANSSON, S. G. O. (1969) Immunological mystery of coeliac disease. *Lancet 2*, 649-650

HOUSLEY, J., ASQUITH, P. & COOKE, W. T. (1969) Immune response to gluten in adult coeliac disease. *Br. Med. J. 1*, 159-161

KEUNING, J. J., PEÑA, A. S., VAN LEEUWEN, A., VAN HOOFF, J. P. & VAN ROOD, J. J. (1976) HLA-DW3 associated with coeliac disease. *Lancet 1*, 506-507

KIVEL, R. M., KEARNS, D. H. & LIEBOWITZ, D. (1964) Significance of antibodies to dietary proteins in the serums of patients with nontropical sprue. *N. Engl. J. Med. 261*, 769-772

LOSPALLUTO, J., DORWARD, B., MILLER, W., JR & ZIFF, M. (1962) Cryoglobulinaemia based on interaction between a gamma macroglobulin and 7S gammaglobulin. *Am. J. Med. 32*, 142-147

MCCARTHY, C. F., FRASER, I. D., EVANS, K. T. & READ, A. E. (1966) Lymphoreticular dysfunction in idiopathic steatorrhoea. *Gut 7*, 140-148

MACDONALD, W. C., DOBBINS, W. O. & RUBIN, C. E. (1965) Studies of the familial nature of celiac sprue using biopsy of the small intestine. *N. Engl. J. Med. 272*, 448-456

MELTZER, M. & FRANKLIN, E. C. (1967) Cryoglobulins, rheumatoid factors and connective tissue disorders. *Arthritis Rheum. 10*, 488-492

PADYKULA, H. A., STRAUSS, E. W., LADMAN, A. J. & GARDNER, F. H. (1961) A morphologic and histochemical analysis of the human jejunal epithelium in nontropical sprue. *Gastroenterology 40*, 735-765

PETERS, T. J., HEATH, J. R., WANSBROUGH-JONES, M. H. & DOE, W. F. (1975) Enzyme activities and properties of lysosomes and brush borders in jejunal biopsies from control subjects and patients with coeliac disease. *Clin. Sci. Mol. Med. 48*, 259-267

RIECKEN, E. O., STEWART, J. S., BOOTH, C. C. & PEARSE, A. G. E. (1966) A histochemical study on the role of lysosomal enzymes in idiopathic steatorrhoea before and during a gluten-free diet. *Gut 7*, 317-332

ROSSIPAL, E. (1972) Die Bedeutung präzipitierender Antikörper gegen Kleberproteïne in der Pathogenese der Coeliakie. *Pädiatr. Pädol. 7*, 253-258

Rubin, C. E., Brandborg, L. L., Phelps, P. C. & Taylor, H. C., Jr (1960) Studies of celiac disease. I. The apparent identical and specific nature of the duodenal and proximal jejunal lesion in celiac disease and idiopathic sprue. *Gastroenterology* 38, 28-49

Rubin, C. E., Brandborg, L. L., Flick, A. L., Phelps, P. C., Parmentier, C. & van Niel, S. (1962) Studies of celiac sprue. III. The effect of repeated wheat instillation into the proximal ileum of patients on a gluten free diet. *Gastroenterology* 43, 621-641

Rubin, W., Fauci, A. S., Marvin, S. F., Sleisenger, M. H. & Jeffries, G. H. (1965) Immunofluorescent studies in adult celiac disease. *J. Clin. Invest.* 44, 475-485

Rubin, W., Ross, L. L., Sleisenger, M. H. & Weder, E. (1966) *Lab. Invest.* 15, 1720

Shiner, M. (1967) Ultrastructure of jejunal surface epithelium in untreated idiopathic steatorrhoea. *Br. Med. Bull.* 23, 223-225

Shiner, M. (1973) Ultrastructural changes of immune reactions in the jejunal mucosa of coeliac children following gluten challenge. *Gut* 14, 1-12

Shiner, M. & Ballard, J. (1972) Antigen-antibody reactions in jejunal mucosa in childhood coeliac disease after gluten challenge. *Lancet 1,* 1202

Søltoft, J. (1970) Immunoglobulin-containing cells in non-tropical sprue. *Clin. Exp. Immunol.* 6, 413-420

Stewart, J. S., Pollock, D. J., Hoffbrand, A. V., Mollin, D. L & Booth, C. C. (1967) A study of proximal and distal intestinal structure and absorptive function in idiopathic steatorrhoea. *Q. J. Med.* 36, 425-444

Stokes, P. L., Asquith, P., Holmes, G. K. T., MacKintosh, P. & Cooke, W. T. (1972) Histocompatibility antigens associated with adult coeliac disease. *Lancet 2,* 162-164

Taylor, K. B., Truelove, S. C. & Wright, R. (1964) Serologic reactions to gluten and cow's milk proteins in gastrointestinal disease. *Gastroenterology* 46, 99-108

Wattiaux, R. & de Duve, C. (1956) Tissue fractionation studies. 7. Release of bound hydrolases by means of Triton X-100. *Biochem. J.* 63, 606

Discussion

Rosen: The gut epithelium has been demonstrated to be the site of C1 synthesis, which may be germane here. Is the kind of fluid loss that we see in gluten-feeding very like what we see in patients with hereditary angioneurotic oedema, where there is C1 activation in the gut, and where the major involvement is also jejunal, and only very rarely in the ileum or the colon?

Booth: I don't know the answer to that.

Rosen: It seems that C1q, C1r and C1s are all synthesized in the gut. But do these patients get massive fluid loss into the gut lumen?

Booth: I don't know. They certainly lose fluid if they are untreated.

Rosen: Falchuk (Katz *et al.* 1976) can also induce the lesion *in vitro*, by taking a biopsy of intestine from a coeliac patient in remission and adding gluten to the culture. He can prevent the change by adding steroids. What is the mechanism of that?

Booth: I think steroids are simply lysosomal stabilizers. If you study the response to steroids in coeliac patients histochemically, as Wall working with us has done, you can show the punctate appearance of the lysosomes becoming clearly re-established (Wall *et al.* 1970). I would have said it was a non-specific response to steroids.

Pierce: It has been shown that gut biopsies from coeliac patients in remission challenged *in vitro* with gluten do not show an increased synthesis of IgA and IgM. How does this fit with what Dr Rosen has just said about induction of flattening *in vitro*? It seems either to be contradictory, or to exclude a role for antibody, since you are saying that antibody may play some role in mediating the response yet it cannot be induced *in vitro* by gluten challenge.

Rosen: But who knows what is in the biopsy material? There may be plenty of antibody there all the time, and you are adding the antigen.

Evans: Those findings are different from those originally reported by Falchuk. If he had a patient in good remission from coeliac disease and cultured a biopsy with gliadin he could not produce an impairment of brush-border height. If on the other hand he gave the patients a small challenge with gliadin beforehand, and then cultured their biopsy tissue, they were sensitive to gliadin. If he co-cultured a biopsy from a patient in complete remission with a biopsy from a patient with untreated coeliac disease, and then challenged with gliadin, there was shrinkage of the brush border in the biopsy of the patient in remission.

Booth: The technical differences between different groups are enormous here. The work David Evans is referring to is based on estimates of alkaline phosphatase activity as a measure of brush-border activity and when you do that, in terms of measuring tissue phosphatase or that in the surrounding fluid, you can get all sorts of results. Conclusions based solely on alkaline phosphatase activity are hard to interpret.

Evans: Falchuk has also stated that there are alterations in brush border morphology (see Katz *et al.* 1976).

Rosen: It comes back to the point that there is probably pre-existing antibody in the biopsy.

White: I am trying to compare your findings with nephritis induced by say serum sickness, Professor Booth. You have an antigen–antibody reaction and this leads to separation of the endothelial cells—that is, histamine or another agent separates them. Therefore antigen–antibody complexes are presumably let out and they sit on the basement membrane. You have evident damage to the basement membrane, which can be gross. That should mean that most biopsies ought to show complexes sitting on the basement membrane and easy to demonstrate. Are they?

Booth: No, they are not. This is the practical point. When you take a biopsy and look for immune complexes, in fact you are looking for antibody in punctate form such as you would find in a renal glomerulus. Nobody has yet found that. I hope Anne Ferguson is going to do so!

Ferguson: One point we tend to forget is that intestinal biopsies are usually taken after a fairly long fast. The patient comes to the hospital without breakfast and the biopsy is obtained a couple of hours later. Thus the intestine of the patient has not been exposed to foods for 15–20 hours before the biopsy is taken—that is, it has been gluten-free for at least this length of time.

Booth: The problem remains that even when you challenge with gluten, it is hard to detect complement. In the Norwegian data on complement in the mucosal biopsies, can you see anything like an immune complex?

Brandtzaeg: I don't think we should expect to see immune complexes in tissues like the lamina propria, which cannot be compared with the kidney.

White: It is a bewilderingly constant thing that if you inject a small dose, say 1 mg, of a protein antigen into an animal it segregates antigen–antibody complexes through the walls of blood vessels throughout the body and they sit as circumscribed foci on the basement membrane.

Rosen: That is intravascular antigen and an intravascular model. This is different.

Brandtzaeg: I have one question about the pathogenetic immunoglobulin class. You suggested that it was IgM.

Booth: Mietens (1967) showed that anti-gluten antibodies in the lumen of the gut were IgM.

Brandtzaeg: In the lumen you may expect the antibodies to be IgM or IgA but in serum most people agree that they are mainly IgG, and this IgG must be distributed extravascularly in the lamina propria. In one patient we succeeded in picking out an antigen from gluten which could be used in the indirect immunofluorescence technique to show local antibody-producing cells. We found that of the IgG class, almost 6% of the cells were involved in antibody production against this gluten antigen. Only 1.5% of the local IgA cells showed this activity and almost none of the local IgM cells. The problem was that the particular antigen that we used successfully didn't work in other patients. This emphasizes the heterogeneity of the immune response to gluten antigens.

Lachmann: A study by Sikora *et al.* (1976) has shown that the B2 subfraction of Frazer's fraction III of a gluten digest gives impressive lymphocyte stimulation in patients with coeliac disease, more so than with crude antigens. One obviously needs to have the right antigen, both in looking for antibodies and in looking for cellular immune reactions in these patients.

André: To come back to *in vitro* biopsy cultures, Dr Ferguson has evidence that if the biopsy is challenged with α-gliadin, the lymphocytes in the biopsy produce MIF (Ferguson *et al.* 1975).

Ferguson: That was work which I have referred to as being only preliminary, and it has not yet been repeated.

André: The shortening of the villi not only occurs after challenging biopsies with gluten but also with casein. This has been shown by Jos *et al.* (1975) at the Enfants-Malades Hospital in Paris.

Ferguson: Jos *et al.* (1974) have shown that casein may cause damage to cultured jejunal biopsies from some children with coeliac disease. They have also shown that the lymphocytes of children with coeliac disease may be stimulated to mitosis by casein extracts.

Porter: Over a number of years there has been evidence in calves of an intestinal sensitivity to an antigen of soya. Dutch workers (Van Adrichem & Frens 1965) showed high levels of serum antibodies against undefined soya antigen in calves fed soya proteins in a milk-replacement diet. Recently Smith & Sissons (1975) showed that after feeding soya proteins to fistulated calves there were physiological changes in the gut in terms of flow rates. There was an increase in the time taken for markers to move between the duodenum and ileum, and yet there was a massive influx of electrolytes, so that the volume passing through the ileum was increased.

We have looked at this syndrome and have demonstrated in Thiry-Vella loop pigs that once animals are sensitized with the soya antigen, the action of the antigen within the loop produces a dramatic decrease in flow through the loop only while the antigen is present. Thus within the experimental model you could apply the antigen at any time and get an immediate decrease in flow rate, remove it and return to the normal rate.

Booth: It would be interesting to know what is happening to the mucosa.

Porter: Coming back to the immunopathogenic component, the immunoglobulins involved in the development of these responses are almost exclusively IgG1, which is both a precipitating and a complement-fixing antibody. I do not believe that that type of Arthus response is immediately responsible for the decrease in flow within the loop in response to the antigen. It is more likely to be an immediate type hypersensitivity mechanism.

Booth: A case has been recorded in man of soya flour sensitivity (Ament & Rubin 1972). I don't know the timing of the response.

Porter: It is very fast in calves. We do not get the physiological response without sensitization. It takes 7–10 days to achieve sensitization. I wonder if this could be a reasonable model system for studying gluten sensitivity?

Pepys: A significant proportion of patients with bird-fancier's lung, a form of extrinsic allergic alveolitis, have recently been found to have jejunal villous atrophy histologically indistinguishable from coeliac disease (Berrill *et al.* 1975). This raises the possibility that similar immunological mechanisms directed against a variety of inhaled or ingested antigens might cause the intestinal lesion seen in coeliac disease.

White: Is there any evidence that villi can actively contract? Are there contractile cells or particular sorts of fibroblasts susceptible to the action of pharmacological agents?

Booth: The best cine pictures of this are in the dog and have been published by Verzar (Verzar & McDougall 1936). The villi can be seen pumping up and down. But it depends on the species: in the rat the villi are mostly leaf-shaped and do not pump. In the dog they do. Whether they pump in man has not been satisfactorily shown.

White: Perhaps smooth-muscle contractant drugs could flatten them.

Ferguson: Villi can readily be made to contract or shrink considerably. In an ordinary biopsy processed for conventional histology they contract by around 50% (A. Ferguson, A. Sutherland & T. T. MacDonald, unpublished work 1976). By altering various aspects of the fixation and embedding procedures it is possible to make the villi long and smooth or short and irregular. However, the number of cells along the sides of each villus remains the same. In the so-called villous atrophy under discussion here, the number of epithelial cells is only about a tenth that of the normal value.

Booth: I do not think contraction has anything to do with coeliac disease, but it is an interesting point whether human villi contract.

Rosen: What is the HLA association of coeliac disease?

Booth: The original observation made in 1972 was of an 80% incidence of HLA-B8, made simultaneously in the USA and in the UK. A recent paper from Holland (Peña et al. 1976) suggests that the true association is with the HLA-DW3. The difficulty is that the DW3 linkage is not absolute. You still have some cases without that particular lymphocyte configuration. It is an interesting association and suggests the possibility of an immune-response gene abnormality of some sort, which probably means that coeliac disease is a genetic reaction to the entry of the small amounts of antigen which get across the mucosa under normal circumstances.

Rosen: The association at D is no more firm that it was at B.

Pepys: There has been one report in which unique B lymphocyte surface antigens were found in almost all the patients studied with either dermatitis herpetiformis or with coeliac disease and were not found in any of the normal population (Mann et al. 1976). It is suggested that these B cell antigens are analogous to the Ia antigens in mice.

References

AMENT, M. E. & RUBIN, C. E. (1972) Soy protein – another cause of the flat intestinal lesion. *Gastroenterology 62*, 227-234

BERRILL, W. T., EADE, O. E., FITZPATRICK P. F., HYDE, I., MACCLEOD, W. M. & WRIGHT, R. (1975) Bird-fancier's lung and jejunal villous atrophy. *Lancet 2*, 1006-1008

FERGUSON, A., MACDONALD, T. T., MCCLURE, J. P. & HOLDEN, R. J. (1975) Cell-mediated immunity to gliadin within the small-intestinal mucosa in coeliac disease. *Lancet 1*, 895-897

JOS, J., LENOIR, G., DE RITIS, G. & REY, J. (1974) *In vitro* culturing of biopsies from children, in *Coeliac Disease* (Hekkens, W. T. J. M. & Peña, A. S., eds.), pp. 91-106, Stenfert Kroese, Leiden

JOS, J., LENOIR, G., DE RITIS, G. & REY, J. (1975) *In vitro* pathogenic studies of coeliac disease. Effects of protein digests on coeliac intestinal biopsy specimens maintained in culture for 48 hours. *Scand. J. Gastroenterol. 10*, 122-128

KATZ, A. J., FALCHUK, Z. M., STROBER, W. & SHWACHMAN, H. (1976) Gluten-sensitive enteropathy. Inhibition by cortisol of the effect of gluten protein in vitro. *N. Engl. J. Med. 295*, 131-135

MANN, D. L., KATZ, S. I., NELSON, D. L., ABELSON, L. D. & STROBER, W. (1976) Specific B cell antigens associated with gluten-sensitive enteropathy and dermatitis herpetiformis. *Lancet 1*, 110-111

MIETENS, C. (1967) *Z. Kinderheilkd. 99*, 130

PEÑA, A. S., VAN LEEUWEN, A., VAN HOOFF, J. P. & VAN ROOD, J. J. (1976) HLA-DW3 associated with coeliac disease. *Lancet 1*, 506-507

SIKORA, K., ANAND, B. S., CICLITIRA, P. J., OFFORD, R. E. & TRUELOVE, S. C. (1976) Stimulation of lymphocytes from patients with coeliac disease by a subfraction of gluten. *Lancet* 389-391

SMITH, R. H. & SISSONS, J. W. (1975) The effect of different feeds, including those containing soya bean products, on the passage of digesta from the abomasum of the preruminant calf. *Br. J. Nutr. 33*, 329-349

VAN ADRICHEM, P. W. M. & FRENS, A. M. (1965) Soya protein as an alimentary tract allergen in fattening calves. *Tijdschr. Diergeneeskd. 90*, 525-531

VERZAR, F. & MCDOUGALL, E. J. (1936) *Absorption from the Intestine*, p. 58, plate V, Longmans Green, London

WALL, A. J., DOUGLAS, A. P., BOOTH, C. C. & PEARSE, A. G. E. (1970) Response of the jejunal mucosa in adult coeliac disease to oral prednisolone. *Gut 11*, 7-14

General discussion

HOMING OF T BLASTS

Parrott: Until recently little emphasis has been placed on the functions of T lymphocytes in the gut mucosa but Dr Rosen (Katz & Rosen, this volume, pp. 243–261) has suggested that they have a protective function whilst Dr Ferguson has emphasized their destructive function (Ferguson & MacDonald, this volume, pp. 305–327). I will summarize the basic data on the location of T cells before describing our recent work on the homing of T blasts to the gut mucosa.

There is good evidence that T like B cells are sensitized to intraluminal antigen and that they become sensitized in Peyer's patches. For example, Müller-Schoop & Good (1975) demonstrated that after oral immunization of guinea pigs with live *Clostridia* or BCG, preparations of T cells from Peyer's patches responded by proliferation to *in vitro* stimulation with killed organisms.

There are clearly defined T and B areas in Peyer's patches and the preparation of T:B cells varies according to age and antigenic challenge (for literature review see Parrott 1976). The area of particular interest in Peyer's patches is that referred to as the 'dome', since this is immediately below the area of specialized epithelium which allows transport of antigen (Bockman & Cooper 1973). In germ-free thymus-deprived mice the dome is depleted of lymphocytes as well as recognized T areas (Parrott & Ferguson 1974). After staining with an anti-T antiserum (Lamelin *et al.* 1972) T cells can be demonstrated in both the dome and in the T areas (D. Guy-Grand, personal communication) and after infusion of [^{3}H]adenosine or [^{3}H]uridine-labelled B or T cells the one place in Peyer's patches where one finds intermingling of both cell types is in the dome (Parrott & Ferguson 1974). Perhaps this is where both cell types meet antigen and immune responses are initiated?

TABLE 1

The 24-hour localization of [^{125}I]iododeoxyuridine-labelled mesenteric lymph node cells (MLN) in the small intestine of normal NIH mice and mice infected with *Trichinella spiralis*[a]: a comparison of mesenteric node T and B blasts

Cell inoculum	Mean % injected dose ± S.D.	
	Uninfected	Infected
Whole MLN[b]	6.3 ± 1.0	9.9 ± 1.9
T-MLN[c]	6.4 ± 0.6	12.1 ± 0.5
B-MLN[d]	4.6 ± 0.6	5.3 ± 1.4

[a]Cells transferred four days before infection by oral intubation with approximately 450 larvae.
[b]Whole MLN contains 45% T cells.
[c]MLN separated on a nylon wool column contains more than 95% T cells as determined by anti-T antiserum cytotoxicity.
[d]From adult thymectomized, lethally irradiated, bone marrow-reconstituted mice; contains less than 15% T cells.
(Data from Rose *et al.* 1976a,b.)

After antigen-induced proliferation it would seem reasonable to suppose that the dividing T cells leave Peyer's patches and travel by the same mesenteric and thoracic duct routes as B immunoblasts (see Cebra *et al.* and Husband *et al.*, this volume, pp. 5–28 and 29–54) to reach the lamina propria. If one separates mesenteric lymph node cells so as to get an almost pure preparation of T cells and then incubates them with [^{125}I]iododeoxyuridine so as to label only immunoblasts, then these T immunoblasts home to the gut (Table 1) in the same purposeful way as has been described by Professor Gowans for B immunoblasts (Husband *et al.*, this volume, pp. 29–54). Sprent (1976) has recently shown that activated T blasts taken from the thoracic duct lymph also home to the gut. Guy-Grand *et al.* (1974) demonstrated by immunofluorescence that there are cells with a T cell surface antigen in the lamina propria and between the epithelial cells of the villi and I have shown by autoradiography (unpublished) that after infusion of labelled T blasts there are labelled cells in both these sites. T blasts therefore normally migrate to the gut, possibly to perform the protective functions described by Dr Rosen. In situations where the gut is inflamed after infection with *Trichinella spiralis*, increased numbers of T mesenteric blasts (but not B blasts) migrate to the gut (Table 1; Ogilvie & Parrott, this volume, pp. 183–195). The increased migration is coincident with villous atrophy and the onset of inflammation and it may be that this experimental model, like Dr Ferguson's allografts, will prove useful in studying the destructive effects of T cells in the gut, particularly in relation to the mechanism of villous atrophy.

I have been interested for some time in what promotes the extravasation of

TABLE 2

The 24-hour localization of [^{125}I]iododeoxyuridine-labelled mesenteric (MLN) and peripheral (PLN) lymph node cells in the small intestine of NIH mice infected with *Trichinella spiralis*

Cell inoculum	Mean % injected dose ± S.D.	
	Uninfected	Infected
MLN	7.0 ± 0.8	11.4 ± 0.6
Ox-PLN[a]	2.0 ± 0.4	6.1 ± 0.9

[a]Ox-PLN: blast cells from lymph nodes four days after the application of oxazolone (10 mg in acetone).
(Data from Rose *et al.* 1976*b*.)

lymphoid cells into the gut and skin and other epithelial tissues and whether cells destined for one site can be diverted to another. Normally blast cells taken from peripheral lymph nodes will not migrate to the gut (Griscelli *et al.* 1969; Guy-Grand *et al.* 1974; Parrott & Ferguson 1974). It seemed possible, however, that the inflamed or infected gut would prove to be more accessible to cells from other sources as well as those which directly drain the gut. We know that T blasts from sites draining a contact sensitizer such as oxazolone migrate in a non-specific way to any site of inflammation on the skin, whether induced by the contact sensitizer or an unrelated sensitizer (such as picryl chloride) or any inflammatory agent such as croton oil or turpentine (Asherson *et al.* 1973). Accordingly, we labelled the blast cells which are produced in lymph nodes 3–4 days after the application of the contact sensitizer with [^{125}I]iododeoxyuridine and injected them into normal mice and mice infected with *T. spiralis*. Such cells, which are almost all T blasts, do go to the gut which is inflamed by the parasite but not to normal gut (Table 2). If, however, infected mice are also treated with oxazolone on the ear skin, localization to the gut returns to normal and the blast cells are located in the treated ears and auricular lymph nodes (Rose *et al.* 1976*b*). Mesenteric lymph node blasts, even pure T blasts, cannot, however, be persuaded into inflamed skin (Rose *et al.* 1976*b*). Splenectomy (unpublished observations) does increase slightly the tendency of both peripheral and mesenteric blasts to migrate to the gut. Can the clinicians tell us whether the presence of an atrophied spleen, which occurs in some patients with coeliac disease, exacerbates the disease?

In summary, we have shown that T blasts of the mesenteric node normally migrate to the gut and that they go there in increased numbers when the gut is infected by the nematode *T. spiralis*. We have shown that peripheral blasts which go to sites of inflammation can be diverted to the infected but not to the normal gut. Now we must investigate whether this increased and diverted migration of T blasts has a clinical significance not only in relation to worm expulsion but also in relation to non-specific exacerbation of inflammation in the gut.

Finally, to bring us back to the problem of what persuades blast cells to extravasate, Peter Wilkinson and his group (Wilkinson *et al.* 1976; Russell *et al.* 1975) in our laboratory have shown recently that activated lymphocytes and immunoblasts (T and B) will 'chemotax' in a Boyden chamber towards endotoxin, casein and altered human serum albumin (HSA). This would seem to offer a good explanation of how one finds lymphocytes as well as monocytes in an inflammatory site. Perhaps chemotaxis will explain why immunoblasts extravasate into the gut wall. In the normal gut endotoxin and perhaps casein would be present. This would not apply to the antigen-free gut grafts which blast cells nevertheless enter (Guy-Grand *et al.* 1974; Parrott & Ferguson 1974) but maybe in an antigen-free gut there might be some altered serum albumin.

Bienenstock: Delphine Guy-Grand & Claude Griscelli have mice of the C3H strain which have no epithelial lymphocytes at all in their guts (C. Griscelli, personal communication 1976). These animals live a normal life, apparently, and reach normal old age. Guy-Grand & Griscelli tried to find out whether normal blasts go into this gut epithelium, doing the same experiments as Delphine Parrott described, and so far have been unable to discover what is wrong with these mice. Therein may lie a key to what is going on.

Gowans: Is secretory IgA produced in this strain?

Bienenstock: The IgA is there, but no T blasts homing to the epithelium. However, T blasts from a syngeneic animal home to the fetal gut of these animals transplanted under the kidney capsule.

Vaerman: Professor Parrott, was the T antigen against which the antibody was made a surface antigen? I was surprised how brightly the sections of Peyer's patches stain. Some cells appear to have their cytoplasm stained—of course, the membrane can be there too. But recalling Dr Mayrhofer's pictures of mesenteric lymph node cells at the periphery of the node, which have surface IgE labelling which distinguishes them from those in the gut epithelium, I am surprised by the intensity of the staining and its appearance, for a surface antigen in sections.

Parrott: I am also surprised, but there are two previous papers (Lamelin *et al.* 1972; Matter *et al.* 1972) in which the same antisera were used to identify T cells and a different antiserum for B cells.

THE INDUCTION OF TOLERANCE TO ORALLY ADMINISTERED ANTIGENS

André: A study of tolerance in mice was started several years ago with

Professor J. F. Heremans and others. Mice were immunized by the intragastric administration of sheep red blood cells. The response was studied in terms of plaque-forming cells in the spleen. This response peaked at about day 9. Plaque-forming cells of the IgA class predominated over a moderate IgM cell response and a smaller number of IgG cells. In the same mice, after a second intragastric immunization of red cells three months later, the response was similar to the first response: there was no memory. This experiment was repeated with two intragastric administrations of antigen only two weeks apart. There was almost no response in the spleen (André et al. 1973). One explanation of this result is that an immune inhibition of absorption of the antigen by the gut occurs (André et al. 1974). This does happen, but it wasn't the sole explanation for this phenomenon.

We then studied the reciprocal influence of parenteral and oral immunization. Mice were immunized with sheep red cells by the intraperitoneal route and two weeks later by the intragastric route. The response in the spleen was the same as that in mice primed only intragastrically, the difference being that the base-line level of plaque-forming cells of the IgM class was raised; this was a carry-over from the intraperitoneal administration 14 days earlier. The reverse is *not* true. When mice were first immunized intragastrically and two weeks later received an intraperitoneal injection of the same antigen, they failed to respond, either at the level of plaque-forming cells in the spleen or at the level of haemolytic IgM antibody in the serum.

We then collected serum from mice that had received antigen intragastrically, two weeks previously. Serum was injected intraperitoneally into virgin mice which eight hours later received a single intraperitoneal injection of sheep red blood cells or an intragastric injection of the antigen. The priming of pretreated animals by the oral or parenteral route did not induce any antibody, although a small number of IgM plaque-forming cells were found. The same results were observed by studying IgA antibody against sheep red blood cells, and IgA plaque-forming cells. So there seems to be a factor in the serum which induces immunological tolerance. No IgM antibody against sheep red blood cells was found in the injected sera, or any IgG, and only a small amount of IgA antibody (maximum 1:8 titre).

At that time Dr P. Masson in Brussels had developed a method for detecting immune complexes, using latex particles covered with human IgG which are normally agglutinated by C1q or by rheumatoid factor. Immune complexes can be shown by inhibition of this agglutination. No evidence of immune complexes could be demonstrated in our serum with C1q but such complexes were shown using rheumatoid factor. As IgA doesn't fix C1q, we concluded that the complex involved some part of the membrane of the sheep red blood cells and IgA.

We now turned to *in vitro* experiments. Mice were immunized intraperitoneally and their spleen cells were incubated four days later with serum—either normal mouse serum, or serum from mice immunized two weeks previously with sheep red blood cells, or serum from mice immunized with a large dose of sheep red blood cells one day earlier.

In such conditions the incubation of the spleen cells in normal mouse serum doesn't modify the IgM plaque-forming cell response. Serum from mice immunized only 24 hours previously doesn't alter the normal IgM response, so we concluded that the tolerogenic factor cannot be a tolerogenic form of the antigen itself. Using serum from mice immunized two weeks previously decreased the normal number of plaque-forming cells of the IgM type.

In our latest experiments done with Dr Vaerman the tolerogenic factor in this serum was removed by immunosorbents; one of these was rheumatoid factor, which completely abolished the tolerogenic properties of the serum *in vitro*. We also used as an immunosorbent antibody against IgA. By removing all IgA from the serum, and presumably all antigen—antibody complexes with IgA, the tolerogenic *in vitro* influence of this serum was also completely abolished. This was not found if we used antibody against IgM as an immunosorbent. The tolerogenic *in vitro* influence of the serum was also abolished when we used antibody against sheep red blood cells as immunosorbent (André *et al.* 1975).

Lachmann: Is it correct to call this tolerance? Tolerance usually describes the failure of *induction* of cells. You are taking cells and stopping them expressing their capacity to make antibody *in vitro*.

André: The *in vivo* process could be different from the *in vitro* system.

Vaerman: The *in vitro* system could be called effector cell blocking.

Davies: Was there a response to the original intragastric injections of antigen in the Peyer's patches and mesenteric lymph nodes?

André: I haven't looked at them.

Davies: We did some experiments which were in essence similar (O'Toole & Davies 1971). We gave intraperitoneal or intravenous injections of sheep red blood cells to mice and at various times later tried to stimulate, by injection of the antigen in the forepaws of the mouse, the lymph nodes draining the site of injection. We found an initial non-specific failure to respond; after four days we found a specific failure to respond which lasted for 14 or 15 days, and this is similar to what you found. This phenomenon was spleen-dependent. In other words, you need an active response in the first instance. If the spleen was removed within about a day of the first intraperitoneal or intravenous injection we didn't get the blocking in these lymph nodes.

In such experiments, having not found an antibody, one must be careful to show that there is not enough antibody to block by passive immunization. You can take hyperimmune serum which contains IgG, dilute it beyond any detectable titre, and still find an almost absolute block on the capacity of a mouse to produce anti-sheep red blood cell antibody. This possibility has to be ruled out. This particular phenomenon was subsequently studied by others who confirmed our findings but did not elucidate the mechanism. The kind of result you have shown, suggesting that a complex may be involved, is the most interesting I have seen as an explanation of that kind of observation.

Soothill: What happens if you go on feeding the antigen to the mice and immunize while you are still feeding the antigen?

André: I have done only a few experiments of this type, and there was no response at all, but I was giving a large dose of antigen. In a similar experiment by Bazin *et al.* (1970) several years ago mice were immunized with sheep red blood cells in the drinking water. They observed a plaque-forming response in the spleen and in the mesenteric lymph node. The experiment went on for about three months, and there was a progressive decay in the IgA response in the spleen.

Pepys: We have been repeating these experiments of Dr André with essentially the same results, although we haven't done transfer or *in vitro* studies. We have looked at numbers of rosette-forming cells (RFC) to sheep erythrocytes in the Peyer's patches and mesenteric nodes at different times after the initial oral immunization (M. B. Pepys & A. H. L. Fielder, unpublished observations). We find a brief peak of RFC which precedes the plaque-forming cell (PFC) response in the spleen, but our results in the spleen are much more variable than André's and we don't find the regular peak of PFC in the spleen at day 9.

Lachmann: Is there a possibility that two weeks later the cells which you would like to find in the spleen making plaques are in the lamina propria not doing anything in particular?

Gowans: I would like to know whether, when you challenge intraperitoneally and get no response in the spleen, you nevertheless find a response in the mediastinal lymph nodes?

André: I don't know. However, on intraperitoneal challenge after intragastric immunization there is no response at the plasma level. As there is no IgM antibody at the plasma level, I think there is no response in the mesenteric and mediastinal lymph nodes.

Lachmann: Do the mice make antibody in the intestinal secretion instead?

André: I haven't looked there.

Bienenstock: Rothberg *et al.* (1973) showed a similar situation in bovine serum albumin (BSA) feeding experiments in rabbits. If he splenectomized the animals or gave them a big dose of BSA intravenously (100 mg), he found lymphocytes in the circulation which were proliferating in response to that particular antigen, whereas before he couldn't show that. Have you given a big dose of antigen intravenously?

André: No, but I have done an experiment in rats using human serum albumin (HSA) as a soluble antigen. We found exactly the same situation. An intragastric administration of 200 mg of HSA was followed by an intramuscular injection of the same antigen. Anti-HSA antibody in sera was assayed by its antigen-binding capacity. By comparison with control animals there was a big reduction in the anti-HSA antibody titres of rats immunized by both routes.

Pierce: Are you referring to the local response?

André: In this experiment there was a local response dependent on IgA. In the serum there was antibody against HSA of IgA and IgM class. In this system, antigen–antibody complexes probably involved both kinds of antibody, because both our systems, based on C1q and on rheumatoid factor, were inhibited.

Pierce: Did you fail to see a local response after the subsequent parenteral challenge?

André: There was a local response after oral immunization. I haven't looked for a local response after the parenteral challenge.

Pierce: The experiment is similar to one we have done with cholera toxoid in rats in which oral priming followed by intraperitoneal boosting does produce a local response (Pierce & Gowans 1975). If the systemic immune response to parenteral antigen is being modified by prior oral exposure, it may be that the gut immune response to the parenteral booster remains intact.

Parrott: In experiments with Howard Thomas we fed BSA to rats in large amounts (Thomas & Parrott 1974). We got a transitory, small amount of serum antibody to BSA but couldn't find any local production—that is, specific antibody-forming cells in the lamina propria or in the lumen of the gut—and neither did they respond to challenge with BSA in Freund's adjuvant given intramuscularly.

Pierce: Did you try a later oral challenge? Under these circumstances we have seen what appears to be inefficient oral priming but much more efficient oral boosting (Pierce & Gowans 1975).

Parrott: No, we didn't challenge orally. But normally you get a nice response to BSA in Freund's adjuvant given intramuscularly.

Lachmann: BSA is a very different antigen from cholera toxoid. When used in monomeric form at appropriate concentrations it induces tolerance so that one cannot get a subsequent response even to BSA in complete Freund's adjuvant (see Dresser & Mitchison 1968).

Parrott: We looked at the state in the serum of the small amount of BSA that had been absorbed. It wasn't the tolerogenic form of BSA. It was native BSA.

Lachmann: Were you getting the phenomenon that the antigen which comes through the liver is monomeric and tolerogenic?

Parrott: We thought we would get that, but we showed that we didn't.

Brandtzaeg: I am curious about your test system, Dr André. Are you suggesting that human rheumatoid factor has affinity for rat IgA and can be used to remove the IgA?

André: Yes. There is no animal species specificity, as P. Masson showed.

IMMUNIZATION WITH ESCHERICHIA COLI HYBRIDS

Schmidt: I would like to describe briefly our attempts to immunize mice orally against salmonellosis with *Escherichia coli* hybrids. It is well known that living cells or live vaccines immunize more efficiently against salmonellosis than do killed cells. For oral vaccination we used a live vaccine consisting of avirulent *E. coli* hybrids which express the O antigens of *Salmonella typhimurium* or *Salmonella typhi*. (We introduced the genetic information for O antigen synthesis from a *Salmonella* Hfr donor into *E. coli* by conjugation. The *E. coli* recipient was a non-enteropathogenic strain isolated from human faeces.) The oral vaccination of adult mice with hybrids resulted in a rather low protection rate against *Salmonella* infections. We found that in adult mice the hybrids were eliminated from the intestine within two days. This may explain the poor efficiency of the vaccine.

In other experiments we vaccinated 4–5-day-old baby mice orally with a drop (containing about 10^8 cells) of hybrid suspension. We found that the hybrids colonized the intestine and persisted for 14 days and in some cases longer. When we challenged these mice four weeks after immunization they were well protected.

To achieve protection of adult mice it appears necessary to start hybridization with *E. coli* strains which can colonize the adult mouse intestine. Experiments of that kind are in progress.

Soothill: Was the protection against oral infection by salmonella organisms, or did you also get protection against parenteral administration of salmonella?

Schmidt: Protection was measured by the rate of elimination of challenge bacteria from liver and spleen. As compared to untreated mice the numbers of challenge bacteria recovered from the organs were also very low in mice infected intraperitoneally.

White: Are there any factors such as the adherence of these *E. coli* organisms to the gut wall which are responsible for their success?

Schmidt: This is what we have to test now.

Cebra: It would certainly be advantageous to isolate an *E. coli* from the mouse for your immunization studies. Although you did succeed in colonizing the neonates, and one presumes that the bacterial organisms used were adherent to cell surfaces, a naturally occurring organism would more surely have been selected for adherence and successful colonization. Have you tried to clean up the gut of the adult mice before you try to colonize them with the hybrid by using antibiotics, in order to cut down competition from the resident bacterial flora?

Schmidt: We haven't done this.

Mayrhofer: If you used native *E. coli*, not hybridized, did it colonize?

Schmidt: The native *E. coli* colonized the intestine of very young mice, but not that of adult mice.

Pierce: It would be important to know whether the colonization you achieved in infant mice was in the small bowel or colon. If it were in the colon you might have induced local colonic protection and perhaps even systemic immunity without neccessarily protecting the small bowel. This could be very important in your attempts to immunize orally with a living hybrid strain, since the major site at which *S. typhimurium* invades the gut is probably the distal ileum (Carter & Collins 1974). Your measure of protection was the duration of survival of the challenge strain in liver and spleen, so systemic invasion had obviously taken place. If you had achieved small bowel protection by oral immunization, you might have prevented invasion by the challenge strain altogether.

Schmidt: It may be that in oral vaccination of baby mice the hybrids penetrate the epithelial cells of the intestine and spread through the whole organism, thus evoking systemic immunity. Whether intestinal immunity is also achieved remains to be tested.

Lachmann: Have you looked to see if you get anti-salmonella antibodies in the milk of the mice infected with the hybrid organism?

Schmidt: No.

Lachmann: One can see fascinating possibilities if you could parasitize a cow with hybrids of the enteric organisms of man and could use the milk to give passive immunity in humans.

ANTIGEN ENTRY IN GUT

Lachmann: The question arises of how much antigen normally goes across the bowel mucosa. We have been told on the one hand that all orally given antigen is digested; on the other hand, various contributors to the symposium have given us to understand that orally administered material, whether sheep red cells, bacteria or food, is adequately immunogenic and presumably does cross the mucosa. Can a quantitative statement be made about what macromolecular material, and where, goes across the gut?

Gowans: Can we add to your questions the possibility that, in pathological conditions, defects of digestion may lead to the chronic exposure of the gut to immunogenic residues?

Bienenstock: Rothberg showed that if rabbits were given 0.1% BSA in the drinking water it did not produce systemic immunization or systemic antibody formation and the level of circulating antigen did not rise above 0.06 μg protein N per ml (Rothberg *et al.* 1970). These levels in the circulation were not immunogenic, as judged by subsequent attempts at parenteral immunization with those amounts. However, those quantities were never systemically infused.

Porter: When we were developing oral vaccination in pigs with *E. coli* we used heat-stripped bacteria which yield endotoxin. We measured the endotoxin in terms of haemagglutination inhibition, but we did a dilution study in which we fed 1 ml doses containing 10^{10}–10^6 organisms. There was a definite threshold at about 10^6 or 10^7 for a local immune response. In none of those was there evidence of a systemic stimulus in terms of circulating antibody.

Gowans: The experiments I am thinking of are not studies on systemic antibody responses but measurements of the transport of immunogenic proteins from the gut into the intestinal lymph.

Bienenstock: Rothberg has looked at the molecular size of BSA in the circulation after oral feeding. Much of what goes across into the circulation is normal intact BSA; about 0.01% of the administered dose gets across and a considerable portion of that is native BSA.

Brandtzaeg: We have an *in vitro* model in which the rabbit colon (the whole gut wall) is used as the membrane in a diffusion chamber (K. Tolo & P. Brandtzaeg, unpublished). After two hours at room temperature we recover in the order of 0.1% of the antigenic material (HSA) applied on the epithelial side.

Pierce: One has to be cautious when interpreting results from a model like that, because the slightest handling of gut considerably alters the diffusion of macromolecules across the mucosa.

Brandtzaeg: Yes. There is a considerable difference between various membranes and various animals and *in vivo* the penetration through the gut epithelium would probably be much less than 0.1%.

Lachmann: Is it clear that the amount absorbed is a percentage of the amount given rather than a function of the time available for absorption? Does the amount absorbed show a dose–response relationship, with the amount present on the epithelial side and, if so, does the curve flatten out at higher concentrations?

Brandtzaeg: I don't know, but at the concentration we have used (30 mg/ml) the serosal concentration after two hours has been in the order of 0.1%.

Soothill: Lippard *et al.* (1936) observed the complement-fixing bovine milk antigen and complement-fixing anti-milk antibodies in normal children when they were weaned, at whatever age. First he detected the antigen and then antibody, after conventional feeding of normal children. I know of no faults in that study. The more recent work includes studies of inverted gut sacs (Walker *et al.* 1972), and the work of Heremans' group on antigen in mesenteric blood after feeding. Immunodeficient children, particularly those with primary immunodeficiency (Buckley & Dees 1969) and those with secondary immunodeficiency due to severe malnutrition, have a high incidence of anti-food antibodies in their blood, so they appear to have been sensitized (see Chandra 1976).

Lachmann: The formation of anti-milk antibodies in children is likely to be due at least in part to regurgitation of milk into the lung, where it should be fully immunogenic.

Pepys: Gruskay & Cooke (1955) gave infants one gram of ovalbumin per kilogram body weight as a 10% solution by gavage after 4–8 hours fasting. Venous blood was drawn one and two hours later and ovalbumin in the serum was measured by a quantitative precipitation technique. The normal absorption was found to be 0.02% of the ingested dose, whilst in children with various sorts of diarrhoea this increased to 0.1%.

White: Delphine Parrott mentioned the idea that antigen goes to and through the domes of the Peyer's patches (p. 347). We attempted to put antigens, not over Peyer's patches, but over the follicles of the caecal tonsils in the chicken, one caecum being used as the control of the other. We failed with several antigens to find penetration of antigen into these follicles, but the follicles have a beautiful dendritic network. This is shown not by the pattern of the antigen, which we couldn't demonstrate, but by using a fluorescent conjugate against 7S chicken immunoglobulin. This demonstrates a pattern very similar to what you see in Malpighian bodies in the spleen: that is, antigen–antibody complexes localized to the surface of dendritic cells scattered uniformly throughout the germinal centre.

Bienenstock: The chicken caecal tonsil is not the same as a mammalian Peyer's patch. Synthetic studies using radio-labelled amino acid precursors show that chicken caecal tonsils are characterized more by the production of IgG than IgA, whereas the bursa produces mainly IgM (Bienenstock *et al.* 1973).

It looks more like peripheral lymphoid tissue than would appear from its position in the bowel.

Gowans: Professor R. R. Wagner and I have recently examined the ability of viable bacteriophage R17 to pass from the intestinal lumen into the thoracic duct lymph. Since this phage is easy to assay by conventional plaquing techniques we could obtain quantitative estimates of the amount of 'undegraded' material which passed across the normal intestinal epithelium into the draining lymph. Phage was injected into the lumen of the duodenum of rats in which a thoracic duct cannula had been inserted on the previous day and, in a number of experiments, 0.03–0.1 % of the administered PFU were recovered in the lymph; most was recovered in the first hour. We do not know whether the phage penetrated the Peyer's patches or passed through the epithelium elsewhere. The total recovery was small but the experiments show that the small gut and the draining mesenteric nodes could not prevent some living virus from entering the efferent lymph and thus the blood. Whether the penetration of the gut by microorganisms and macromolecules occurs normally and on a scale which is potentially hazardous to the animal remains to be established.

Porter: The quantity is a question of the initial load. If you had fed only 0.1 % of what you in fact fed, would any have got across?

Gowans: I don't know. We certainly gave huge quantities of phage (about 10^{11} PFU) and the assay is very sensitive so the physiological significance of these observations is unclear. At the moment we are simply interested in finding out whether the phage passes through the Peyer's patches or elsewhere; our methods should enable us to do this.

Lachmann: If you think of eating a 12 oz steak, 0.01 % is about 34 mg, which could be a substantial dose of antigen!

Gowans: Presumably information on this point can be obtained by feeding radiolabelled antigens and assaying in the intestinal lymph. On the other hand, I don't know the extent to which fragments large enough to be immunogenic would be absorbed into the portal blood.

Soothill: There is the problem of digestion, leading to detection of the label on small peptides, and of free label sticking to endogenous proteins.

André: We have now measured the total human albumin transmitted by the gut in the rat (André *et al.* 1974). In this system we had evidence that local immunization of the gut with human albumin impairs its capacity to absorb the corresponding antigen and that immune intestinal secretion also blocks antigen absorption in non-immune rats. Quantitative data were obtained by Warshaw *et al.* (1971). They observed that around 0.01 % of the administered dose of horseradish peroxidase was transmitted into mesenteric lymph and portal blood of rats. But the same group (Warshaw *et al.* 1974) also observed that a larger percentage of the administered dose of bovine albumin was absorbed.

Lachmann: Do you find whole proteins in venous blood?

André: Yes.

Ferguson: Warshaw et al. (1974) infused ^{3}H-labelled BSA into the duodenum of rats and found that 2% was absorbed as intact BSA molecules. In other experiments they showed that 0.8% was transported away from the gut via the lymphatics and 1.1% via the portal vein (Warshaw & Walker 1974).

Booth: The liver also affects the amount absorbed; there is a difference in the antibody titres to dietary antigens in patients who have a portocaval shunt and those who haven't, suggesting a hepatic sieving of whatever goes up the portal vein. This is well-known for bacteria.

Brandtzaeg: In the *in vitro* system that I referred to (p. 357), the penetrability of the large bowel wall in the rabbit is at least 20 times greater than that of the sublingual oral mucosa. This shows the difference between the various mucous membranes.

Lachmann: This suggests that if people don't digest their food they might absorb more of it further down the gut!

Booth: Insulin given by mouth is absorbed.

THE INTESTINAL BACTERIAL LOAD

Booth: The gut is far from sterile. The proximal intestine has broadly speaking an aerobic flora which reaches concentrations of 10^3 to 10^5 organisms per ml. The ileum has something between the jejunum and the colon, and you begin to find an anaerobic flora of various types in the ileum. In the colon the flora is predominantly anaerobic when grown under proper conditions. *E. coli* is less important here. But the flora is there, and the infection following perforation of the duodenum shows that very clearly.

Pierce: It is important to recognize that most of the laboratory animals we work with are quite different from humans. Mice and rats, for example, have a highly developed complex microflora with much larger numbers of bacteria in the small intestine than do humans. This is an important difference when one is considering the antigenic load or the microbiological environment of the small bowel in man, as compared with laboratory animals.

Booth: The so-called normal subjects studied in Calcutta had loads much more like those of experimental animals, in the 'normal' intestine. Western Europeans seem to have greater loads than patients in the USA. One assumes that the more extensive packaging of food in the USA is responsible for that difference.

Gowans: It is interesting that the bacterial load in the various parts of the intestine is not apparently reflected in the local density of IgA-secreting cells in the lamina propria: the density in the large and small gut of rats looks to me to be about the same.

Booth: In patients with huge bacterial loads due to jejunal diverticulosis, there is no evidence of an increase in IgA cells.

Porter: In the pig there is almost a reciprocal arrangement: the bacterial load increases towards the posterior region of the small intestine and the IgA and IgM cell population increases towards the anterior (see earlier discussion, p. 44).

Pierce: There are certainly non-immunological mechanisms which contribute to keeping much of the small bowel 'clean'. These include the 'acid barrier' of the stomach and the continuous distal propulsion of the gut contents. Their importance can be seen in the terminal ileum where stasis apparently contributes to the development of a colon-like microflora, even though the local immune system appears similar to that of the proximal small bowel. It should also be apparent that the 'clean' proximal bowel is repeatedly exposed to a wide variety of microbial and dietary antigens, sufficient to account for a vigorous local immune response even though persistent and heavy bacterial colonization is not seen.

White: Of course, measured loads refer to the content of the bowel and don't take account of bacteria sticking to the wall.

Mayrhofer: In small rodents, the mucus layer of the small intestine contains large numbers of bacteria and these are not necessarily of the same species as those that can be isolated from the luminal contents (Savage *et al.* 1968).

GUT NOT A PRIMARY LYMPHOID ORGAN

Lachmann: One other topic is the possible role of the gut, particularly in the mammal, as a primary lymphoid organ. It hasn't been mentioned so far: is that because there is a general consensus that the idea is exploded?

Gowans: The evidence on this point can be found in the excellent Ciba Foundation Symposium on the Ontogeny of Acquired Immunity (1972). My own view is that the evidence for gut-associated lymphoid tissue having a role analogous to that of the bursa in birds is very weak. In any event we now have excellent experimental support for a special function for the Peyer's patches: to fire off cells into the intestinal lymph which migrate into the lamina propria and synthesize IgA.

Lachmann: Further, Max Cooper and John Owen have now shown that fetal liver is the source of B cells in mammals (see Owen 1972).

FUTURE WORK

Lachmann: The clinicians here are surrounded by many members of the clone of immunologists interested in the secretory immune system. What models of investigation would they (the clinicians) like to suggest that could give more information about the problems exercising them? On the other hand, one could ask the immunologists to suggest appropriate investigations to apply to the clinical problems, ethical considerations being taken into account. Has any line of work become apparent during the symposium which could throw light on the problems of inflammatory bowel disease and of coeliac disease, or establish their immunological origin?

Gowans: And can you produce in experimental animals diseases whose pathology mimics the pictures seen in Crohn's disease and ulcerative colitis?

Ferguson: Many acute infectious diarrhoeas produce changes in the rectal mucosa which are virtually indistinguishable from the appearances of colitis. Also, D. B. L. McClelland & H. Gilmour (personal communication) have seen granulomata in the rectal mucosa in patients with salmonella gastroenteritis. If the mechanisms of tissue damage in infectious diseases are elucidated, this may throw some light on the idiopathic inflammatory bowel diseases such as ulcerative colitis and Crohn's disease.

White: Do you mean that a fully blown epithelioid cell granuloma with giant cells is found in someone who has had salmonellosis?

Ferguson: Yes: classical granulomas (with giant cells) are found in rectal biopsies from patients admitted to hospital merely for the clinical management of diarrhoea associated with proven enteropathogenic infection. These granulomas appear to be due to the infective process, although these patients have not yet been studied for long enough to exclude completely the possibility of underlying Crohn's disease.

Parrott: I am interested in investigating the consequences of the switching or diversion of cells destined for some experimentally induced lesion to the gut. Can Professor Booth tell me whether, when other lesions arise in association with ulcerative colitis—iritis, joint lesions and so on—the colitis gets better or worse, or are they in parallel?

Booth: They can be completed unrelated.

Parrott: And can you give me any leads with the atrophic spleen?

Booth: The spleen is not usually atrophic in children in coeliac disease; this occurs in about 20% of adult patients, if you measure spleen size using chromium-labelled heat-denatured red cells and scanning.

Parrott: Are the other lesions worse in patients with atrophic spleens?

Booth: I can't answer that.

Rosen: I would like to go back to a point of departure which had to do with IgA-producing cells. We didn't discuss the fact that if you look at a population of IgA-deficient children, they are at risk for a list of diseases that is too long to enumerate. The best studied are lupus erythematosus and rheumatoid arthritis. We have much information on the homing of IgA cells but we need more information on what they are doing physiologically, in terms of what their cell products are doing to enhance the barrier function of the gut.

Lachmann: Although these children are IgA deficient, we don't know what their primary defect is. It may lie on a biochemical pathway that has additional manifestations in functions other than IgA synthesis. There is no evidence that they have a defect in the structural gene for the α chain.

Soothill: There is good evidence that they haven't, since they have IgA on the surface of their B lymphocytes.

* * *

Lachmann: This is probably a good point at which to draw the discussion to a close, having got back to where we started from! We have studied three fairly distinct types of problem, starting with the physiology of the immune system as it affects the gut, mainly from the secretory immunoglobulin point of view but also from that of cell-mediated immunity; we have discussed infectious organisms, both bacteria and nematodes; and we have considered the immunopathology of inflammatory bowel disease and some other conditions. A great deal of information has been put about. Nevertheless, it is clear that answers to the immunological problems of gut disease are not yet forthcoming. We don't yet understand the aetiology or even in any detail the pathogenetic mechanisms in inflammatory bowel disease. Perhaps by the time the Ciba Foundation explores this topic again, this will all have changed.

References

ANDRÉ, C., BAZIN, H. & HEREMANS, J. F. (1973) Influence of repeated administration of antigen by the oral route on specific antibody-producing cells in the mouse spleen. *Digestion 9*, 166-175

ANDRÉ, C., LAMBERT, R., BAZIN, H. & HEREMANS, J. F. (1974) Interference of oral immunization with the intestinal absorption of heterologous albumin. *Eur. J. Immunol. 4*, 701-704

ANDRÉ, C., HEREMANS, J. F., VAERMAN, J. P. & CAMBIASO, C. L. (1975) A mechanism for the induction of immunological tolerance by antigen feeding: antigen-antibody complexes. *J. Exp. Med. 142*, 1509-1519

ASHERSON, A. L., ALLWOOD, G. G. & MAYHEW, B. (1973) Contact sensitivity in the mouse. XI. Movement of T blasts in the draining lymph node to sites of inflammation. *Immunology 25*, 485

BAZIN, H., LEVI, G. & DORIA, G. (1970) Predominant contribution of IgA antibody-forming cells to an immune response detected in extraintestinal lymphoid tissues of germ-free mice exposed to antigen by the oral route. *J. Immunol. 105*, 1049-1051

BIENENSTOCK, J., GAULDIE, J. & PEREY, D. Y. E. (1973) Synthesis of IgG, IgA, IgM by chicken tissues: immunofluorescent and ^{14}C amino acid incorporation studies. *J. Immunol. 111*, 1112-1118

BOCKMAN, D. E. & COOPER, M. D. (1973) Pinocytosis by epithelium associated with lymphoid follicles in the bursa of Fabricius, appendix and Peyer's patches. An electron microscopic study. *Am. J. Anat. 136*, 455

BUCKLEY, R. H. & DEES, S. C. (1969) The correlation of milk precipitins with IgA deficiency. *N. Engl. J. Med. 281*, 465

CARTER, P. B. & COLLINS, F. M. (1974) The route of enteric infection in normal mice. *J. Exp. Med. 139*, 1189-1203

CEBRA, J. J., KAMAT, R., GEARHART, P., ROBERTSON, S. M. & TSENG, J. (1977) The secretory IgA system of the gut, this volume, pp. 5-28

CHANDRA, R. K. (1976) Immunological consequences of malnutrition including fetal growth retardation, in *Food and Immunology (Swedish Nutrition Foundation Symposium XIII)*, Almqvist & Wiksell International, Stockholm, in press

Ciba Foundation (1972) *Ontogeny of Acquired Immunity (Ciba Found. Symp. 5)*, Elsevier/Excerpta Medica/North-Holland, Amsterdam

DRESSER, D. W. & MITCHISON, N. A. (1968) The mechanism of immunological paralysis. *Adv. Immunol. 8*, 129

FERGUSON, A. & MACDONALD, T. T. (1977) Effects of local delayed hypersensitivity on the small intestine, this volume, pp. 305-327

GRISCELLI, C., VASSALLI, P. & McCLUSKEY, R. T. (1969) The distribution of large dividing lymph node cells in syngeneic recipient rats after intravenous injection. *J. Exp. Med. 130*, 1427

GRUSKAY, F. L. & COOKE, R. E. (1955) The gastrointestinal absorption of unaltered protein in normal infants and in infants recovering from diarrhoea. *Pediatrics 16*, 763-768

GUY-GRAND, D., GRISCELLI, C. & VASSALLI, P. (1974) The gut-associated lymphoid system: nature and properties of the large dividing cell. *Eur. J. Immunol. 4*, 435

HUSBAND, A. J., MONIÉ, H. J. & GOWANS, J. L. (1977) The natural history of the cells producing IgA in the gut, this volume, pp. 29-54

KATZ, A. J. & ROSEN, F. S. (1977) Gastrointestinal complications of immunodeficiency syndromes, this volume, pp. 243-261

LAMELIN, J.-P., LISOWSKA-BERNSTEIN, B., MATTER, A., RYSER, J. E. & VASSALLI, P. (1972) Mouse thymus-independent and thymus-derived lymphoid cells. I. Immunofluorescent and functional studies. *J. Exp. Med. 136*, 984-1007

LIPPARD, V. W., SCHLOSS, O. M. & JOHNSON, P. A. (1936) Immune reactions induced in infants by intestinal absorption of incompletely digested cow's milk proteins. *Am. J. Dis. Child. 51*, 562

MATTER, A., LISOWSKA-BERNSTEIN, B., RYSER, J. E., LAMELIN, J.-P. & VASSALLI, P. (1972) Mouse thymus-independent and thymus-derived lymphoid cells. II. Ultrastructural studies. *J. Exp. Med. 136*, 1008-1030

MÜLLER-SCHOOP, J. W. & GOOD, R. A. (1975) Functional studies of Peyer's patches: evidence for their participation in intestinal immune responses. *J. Immunol. 114*, 1757

OGILVIE, B. M. & PARROTT, D. M. V. (1977) The immunological consequence of nematode infection, this volume, pp. 183-201

O'TOOLE, C. M. & DAVIES, A. J. S. (1971) Pre-emption in immunity. *Nature (Lond.) 230*, 187-189

OWEN, J. J. T. (1972) The origin and development of lymphocyte populations, in *Ontogeny of Acquired Immunity (Ciba Found. Symp. 5)*, pp. 35-54, Elsevier/Excerpta Medica/North-Holland, Amsterdam

PARROTT, D. M. V. (1976) The gut as a lymphoid organ, in *Clinics in Gastroenterology*, vol. 5, no. 2 (Wright, R., ed.), p. 211, Saunders, Philadelphia
PARROTT, D. M. V. & FERGUSON, A. (1974) Selective migration of lymphocytes within the mouse small intestine. *Immunology 26*, 571
PIERCE, N. F. & GOWANS, J. L. (1975) Cellular kinetics of the intestinal immune response to cholera toxoid in rats. *J. Exp. Med.* 142, 1550-1563
ROSE, M. L., PARROTT, D. M. V. & BRUCE, R. G. (1976a) Migration of lymphoblasts to the small intestine. I. Effect of *Trichinella spiralis* infection on the migration of mesenteric lymphoblasts and mesenteric T lymphoblasts in syngeneic mice. *Immunology 31*, 723-730
ROSE, M. L., PARROTT, D. M. V. & BRUCE, R. G. (1976b) Migration of lymphoblasts to the small intestine. II. Divergent migration of mesenteric and peripheral immunoblasts to sites of inflammation in the mouse. *Cell Immunol.* 27, 36
ROTHBERG, R. M., KRAFT, S. C., FARR, R. S., KRIEBEL, G. W. & GOLDBERG, S. S. (1970) Local immunologic responses to ingested protein, in *The Secretory Immunologic System* (Dayton, D., ed.), pp. 293-307, U.S. Dept Health, Education & Welfare, Bethesda, Maryland, USA
ROTHBERG, R. M., KRAFT, S. C., ASQUITH, P. & MICHALEK, S. M. (1973) The effect of splenectomy on the immune responses of rabbits to a soluble protein antigen given parenterally or orally. *Cell. Immunol.* 7, 124-133
RUSSELL, R. J., WILKINSON, P. C., SLESS, F. & PARROTT, D. M. V. (1975) Chemotaxis of lymphoblasts. *Nature (Lond.) 256*, 646
SAVAGE, D. C., DUBOS, R. & SCHAEDLER, R. W. (1968) The gastrointestinal epithelium and its autochthonous bacterial flora. *J. Exp. Med.* 127, 67-76
SPRENT, J. (1976) Fate of H-2 activated T lymphocytes in syngeneic hosts. I. Fate in lymphoid tissues and intestines traced with ^{3}H-thymidine, ^{125}I-deoxyuridine and ^{51}chromium. *Cell. Immunol.* 21, 278
THOMAS, H. C. & PARROTT, D. M. V. (1974) The induction of tolerance to soluble protein antigen by oral administration. *Immunology 27*, 631
WALKER, W. A., ISSELBACHER, K. J. & BLOCH, K. J. (1972) Intestinal uptake of macromolecules: effect of oral immunization. *Science (Wash. D.C.) 177*, 608
WARSHAW, A. L. & WALKER, W. A. (1974) Intestinal absorption of intact antigenic protein. *Surgery 76*, 495-499
WARSHAW, A. L., WALKER, W. A., CORNELL, R. & ISSELBACHER, K. J. (1971) Small intestinal permeability to macromolecules. Transmission of horseradish peroxidase into mesenteric lymph and portal blood. *Lab. Invest.* 25, 675-684
WARSHAW, A. L., WALKER, W. A. & ISSELBACHER, K. J. (1974) Protein uptake by the intestine: evidence for absorption of intact macromolecules. *Gastroenterology 66*, 987-992
WILKINSON, P. C., ROBERTS, J. A., RUSSELL, R. J. & MCLOUGHLIN, M. (1976) Chemotaxis of mitogen-activated human lymphocytes and the effects of membrane active enzymes. *Clin. Exp. Immunol.*, 25, 280-287

Index of contributors

*Entries in **bold** type indicate papers; other entries are contributions to discussions*

Allen, W. D. **55**
Ahlstedt, S. 42, **115**, 130, 131, 132, 133
André, C. 69, 109, 131, 236, 238, 260, 280, 321, 343, 350, 352, 353, 354, 359, 360
Baklien, K. **77**
Beeson, P. B. 150, **203**, 214, 215, 216, 217, 218, 219, 220, 277
Bienenstock, J. 45, 72, 73, 133, 153, 181, 195, 258, 259, 319, 320, 324, 350, 353, 357, 358
Booth, C. C. 22, 42, 44, 71, 197, 198, 199, 215, 220, 221, 255, 256, 257, 260, 275, 276, 277, 278, 280, 297, 321, 325, **329**, 341, 343, 344, 345, 360, 361, 362
Brandtzaeg, P. 42, 43, 52, 69, **77**, 108, 109, 110, 111, 112, 130, 133, 150, 151, 177, 178, 219, 237, 258, 259, 260, 277, 278, 303, 343, 355, 358, 360
Carlsson, B. **115**
Cebra, J. J. **5**, 22, 23, 24, 25, 26, 27, 43, 46, 47, 48, 49, 50, 51, 72, 103, 109, 110, 131, 178, 240, 278, 323, 324, 325, 326, 356
Dash, A. C. **283**
Davies, A. J. S. 50, 51, 150, 177, 217, 218, 257, 258, 275, 276, 352
Doe, W. F. **329**
Druguet, M. **283**
Evans, D. J. 27, 110, 111, 131, 179, 180, 196, 216, 236, 257, 277, 279, 297, 322, 342
Fällström, S. P. **115**
Ferguson, A. 111, 152, 181, 198, 199, 218, 254, 257, 260, **305**, 319, 320, 321, 322, 323, 324, 325, 326, 343, 344, 345, 360, 362
Gearhart, P. **5**
Gowans, J. L. 23, 24, 25, **29**, 42, 43, 44, 45, 47, 49, 71, 109, 110, 131, 153, 177, 181, 217, 256, 276, 279, 297, 320, 321, 350, 357, 359, 361, 362
Hanson, L. Å. **115**
Holmgren, J. **115**
Husband, A. J. **29**
Jodal, U. **115**
Jones, J. V. 299, 300, 301
Kaijser, B. **115**
Kamat, R. **5**
Katz, A. J. **243**
Klass, H. J. **283**
Lachmann, P. J. **1**, 47, 48, 49, 52, 70, 71, 72, 73, 109, 112, 131, 132, 133, 150, 181, 213, 214, 215, 218, 219, 220, 239, 255, 259, 280, 298, 299, 300, 302, 323, 343, 352, 353, 354, 355, 356, 357, 358
Lehner, T. 23, 68, 73, **135**, 150, 151, 152, 153, 180, 185, 195, 196, 199, 216, 239, 301, 325
Lidin-Janson, G. **115**
Lindblad, B. S. **115**
MacDonald, T. T. **305**
Mayrhofer, G. 49, 69, **155**, 176, 177, 178, 179, 180, 181, 196, 197, 216, 219, 220, 280, 356, 361
Mirjah, D. D. **283**
Monié, H. J. **29**
Ogilvie, B. M. 175, 176, **183**, 195, 196, 197, 198, 199, 200, 213, 214, 215, 216, 220, 221, 222, 257
Parrott, D. M. V. 26, 27, 44, 69, 74, **183**, 195, 199, 325, 347, 350, 354, 355, 362
Parry, S. H. **55**
Pepys, M. B. 26, 44, 45, 49, 73, 131, 215, 217, 237, 256, 260, **283**, 297, 298, 299, 300, 301, 302, 303, 323, 344, 345, 353, 358

Peters, T. J. **329**
Petrie, A. **283**
Pierce, N. F. 25, 26, 46, 67, 68, 130, 131, 199, 255, 323, 324, 342, 354, 356, 357, 360, 361
Porter, P. 22, 24, 25, 44, 51, 52, **55**, 68, 69, 70, 71, 72, 73, 111, 112, 129, 130, 199, 200, 240, 256, 344, 357, 359, 361
Robertson, S. M. **5**
Rosen, F. S. 43, 73, 152, 214, 215, 217, 218, 219, 240, **243**, 255, 256, 257, 258, 260, 276, 278, 279, 303, 341, 342, 343, 345, 363
Schmidt, G. 196, 200, 355, 356

Seligmann, M. 43, 50, 52, 217, 257, 259, **263**, 275, 276, 277, 279, 280
Sohl-Åkerlund, A. **115**
Soothill, J. F. 22, 23, 72, 131, 176, 219, 221, **225**, 236, 237, 239, 240, 241, 257, 258, 259, 301, 353, 355, 358, 359, 363
Tseng, J. **5**
Vaerman, J. P. 109, 111, 133, 219, 220, 350, 352
Wadsworth, C. **115**
White, R. G. 26, 52, 70, 71, 74, 151, 178, 197, 217, 220, 222, 238, 239, 277, 279, 301, 342, 343, 345, 356, 358, 361, 362

Indexes compiled by William Hill

Subject index

adhesion, bacterial
  64, 71
adjuvants
  238
  dental plaque as 140
  macrophages and 138, 230, 232
  mechanism of action 141
agammaglobulinaemia
  B cells in 249
  pernicious anaemia and 246
allergic reactions
  3, 227
allograft rejection
  as delayed hypersensitivity 306
  intestinal effects 308
alpha chain disease
  antibiotics and 277, 280
  cellular studies 267
  gastrointestinal infection and 271
  geographical incidence 271, 275
  hygiene and 271, 272
  immunoglobulin abnormality in 264
  malignancy in 269, 276
  natural history 268
  plasma cell proliferation and 272
  protein in 266
  respiratory form 263, 276
amniotic fluid
  58

antibodies
  in serum and milk 115, 118
antibody response
  to *E.coli* 116, 117
  to food proteins 122
  macrophages and 239
  protective effect 124
antigens
  entry into gut 356
  E.coli 62
antigen absorption
  69
antigen elimination
  defective 228
  genetic differences 231
antigen exclusion
  226, 231
antigen handling
  225, 232
antigen-sensitive precursors
  11
anti-milk antibodies
  358
aphthous ulcers
  301
asthma
  204, 284, 285
atopy
  284

bacteria
  load in intestine 360
  mucus wrapped 71
  overgrowth in immunodeficiency 250
bacterial adhesion
  64, 71

bacterial plaque
  acting on lymphocytes 140, 141
  as adjuvant 140
  caries and gingivitis and 142
  components 136, 141
  deposition 136
  diet and 150
  effect on immunological memory 144
  immunopotentiation by 140, 142
  lymphoproliferative response to 136
  origin 153
  stimulating macrophages 139
bacteriophage R 17
  359
bacteriophage φ X 174
  antibodies to 300
bacteriostasis
  65
basement membrane
  92, 110
Behçet's syndrome
  301
Bence-Jones protein
  270
benign monoclonal gammopathy
  280
bird fancier's lung
  344
blast cells, homing
  31-35, 38-40, 43, 195, 347

bone marrow
    cell differentiation in 51
    eosinophil formation in 203, 206, 217
    IgA cells in 47, 82
breast-feeding
    124, 232
Brunner's glands
    95

Candida albicans
    246
carcinoma
    eosinophilia in 205
cell-mediated immune reaction
    306
    damage from 314
    in parasite enteropathy 315
    malnutrition and 318
Charcot-Leyden crystal
    204
cholera enterotoxin
    64
    immunization with 68
    milk antibody against 121
    response to 35, 39, 67, 116, 323, 354
clonal analysis
    11
clonal precursor cells
    11
coeliac disease
    303, 322, 324, 329-346
    alpha chain disease and 280
    antibodies against food proteins 122
    B cell antigens in 345
    T cell function in 258
    complement in 334, 341
    cryoglobulinaemia and 337
    cytochemistry 331
    definition 330
    glandular immunoglo-bulin transport in 101
    gluten challenge in 342
    HLA and 345
    histochemistry 330

histology 334
hypersensitivity and 322, 323
immunocytes in 86
IgA deficiency 250, 255
immunological abnormalities in 333, 336, 343
lymphocytes in 326, 337
mechanism 329
morphology 111, 330
nematode infection and 199
secretory component pattern in 101
spleen in 362
steroids in 341
colon
    cells in 44
colostrum
    immunoglobulins in 57
    IgA antibodies in 130
    IgA:IgM ratio in 80
complement
    in coeliac disease 299, 334, 341
    in inflammatory bowel disease 292, 299, 301, 303
contact hypersensitivity
    314
cot death
    103, 258
cow's milk proteins
    122, 226, 234
C-reactive protein
    in Behçet's syndrome and aphthous ulcers 301
    in inflammatory bowel disease 288, 298
    interactions 299
    interaction with lympho-cytes 292
    properties 289
Crohn's disease
    283, 362
    atopy in 284
    compared with ulcerative colitis 287
    complement in 292, 299, 301, 303
    C-reactive protein in 288, 298

glandular immunoglobulin transport in 101
immunoglobulins in 111
IgG in 87, 104
incidence 283
in immunodeficiency 251
cryoglobulinaemia
    337
crypts
    IgA in 324
    in graft-versus-host reaction 311
    in intestinal allografts 210
cystic fibrosis
    227

dental caries
    142, 150
diarrhoea
    246
    B cell deficiency and 255
    T cell deficiency and 245, 254
    immunodeficiency and 240
digestion
    359
disaccharidase deficiency
    251
dysentery
    255

EB virus
    303
eczema
    204, 227
enteric infections
    immune mechanisms 55-75
    oral immunization 60
enterocyte transit
    317
enteropathic lymphokines
    314, 325, 326
enterotoxin production
    64
eosinophils
    adherence to parasites 215
    clinical associations 204
    Fc receptors on 215

SUBJECT INDEX

formation in bone marrow 203, 206, 217
immunosuppression and 207
in diseases of gut 205
in fungal infection 215
in immune response 209
lymphocytes and 208, 217
mast cells and 208, 213
role 203-223
tissue injury and 210
eosinophil chemotaxis 205, 210
eosinophilic gastroenteritis 205, 210
eosinophilic granulocytes 178
eosinophilic granuloma 216
Escherichia coli 56
antigen response to 59
K antigens of 120, 124
breast-feeding and 124, 232
enterotoxin 64
filamentous surface antigens 62
host resistance to 62
intestinal stasis and 200
milk antibody response to 117, 124
serum antibody response to 116
synthesis and secretion of antibodies 60
E.coli **hybrids**
immunization with 355
exocrine glands secreting immunoglobulin 81

flat-gut lesion 250
food allergies 126, 205, 233
food proteins 122, 230, 231
fungal infection 215

gastroenteritis
eosinophilic 210

Giardia lamblia **infestation** 236
age incidence 257
B cells in 251
effect on lymphocytes 316
immunodeficiency and 246 257
protective immunity 324
villous flattening in 250
gingivitis 150
dental plaque and 142
effect of drugs 146
immune response to 139
incidence 152
glandular immunoglobulin transport 99, 101, 103
globule leucocyte 161, 169, 220
gluten challenge in coeliac disease 336, 342
gluten-sensitive enteropathy 250
goblet cells 92
Golgi complex 95, 110
graft-versus-host disease 311, 321
granulomas 138, 362

Haemonchus **infestation** 222
Hassall's corpuscles 95
heavy chain disease 263 *et seq.*
hepatitis 252
histocompatibility antigens 345
histiocytosis X 216
Hodgkin's disease 255, 269
homocytotropic antibody 158, 172, 179
host–pathogen interaction 65

humoral immunity 16
hypersensitivity, contact 314
hypersensitivity, delayed
allograft rejection as 306
antigens producing 323
effects 305-327
hypersensitivity, immediate
IgE and 156, 170
hypogammaglobulinaemia 98

immune complexes, detection 351
immune elimination
mechanisms 227
immune exclusion 226, 237
immune mechanism
enteric infection and 55-75
immune reaction, cell-mediated
see cell-mediated immune reaction
immune response 22
adjuvant effect 23, 138
biphasic 26
enhanced 23
eosinophils in 209
initial phase 103
maturation 238
priming and 44, 45, 46
sequence 195
to bacterial plaque 135
to cholera toxoid 67
to gingivitis 139
immunization
antibody and 70
oral *see oral immunization*
with cholera toxoid 68
immunoblasts
parasites affecting traffic 189
immunoconglutinin 292, 294
immunocyte populations
characteristics 86
coeliac disease and 86
origin 87

immunodeficiency
2
  classification 243, 244
  Crohn's disease and 251
  diarrhoea and 240, 245
  disaccharidase deficiency
    and 251
  gastrointestinal complications of 243
  gastrointestinal malignancy and 252
  Giardia lamblia and 246, 257
  liver disease and 252
  lymphoid nodular hyperplasia and 248
  protein-losing enteropathy in 253
  secretory component in 259
  ulcerative colitis in 251
  underlying immunopathy 226
  villous flattening in 250
immunoglobulins
  abnormality in alpha chain disease 264
  Crohn's disease and 111
  glandular transport of 101
  in milk 57
  mucosal distribution 89
  quantitation 80
  receptors for 27
  synthesis 260
immunoglobulins, maternal
56
immunoglobulin A (IgA)
2, 5-28
  binding with SC 80, 83, 87, 95, 132
  concentration 237
  development with age 237
  dimeric and monomeric 133
  distribution 94
  epithelial uptake 99
  Fc receptors 73
  glandular transport 78, 95
  in amniotic fluid 58
  in crypt cells 324
  in lamina propria 90

  in maternal immunity 57
  in treatment of alpha chain disease 278
  inhibiting K cell cytotoxicity 73
  J chains in 85, 109
  mediating tolerance 237
  memory in 68
  mucin complexes 71, 72
  preventing antigen absorption 69
  protective role 7
  receptor 78, 112
  survival in gut 130
  synthesis 6, 7, 94, 236, 350
  transport 98, 103, 111, 133
IgA antibodies
  against food proteins 122
  in milk 118
  passage along intestine 130
  production 49, 125
  protective role 124, 130
  transport 6
IgA cells
10
  homing 43
  in bone marrow 47
  in lamina propria 46, 108
  in lymph 35
  in milk 16, 131
  in neonatal lamina propria 58
  in Peyer's patches 22, 36, 37, 47
  in villi 27
  maintenance 29
  natural history 29-54
  numbers 86
  origin 30, 33, 36, 37, 47, 48
  production 48, 49
  precursors 24, 27, 42
  repopulation with 14
IgA deficiency
77, 227, 236, 250
  allergy and 232-234
  coeliac syndrome and 255

  cot death and 259
  genetics 256
  in alpha chain disease 265
  selective 253, 260
IgA secretion
77-113
  cells responsible 6
  immunochemical observations 80
  immunohistochemical observations 86
  physicochemical observations 80
immunoglobulin D cells
  detection 43
immunoglobulin E (IgE)
3
  immediate hypersensitivity and 156, 170
  in coeliac disease 334
  in Crohn's disease 288
  in cot death 259
  in eosinophilic gastroenteritis 205
  in thoracic duct lymph 168
  in ulcerative colitis 288
  localization 155
  mast cells and 155, 163, 169, 178, 180, 219
  measurement 286
  N. brasiliensis and 155, 185
  parasite immunity and 172
  Peyer's patches and 163
  physiological function of 220
  secretion 99
  self-cure and 221
  specificity 179
IgE antibodies
286
  anaphylactic reactions 188
  effect on nematodes 188
  immediate hypersensitivity and 155, 156
  in inflammatory bowel disease 284, 287
  production 45
IgE cells
  in medullary cords 166

in spleen 166
in thoracic duct lymph 167
IgE synthesis
175
increased 160
in lymph nodes 176, 180
in mast cells 177
in mesenteric lymph nodes 163
site 155, 156, 163, 168, 169
immunoglobulin G (IgG)
2
catabolism 111
food protein antibodies 122
in Crohn's disease 104
in lamina propria 90
in myeloma 50
in ulcerative colitis 104
location 111
production 51
IgG deficiency
265
immunoglobulin M (IgM)
combination with SC 83
distribution 82, 94
glandular transport 78
in amniotic fluid 58
in coeliac disease 333, 343
in maternal immunity 57
J chain 85
membrane receptors 78
mucin binding and 72
myeloma cells and 50
transport 103
IgM cells
development 52
immune response and 24
in neonatal lamina propria 58
IgM secretion
77-115
immunochemical observations 80
immunohistochemical observations 86
physicochemical observations 80
immunopotentiating drugs and gingiva
146

immunopotentiation by dental plaque
140, 142
immunosuppression
by B cell mitogens 144
eosinophil response and 207
on gingivitis 146
infant feeding
122, 126, 231, 234
infection
malnutrition and 233
inflammatory bowel disease
283-304
intestinal allografts
crypts in 310
destruction 320
lymphocytes in 320
rejection 316, 321
villi in 309
intestinal secretory immunity
58

J chains
7, 78
alpha chain disease and 277
binding site for SC 85, 109
synthesis 109

Kurloff cells
180

lamina propria
IgA cells in 7, 14, 42, 46, 80, 108
IgE cells in 158
immobilization of lymphocytes in 40
in alpha chain disease 268
lymphoid cells in 321
mast cells in 161, 176
migration of lymphocytes to 31, 38
neonatal 58
origin of IgA cells in 33
repopulation 16
leukaemia
252
liver
B cells in 361

immunodeficiency and 252
Loeffler's endomyocarditis
210
lung
in *N. brasiliensis* infection 165, 168
lymph
origin of IgA cells 35
lymph nodes
IgE in 163, 166, 169
B lymphoblasts
homing 195
maturation defect 103
T lymphoblasts
190
homing 195, 347
lymphocytes
antigen and localization 39
complement activation and 301, 302
eosinophil response and 206, 208, 217
Giardia lamblia affecting 316
immobilization in lamina propria 40
in coeliac disease 326, 337
interaction with C-reactive protein 292
migration to lamina propria 22, 31, 38
modulation of activity 137
relation to mast cells 177, 181
stimulation by antigen 45
worm expulsion and 196
B lymphocytes
320
becoming IgA plasma cells 48
dental plaque acting on 137, 140, 141, 144
dissociation of intestinal and circulating 251
division in Peyer's patches 14, 47-48
generating response 49
in agammaglobulinaemia 249
in α chain disease 279

SUBJECT INDEX

B lymphocytes, *continued*
  in fetal liver 361
  in Peyer's patches 8, 9, 47, 347
  site of early response 16
B lymphocyte antigens
  in coeliac disease 345
B lymphocyte deficiency 255
B lymphocyte mitogens 152
  immunosuppression by 144
  lymphoproliferative response to 137
T lymphocytes 320
  deficiency 232, 245, 254
  dental plaque acting on 137, 140, 144
  eosinophils and 217
  immune elimination and 230
  in bone marrow 217
  in coeliac disease 258, 337
  in Peyer's patches 8, 26, 347
  lymphokines in 326
T lymphocyte cytotoxicity 314
lymphocyte homing 38, 42, 47, 195
  SC and 42
lymphocyte trapping 191
lymphoid nodular hyperplasia 248, 256, 260
lymphokines
  enteropathic 314, 325
  on T lymphocytes 326
lymphoma 252
  immunoblastic 268-270, 278
lysosomes 333
  adjuvants and 238
  immune elimination and 230
  immune reponse and 138-139, 239

protein malnutrition and 232
stimulation by dental plaque 139
worm expulsion and 196

macrophage migration inhibition factor 138
malabsorption 246
malignant disease 252
malnutrition 232, 318
mast cells
  degranulation 171, 209
  distribution 181
  eosinophils and 208, 213
  IgE and 155, 163, 169, 177, 180, 219
  in lamina propria 161, 176
  in worm expulsion 172
  lymphocyte relation to 181
  membrane affinity for IgE 178
  numbers in intestine 171
  origin 177, 181
  properties 171
  worm expulsion and 197
maternal immunity 56
Mediterranean lymphoma 270
membrane receptors 78
memory, immunological 68, 144
mesenteric lymph nodes
  IgE in 163, 169, 176, 180
  in alpha chain disease 268
  lymphoblasts in 349
microbial growth in gut
  nematodes affecting 185
milk, antibodies in 117, 118, 121, 124
  immunoglobulins in 57
  IgA antibodies in 118
  IgA cells in 131

mitogenic factor 325
mouth, bacterial plaque
  see bacterial plaque
mucin
  IgA complexes 71
mucosa
  IgA plasma cells in 14
myeloma 50, 276, 279

nasal polyp fluid
  IgE in 170, 176
necrotizing vasculitis 216
nematodes
  affecting immunoblast traffic 189
  affecting microbial growth 185
  antibodies on 199
  coeliac disease and 199
  effect of IgE antibodies 188
  effect of immune system of host 185
  eosinophil adherence to 215
  immunological consequences 183
  nutrition affecting infection 198
  pathological changes 184
neonates
  as germ-free animals 256
  intestinal secretory immunity in 58
  maternal immunity in 56
Nippostrongylus brasiliensis 184, 189
  adherence mechanism 199
  effect on host immune system 186
  eosinophils in 214
  homocytotropic antibodies in 158, 172, 179
  IgE and 155, 185
  lung infestation 165, 168
  rejection 324
  tissue effects 317
nodular lymphoid hyperplasia 248, 256, 260

SUBJECT INDEX

nutrition, nematode infection and 198

oral immunization 357
  enteric infection and 60
  host resistance to *E.coli* following 62, 355
  response to 354
  tolerance following 70, 350
  with soluble proteins 49

parasites
  affecting immunoblast traffic 189
parasite enteropathy 315
parasite immunity 172
peripheral lymph nodes
  IgE in 166
pernicious anaemia 246
Peyer's patches
  antigen in 358
  antigen-sampling role 8
  antigen-sensitive precursors in 11
  compared with other lymphoid tissue 13
  graft rejection and 321
  IgA cells in 22, 47
  IgE in 163
  in alpha chain disease 279
  lymphocytes in 8, 347
  B lymphocytes in 9, 14, 47, 347
  T lymphocytes in 26, 34
  migration of cells from 25, 248
  origin of IgA cells in 37
  transfer of cells from 50
phagocytosis 43
platelets 300
polyclonal stimulation 151
prostaglandin E 188

protein calorie malnutrition 120, 232-234
protein-losing enteropathy 253
rheumatoid factor 355
schistosomiasis 213, 216
secretory component (SC) 77
  affinity with IgA 87, 132
  as membrane component 108
  binding 83, 108, 131
  combination with IgA and IgM 80, 83, 95, 132
  deficient synthesis 101
  distribution 94
  in Brunner's glands 95
  in Crohn's disease 101
  in Golgi zone 95
  in immunodeficiency 259
  location 89, 110
  lymphocyte homing and 42
  origin 92, 98
  synthesis 95
self-cure 221
serotonin 189
Shigella 124
soya antigen 344
spleen
  compared with Peyer's patches 13
  IgE cells in 166
  in coeliac disease 362
  Peyer's patch cells in 25
  repopulation with IgA cells 15
steroid
  in coeliac disease 341
sudden infant death syndrome 103, 258
Syphacia 185

Thiry-Vella loops 39, 44, 321

thoracic duct 35
thoracic duct lymph
  IgE in 167, 168
thoracic duct lymphocytes
  as origin of IgA cells 30
  response to cholera toxin 35, 36
tolerance
  after oral immunization 70
  IgA and 237
  induction 350
transmissible gastroenteritis virus 129, 319
Trichinella spiralis 184, 189, 191, 348
  effect on host immune system 186
  eosinophils and 206, 214
Trichostrongylus colubriformis 187, 189

ulcerative colitis 234, 283, 362
  atopy in 284
  C-reactive protein in 288, 298
  compared with Crohn's disease 297
  complement in 292, 299
  eosinophilia in 205
  glandular transport of immunoglobulin 101
  immunodeficiency and 251
  IgG cell response 87, 104
  mucosal appearance in 111

vasculitis 234
Vibrio cholerae 255
  antibodies 125
villi
  atrophy 190
  contraction 345
  flattening in immunodeficiency 250

villi, *continued*
  IgA cells in 27
  in coeliac disease 330
  in graft-versus-host
    reaction 311
  in intestinal allografts
    309
  in nematode infection
    198

Wegener's granulomatosis
  216
Wiskott-Aldrich syndrome
  252
worm expulsion
  eosinophils in 214
  lymphocytes in 196

  macrophages in 197
  mast cells and 172, 197
  mechanism 187, 196
  serotonin 189
  types 221
Wuchereria bancrofti
  214

HOME AT LAST

HOME AT LAST

Elsa K. Hummel

Copyright © 2012 Elsa K. Hummel
All rights reserved. No part of this book may be reproduced, scanned, or distributed in printed or electric form without permission.

ISBN-13:978-1470095703
ISBN-10:147009570X

All characters appearing in this work are fictitious. Any resemblance to real persons, living or dead, is purely coincidental.

This book is dedicated
With love
To my husband Franz,
My children:
Heidi, Hannelore, Martin, and Andy,
And my grandchildren:
Henry and Isabel,
Andrew, Lauren, and Dominic,
Gretchen and Davis,
Audrey, Andrew K., and Teddy

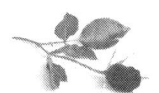

A house is made with walls and beams.
A home is made with love and dreams.
-Unknown-

Prologue

1936

On a crisp October morning, the freighter *Neue Welt* was plowing steadily from its port of Hamburg through the choppy waters of the English Channel, heading out into the open Atlantic. Laden with industrial machinery, chemicals and pharmaceuticals, it was beginning a lengthy voyage, across the equator, en route to its final destination, Buenos Aires, Argentina.

The few passengers who occupied the six cabins on board were crowded on the small rear deck. In the back corner, a young woman reclined on a chaise, covered by a blanket to ward off the early morning chill. Through half-closed eyes, she observed the small group gathered there. At the far end, two men were engaged in conversation, an elderly couple stared wordlessly out to sea, a man with his adolescent son, rapidly pacing back and forth, and a young couple, nervously watching their two children playing tag in the small space. Their carefree shrieks brought a smile to the young woman's face.

"At least they seem happy on this adventure," she thought, noting the somber looks of the adults. "Who are these strangers I am traveling with? What are their stories?"

She knew where she was going and why; she had no regrets. She had made her decision happily and willingly, placing her life in the hands of someone she loved. She stroked her shiny wedding band, relishing her new status. Still at this moment, although filled with excitement and anticipation, she could not suppress her anxiety and fear of the unknown. She shivered slightly as a gust of wind blew her long blonde hair into her face. She sat up straight, bravely banning the disquieting thoughts from her mind.

Her musings now wandered back to the past, where she had come from, who she had been until this day. With profound longing she pictured the family she had left behind. In her mind's eye she could see them all back in Hamburg: her beautiful sister, consumed by her music and dreams of a career, her gentle mother, devoted to her family and the love of her rose garden, and old Johann, who had been part of the family for as long as she could remember. But most of all, her beloved father, her Papa, so strong and caring, who, in her estimation seemed omnipotent. Just thinking of him brought a smile and eased her mind. What a perfect provider he was, always taking care of his family, his business, his employees, and especially of her. It was his approval and blessing that meant the most to her, as she was now embarking on the greatest adventure of her young life. Thinking of her family now, she could not dismiss feelings of loneliness and melancholy, but her deep love for them lifted her spirits as she sat, now all alone on the rocking ship, dreaming, yearning, and remembering how it had all begun....

PART ONE

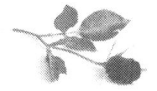

Beginnings

ONE

Hamburg, Germany

1936

When Wilhelm thought about it, years later, he sharply realized, that this was the summer when a number of events occurred, that severely impacted his life, and that of his family, in ways he could not even imagine. Even though these events were imminent, on this beautiful, warm June afternoon, Wilhelm was totally and blissfully unaware of them.

Sitting in his chauffeur-driven black Daimler, Wilhelm seemed quite relaxed, observing the sun's bright rays bathing the city of Hamburg in a soft golden light. Turrets and towers of ancient buildings glistened with magical beauty. A light breeze, coming off the North Sea, rustled the tender green leaves of the many Linden trees, for which the city had become famous. Along the many boulevards, the traffic was moving at a leisurely pace, as if nobody was in a hurry. The streetcars, clanking along their metal tracks, seemed to make friendly sounds, as they stopped to pick up many tourists and shoppers, laden with bags. Even the pedestrians, strolling along the wide sidewalks, seemed to be caught up in the beauty of the day, in no rush to get inside. A small group of young soldiers, on leave from the nearby barracks sauntered along, laughing, apparently without a care in the world.

As the Daimler crossed the bridge from the low-lying, bleak industrial area onto the hilly street leading to the city center, the chauffeur smiled with great pride. How Johann enjoyed driving this beautiful car for his beloved employer, Wilhelm Lindemann. Johann stole a backward glance at him, sprawled relaxed in the backseat, surrounded by his open briefcase and scattered papers. Smiling indulgently, he drove on, enjoying the slow pace of a peaceful afternoon.

Wilhelm did not see all the activities on the streets, nor did he notice the magic of the first really warm day of summer. Hard as he tried, he could not concentrate on the business at hand. He sighed, leaning back and closing his eyes; he seemed to be dozing. However, behind the peaceful exterior, many worrisome thoughts were crowding his brain. First and foremost, Wilhelm was extremely tired today. For the first time in years, he was actually happy to have a driver. So often he had felt like taking the wheel into his own hands, and going wherever the road would take him. But how could he retire old Johann, after so many years of faithful service to his father? After his father's death, it had seemed only natural to keep Johann, who loved the car and the entire Lindemann family like his own. He performed so many useful tasks around the house and garden, and drove Wilhelm to and from his office. Johann was so proud to be working at his age, and Wilhelm did not have the heart to suggest retirement.

Today, however, Wilhelm was very thankful to have Johann at the wheel. He could lay back his head and think about the many problems that were on his mind. Another surprise resignation of a most valuable employee, a large order that proved particularly difficult to finish on time, the well-deserved vacation his general manager, Kurt Walter, had had to cancel today. The loud whistle of a fire truck woke him from his reverie, just as Johann turned into the street where Wilhelm lived. As they drove down the quiet, tree-lined avenue to his home, his mood lightened. It always gave him a tremendous feeling of well-being, seeing his beautiful home and thinking of his loving family within.

As was his habit, Johann stopped in front of Burgstrasse #47, as Wilhelm eased out of the car, and with a friendly wave, turned and walked up to his front door. As Johann drove the car around the back to the garage, his thoughts lingered with Wilhelm. He loved his employer even more than he had loved the father, Wilhelm, Sr. whom he had served all his working days. He was very proud to be working for the Lindemanns. Especially Wilhelm, who, to him, was the epitome of everything that is honorable and worthwhile in a human being. He greatly respected Wilhelm's business acumen, reveled in his successes, adored his family, but more than that, he valued him as a fair and kind man, a true friend. He would do anything for him, of that he was certain.

After parking the Daimler in the garage, Johann mounted the stairs to his small apartment above. He had lived there happily with his wife, Trudi, until her death two years ago. Sadly they never had a family of their own, but having each other and the Lindemann children around, had been enough for them. Although Johann still missed her terribly, he somehow felt part of the family he served. Looking out of his window across the spacious garden to the main house, he felt secure and happy.

"Life is good," Johann said out loud, as he settled himself in his old easy chair to finally read today's newspaper.

Wilhelm opened the wrought iron gate, and walked up the steps to his front door. A broad smile crossed his face, as he heard from an open window above him the delightful voice of his oldest child, his daughter Margarete. Practicing again, he thought, always practicing, when, to him, she sounded perfect enough. With a final glance at the well-kept grounds around him, he turned the key and entered. The entry hall was cool and dim, and except for the sounds coming from upstairs, the house seemed deserted.

Setting down his briefcase and hanging up his coat, he looked through a stack of mail lying on the hall table. Above hung a huge mirror, framed with a gilded, antique Biedermeier frame, reflecting a crystal vase filled with fragrant pink roses. Wilhelm caught himself looking into the mirror, and it suddenly occurred to him that this mirror, as well as the roses, symbolized his whole life. The mirror represented his life's work, and the roses his family, his wife Marianne the gardener, his daughters Margarete and Lisbeth. Both girls were adults now, and yet he felt they all needed his care and protection, his watchful eye and his total devotion. His business, as well, required his time and attention.

Wilhelm's father had owned a small glass factory on the outskirts of Hamburg, but with Wilhelm's innovative ideas and tireless work, the business had grown into a sizable company. It had been his idea to add the manufacture of mirrors, and under his strong leadership, Lindemann Glass & Spiegelwerke (Glass and Mirrorworks) had become one of the best known factories of its kind in all of Germany. It continued to amaze him, how many stores, hotels, restaurants, theatres, and opera houses were continually in need of more mirrors. In time the production of crystal for elaborate chandeliers was added. With great pride Wilhelm could name all the famous locations where "his" chandeliers hung, including a few foreign countries. In some ways Wilhelm's success surprised him, as he was a very modest man. He was quick to give credit where it was due, and he truly felt that much of the firm's success stemmed from the excellent creativity and devotion of his young general manager, Kurt Walter. Kurt was largely responsible for the firm's expansion, as well as the export business. "I'm thankful every day that I hired that young man five years ago," Wilhelm thought, suddenly realizing that he was still standing in the front hall, staring at himself in the mirror. "I am really tired," he said quietly, as he went into the living room and settled himself in his favorite chair. Before he knew it, his eyes fell shut, and Wilhelm was sound asleep.

With a start, Wilhelm awoke. Suddenly there were

noises coming from all directions. Margarete was running down the steps, and almost at the same time, the front door slammed, as Lisbeth arrived home, calling: "Is anyone home?"

"Yes, yes, everybody is home," he heard Marianne's voice coming from the kitchen. "Even Papa is home early today. But he must be very tired; he's resting. Try not to be so loud, you two—"

But Wilhelm was awake and happy to see his family. "Hello girls." He smiled as both girls hugged and greeted him.

"You're home early today. Are you alright, Papa?" Lisbeth asked.

"Yes, everything is fine. I'm just a little tired today."

That seemed to satisfy the girls, as they left the room, chatting with each other. Wilhelm watched them disappearing down the hall toward the kitchen and he realized with a shock, that yes, they had become young women, and that they had grown up in a flash. Where has the time gone?

Wilhelm followed the girls out into the kitchen where Marianne was putting the final touches on their evening meal. Before long they were all sitting on the terrace overlooking Marianne's rose garden having a light supper of cold meats, bread, and cheese. They lingered over fresh strawberries with cream, chatting, and enjoying each other's company.

"So what have you been up to today?" Wilhelm asked the three women.

"Well, I had my voice lesson this morning, then I

stopped at the music store for more sheet music, then I practiced and practiced all day…" Margarete told them as they all nodded.

"And what about you, Lisbeth? Did you have a nice day too?"

"Yes I did, but I did not work all day like Margarete here." She smiled at her sister. "I played tennis this morning, then I went to the library, and after lunch I went over to visit my friend, Brigitte. Nothing as important as a recital coming up in my life," she teased, looking admiringly at her big sister.

Soon they were discussing Margarete's upcoming musical recital that she had been preparing for months. She had just finished her first year at the Conservatory, where she was studying voice. Wilhelm had to admit that Margarete had a beautiful soprano voice and he was very proud of her, but he didn't take her music seriously. He loved hearing about her great talent from her professors, and he was happy to indulge her. Yet, he never considered music as a career for her. For the time being, if she was happy studying and practicing for hours, he was willing to let her pursue her dream to sing at the opera one day. He thought of her singing only as a passing whim of youth, a dream that would surely fade away once she was married and had a family of her own. Yet, not realizing her passion, he could not refuse his daughter anything.

The recital was to take place in one week, and the excitement in the house was mounting. The invitations had been mailed weeks ago, Margarete's new gown had been delivered, the reception afterwards arranged for. Now that the recital was imminent, everyone was slightly apprehensive. Lisbeth, however, seemed carefree as ever. All she wanted was for the recital to be over so that she could enjoy the summer with her sister and her friends. Even now, she was teasing Margarete, saying her sister should take some time to have fun.

"I do take time for fun," Margarete protested. "Just last night Peter and I went to the movies, and last weekend we went dancing. Did you forget that?"

"Yes, I know. Once in a while you and Peter go out and have fun, but you must admit that for the last two months you have done nothing but rehearse and work on your recital. I will be very glad when it is behind you! Then maybe we can spend some time together, go swimming, or shopping, or to the movies, or whatever!"

Margarete laughed with her sweet silver voice, promising that soon, very soon, she would be free to enjoy the summer together.

"I have an idea for you girls," Wilhelm said, looking excitedly at his daughters. "After the recital, why don't you two take a few days and go to the seashore in Cuxhaven. It would do Margarete good to get away after all the stress, and surely you, Lisbeth would love it too. Remember the times we spent at the Strandhotel when you were young, what fun you had building sandcastles and running along the surf?"

"What a great idea, Papa, but why don't you and Mutti come and have a little vacation too?" Margarete said.

"It sounds wonderful, but I really cannot get away right now, there is too much going on at the office. But what about you?" He turned to his wife, "Why don't you go with the girls?"

"Oh no, I have things to do here too. And besides, I think the girls would have a better time without their Mutti tagging along," Marianne commented. "Wilhelm, that is such a good idea. What do you girls think?"

Lisbeth and Margarete looked at each other, grinning happily, and answered almost simultaneously: "It's a wonderful idea!"

"After the recital is over, we'll pack our bags and take off for the shore! What a perfect get-away and a good place for Margarete to unwind," Lisbeth added.

Both girls smiled happily.

"Well, it's settled then, I'll arrange everything for your little vacation. Just don't worry about a thing!"

"Of course, Papa, you always take care of everything for us! Thank you so much! I know we will enjoy the shore, and especially the Strandhotel! Thank you Papa, you always know what to do!"

Wilhelm loved listening to his girls banter back and forth. He smiled contentedly. For the moment all his problems were forgotten and he could relax.

"Marianne, what about your day? Anything exciting happen around here today?" He asked his wife.

"Nothing too exciting, but for me it was a perfect day!" Marianne answered as she leaned back in her chair. It had been the kind of day she truly enjoyed and did not come along too often. She had no obligations today, and was able to spend many hours in her beloved rose garden. There was always something to do, and tending her flowers was one of her favorite pastimes. There were a number of jobs she let

Johann attend to, but her roses were her domain. She loved the many varieties of roses, but working in her garden gave her time for quiet thoughts and contemplation. Spending time with her roses gave her a special peace of mind.

"My roses are like my children, I care for them, I love them, I protect them from harm, and in return they love me by giving their beauty, their fragrance, their trust, giving me the best they can be. How lucky I am to have my Wilhelm and my own two special roses with me here tonight in my garden," she said.

In Marianne's mind, her life was perfect. It had never occurred to her that life might not always continue in the peaceful way she had experienced so far. First her father, then her husband had always taken care of everything for her, and she trusted it would always be so. Her world consisted of her husband, her two beautiful daughters and her many friends. She worked hard to make their lives happy. She loved Wilhelm for creating this sheltered and comfortable life. She just knew that whatever the future would bring, Wilhelm would take care of everything.

After a while the girls rose to take a bike ride in the neighborhood. Wilhelm too, was caught up in his own reverie. He watched them disappear around the corner of the house and was filled with an aching melancholy. How much joy they had brought into his life and how quickly they had grown up! They were different from one another, yet quite similar. They were very close, really best friends. Margarete was almost 21 now, serious and determined, tall and slender with her large blue-grey eyes and light brown hair. At the Hamburg Music Conservatory she had met a young man, Peter von Orb, equally serious and sensible, who had his own dream of becoming a conductor. They were a lovely couple, and Wilhelm hoped they would someday be married. "Some day, but not just yet," he prayed.

Then there was Lisbeth. At 19, she had no plans, no goals for the future. She was very happy to have graduated from *Realschule* (high school) last month, and at her parents' suggestion had applied at the Art Institute to study Interior Design. Until the new term began in January, Lisbeth planned very little, just enjoying life with her friends, of whom there were many. Her greatest talent seemed to be enjoying every moment of her life. Lisbeth, a petite blue-eyed blonde, with a light heart and a quick smile, enchanted everyone she met.

That smile reminded Wilhelm of his own sister, Anni, whom he had not seen in ten years. Yes, Anni had been just like Lisbeth as she was growing up. Full of life and enthusiasm, Anni had married her high school sweetheart against the initial wishes of her parents. But with charm and grace she had persuaded her parents that Josef Bauer was her one and only love, and what was the use of waiting? After a simple family wedding, Anni and Josef had carved out a new life for themselves. They were living happily in New Jersey in the U.S.A. where Josef now owned and operated a garden center and greenhouse. How different Anni's life would have been staying here and marrying someone of her parents' choice! Wilhelm had to admit that he always admired, almost envied, her courage and determination. Anni knew what she wanted in life and was willing to make any sacrifice to achieve her happiness. Going off to a new country and a new life was just the kind of challenge that Anni thrived on. She looked upon life as a great adventure to be enjoyed.

Her greatest sacrifice for love, of course, had been leaving her family behind. When she returned to visit ten years ago, both parents had died. Anni had never made another visit. She maintained the connection to her brother, writing only sporadically, but with great love for him and his family.

In many ways, Wilhelm's little Lisbeth reminded him of Anni, full of enthusiasm and *joie de vivre*, loving but headstrong, sweet yet stubborn. Her smile melted his heart, and he could not refuse her anything.

The first item on Wilhelm's agenda the next morning was a meeting with Kurt. They needed to discuss the sudden resignation of Adam Heller, his chief designer.

"Why is he resigning? What is wrong? What did he tell you?" Wilhelm asked without preamble. "Is he leaving to work for someone else? What is going on here?" he asked impatiently.

"I wish it were that simple." Kurt replied. "Then at least we could negotiate. No, no, it is beyond our control, Wilhelm. Adam and his family are leaving the country."

"Leaving the country?" Wilhelm asked incredulously.

"Have you forgotten Max Vogelsang, our plant manager, who left us six months ago? He cited health reasons, but I heard from his co-workers later, that he too, has left Germany. They are not sure where he went, but the fact is that he left the country too," Kurt added simply.

Wilhelm was stunned. Yes, he had heard some of his business and banker friends speak of sudden departures of valuable employees and clients, but Wilhelm had considered them isolated cases. The truth was that more and more people no longer felt comfortable in Germany's political climate since the advent of the new Chancellor in 1933. What was Wilhelm to do? Today he lost Adam, perhaps next week or next month he may lose six more.

Resolutely he spoke to Kurt. "We must do something! Let me speak with Adam. Perhaps I can persuade him to stay! We can't lose our best people!"

"We will do the best we can with what we have," Kurt replied as he left to find Adam in his office.

A few minutes later, a dark-haired young man wearing glasses entered Wilhelm's office. He stood uncomfortably, not knowing what to say. Wilhelm invited him to sit and dove right into the matter.

"Adam, Adam, how can you think of leaving us? You are the best designer, the very best, and we need you! Please reconsider and stay with us. I'll do whatever I can to help you!"

Sadly, Adam looked up, speaking with difficulty. "It is done, the decision is made. My father may be overly pessimistic, but he feels that we are no longer safe here in Germany. All the documents are ready, our possessions have been sold or packed, our passage booked. Next week we are leaving for Shanghai, China. My mother cries every day. I hate leaving this country, it is my home, it is what I know. Don't you think I would rather stay, do the job I love here, and build a life? Our family is not alone, doing this. Perhaps we are fools, but for now, we must leave. Jewish people are no longer welcome here. Things are not too bad yet, and we have an opportunity to leave. I'm so sorry, Mr. Lindemann, so sorry."

With tears running down both men's faces, they embraced for a final farewell.

Alone again in his office, Wilhelm finally understood. Tiredly, he closed his eyes, remembering Adam and his pain. I wish him well, but what could I have done for him? Wilhelm did not have an answer. All he knew now was that things were changing and there was nothing, nothing he could do about it.

Finally Wilhelm stood and walked to the window. Everything was normal, the traffic was moving, a cool breeze gently rustled the leaves, the red umbrellas at the corner café glistened brightly in the sunshine. A perfect summer day, a blue sky, yet with a feeling of foreboding, Wilhelm watched dark clouds forming on the horizon.

TWO

Cuxhaven, Germany

One week later

The morning sun glowed warmly, bathing everything in its radiant light: the long sandy beach bordering the North Sea, the boat dock in the distance, as well as the wide veranda surrounding the old traditional Strandhotel by the shore. The impressive three-story building sat on a narrow tongue of land as a seagull might perch on a post. Several guests were enjoying the peaceful scene, relaxing with a good book or a cool drink. Near the railing, two young women reclined on their chaises, eyes closed, but not asleep. Each was daydreaming fanciful thoughts of her own as music played softly in the background and the gulls shrieked with abandon as they dipped into the sea.

"Isn't it beautiful here? I wish I could stay forever," sighed the younger one with the blonde hair, to no one in particular.

"Lisbeth, you know we can't. You're right; these last few days have been heavenly, just perfect. But I have to get back," her sister replied.

"Oh, Margarete, you are always the practical one! But at least we still have one more full day. Let's go to the beach early and make the most of it."

"Yes, let's! One more day of fun! But I'm still anxious to get home. Maybe there's a letter or a call about an audition. I know it's wishful thinking, but I can always hope."

Lisbeth sat up straight and looked at her sister. "Know what I think? I'm sure you will get an audition to sing in the Opera Chorus. You know why? Because your recital was fabulous, and unless that talent agent was deaf, he knows that you're the best. I will never forget how beautifully you sang that night and how everybody applauded. You'll get it, you'll see!" Lisbeth said with conviction. And jumping up impulsively, she added, "Now, Margarete, let's go for a swim,"

"Go ahead," Margarete said. "I'll come in a few minutes."

As she lay there in the sun, memories of her recent recital came back to her mind: The auditorium was filled with her conservatory classmates, professors, family, friends and music lovers waiting with keen anticipation. She herself was quite nervous all day. In fact, while getting dressed, she suddenly felt a great panic, convinced that no sound could escape her mouth. However, standing backstage and hearing the reassuring voice of her coach and mentor introducing her, a wonderful calm settled over her. On cue, she stepped on stage to grand welcoming applause.

With the familiar sounds of the accompanying piano, she sang with strength and confidence. She had selected the many pieces to demonstrate her full vocal range, control and sensitivity. She ended the recital with the breathtakingly beautiful aria *Un bel di vedremo* by Puccini. The audience was ecstatic, applauding her with a standing ovation and begging for more. Lastly, she rewarded the appreciative audience with an encore, Franz Schubert's *Liebestraum*. Her head was spinning with excitement as well as relief. After many bows, she was able to calm herself enough to thank her coach, her parents and everyone else who had made the performance possible.

Marianne and Wilhelm Lindemann glowed with joy and parental pride. Lisbeth was totally awed. Margarete realized that her sister looked at her with new appreciation for her gift and was really happy for her success. Old Johann, the family gardener and chauffeur, was moved beyond words, wiping a tear off the corner of his eye. Peter, her boyfriend, was also beaming with happiness and pride. Ordinarily a quiet young man, he could hardly contain himself, jumping, whistling, applauding and calling out bravos with unbridled enthusiasm.

She recalled the special celebration dinner at the Hotel Krone with all her family and close friends assembled. She was toasted with champagne. Her excitement was complete at the news that a Mr. Kühnle, a talent scout for the Hamburg Opera, had been spotted in the audience. Perhaps there was a chance for an audition, maybe even an opportunity to perform in the chorus of the fall season productions.

Still basking in her triumph, she remembered Peter's excitement and pride, and smiled again. When he kissed her good night, looking deeply into her eyes, he told her again and again, "You are on your way. I just know it. You will achieve all you have worked for. You will be famous one day. I love you. I love you! You are simply fantastic."

Margarete smiled contentedly as she let the sun warm her.

Lisbeth ran lightly over the hot sand and quickly jumped in. She was slightly taken aback with the shock of the cold North Sea water. But being a strong swimmer, she moved with swift strokes and was soon far from shore. I'll swim out as far as I can, she thought, and take a good look at the shore from far away.

A sailboat in the distance became her goal as she continued with confidence. She had almost reached the boat when suddenly she felt a piercing pain in her leg, followed by a cold numbness. Paralyzed with fear and helplessness, she yelled out in panic. "Help, Margarete, help me!" she screamed. But Margarete was still dozing far away on shore.

Thrashing about in the cold water, she began to panic. The pain in her leg intensified, and she gasped for air as she came to the surface after doubling up in agony.

The next thing Lisbeth knew, she was lying on the deck of the sailboat. Two men were hovering over her. A blanket covered her, but she was still shivering. Her teeth chattering violently, she grasped the blanket with stiff, blue fingers. In shock and totally disoriented, she stared into the faces of the strange men.

She struggled to sit up, but the men urged her to rest. The stocky blond man handed her a glass of water which she drank slowly. With a shock, Lisbeth realized how close she must have come to disaster. All she remembered was the cramp in her leg and her cry for help. Had she been rescued by these men in the boat?

"There you are, safe and sound. Just rest. Are you feeling better now?" he asked. "What were you doing, swimming out so far? Did you think you were a mermaid? How lucky that we were close enough to help you, and especially that my friend Lorenzo was with me! He jumped right into the water and pulled you out."

With a charming smile, the dark-haired man, Lorenzo, interjected in halting German, "Señorita need help. I fetch Señorita. My pleasure." With that he placed a towel around her shoulder.

A cold shiver ran over Lisbeth again, suddenly understanding what had happened. How foolish she had been, swimming beyond the safety of the shore! "You saved my life. Thank you, thank you." she sputtered. The towel had slipped off her shoulders, and Lorenzo replaced it, putting his arms around her and holding her trembling and miserable form.

The blond man was back at the helm, steering toward a pier at the end of the swimming beach. Margarete, now fully awake and highly alarmed, had been waiting and looking for her sister. Finally she saw Lisbeth on the pier, escorted by two men, and she knew that something terrible had just happened.

"Your sister will be fine," one of the men told Margarete, as she arrived, panting, on the pier. "We were happy to help her. She is a very lucky young lady. By the way, I am Hans Peter, and this is my new friend Lorenzo."

Margarete nodded, too stunned to speak. Hans Peter continued in a calm voice, telling her what had taken place out on the water. "Oh, what great luck you were nearby! How can I thank you both?" she said.

Lisbeth was still too shaken and scared to speak. "Why don't you take the two young ladies home, Lorenzo?" Hans Peter suggested. "I'll take care of the boat." Wordlessly, everyone seemed to agree.

Slowly the three started on their way back to the Strandhotel, each lost in their own thoughts. What had begun as a lovely summer day could have ended in the most tragic way. Fate had intervened and brought her a savior, Lisbeth thought. "I can't believe what happened today! How lucky I am to be alive." She stole an admiring glance at the good-looking young man walking beside her. As the shock of the near tragedy was beginning to wear off, she couldn't help but wonder how or why this new person had come into her life and how he might affect her future. She would be forever beholden to him.

Margarete's thoughts were of concern for their parents, and how she could best relay the eventful afternoon to them. Grateful for the fortuitous outcome, she silently offered a prayer. She would find the right words later.

Lorenzo was smiling happily to himself. What had prompted him to jump into the cold waves of the sea to rescue this young woman? Without thinking, he had just known what he had to do. All his life, he had been swimming in the turbulent Paraná River, but never thought he would have to save a life. Almost surprised at the successful outcome of his impulsive action, he too offered a prayer of thanks. He smiled broadly as he continued to steal glances at the beautiful, though somewhat bedraggled, Lisbeth walking beside him. What a way to meet two lovely young women in a foreign country!

Arriving at the hotel entrance, Margarete once again began thanking Lorenzo for what he had done for her sister. With tears in her eyes she shook his hand, asking him for his full name and address. Surely her parents, too, would want to thank him for his heroic rescue.

"My pleasure, madam, my pleasure," he repeated, and added, "What can I do now to help you? Anything I will do."

Before Margarete could answer, Lisbeth impulsively hugged Lorenzo and amid great wrenching sobs, tried to thank him again. Helplessly Lorenzo smiled and shrugged his shoulders, looking at Margarete over Lisbeth's bedraggled head.

"I just want to go home." Lisbeth raised her head and repeated, "I just want to go home. I don't want to stay here one minute longer!"

Margarete understood. "All right, Lisbeth, we don't have to stay here until tomorrow. We can take the afternoon train back to Hamburg. Let's go in and get our things together and leave today."

Turning to Lorenzo once again, she stated firmly, "Lorenzo, would you be so kind as to come with us. Let's go home together. I know our parents want to meet the man who saved their daughter's life."

"If you wish, Madame, I am happy to go with you.

Whatever I can do to help will be my pleasure."

Again he smiled, his heart beating with joy, hoping that the sisters could not read his mind and see how excited and happy he was to remain in their company a while longer.

The same day, Wilhelm sat behind his desk in his overheated office. The windows were open, but there was no breeze there. The small overhead Casablanca fan whirled slowly, moving heavy, hot air, but not really cooling the room. He was looking over some papers, but his mind was not on the contracts before him. Leaning back in his chair, he closed his eyes and sighed deeply. Oh this heat! His daughters had been right, saying he should take some time off, and spend a few days at the shore. *I used to enjoy that. Actually that is where the girls are right at this moment,* he thought to himself. But there was just too much work to do here. He was thankful the business was doing well and running relatively smoothly, although there were daily problems to contend with. Fortunately, Kurt had been able to replace his plant manager, Max, and had also hired two new bookkeepers to replace Jakob and Alex Liebherr, who were leaving in ten days.

Today, Wilhelm was dealing with yet another resignation. The head of the shipping department, Justin Glasberg had had a serious talk with Wilhelm a few days ago. Much as he loved his work, and the city where he had spent all of his life, he was looking for a way to move his family out of the country as soon as possible.

"If this trend continues, I'll have to close my business,"

Wilhelm thought sadly. He valued his employees and missed them terribly already. Again, he thought fondly of Kurt, his trusted right hand man. Wilhelm knew that without Kurt he would be in great trouble. More and more he had allowed Kurt to take greater responsibility, and he never made a business decision without consulting him.

Wilhelm stretched and tried to concentrate on his paperwork once again, but it seemed impossible today. He was just too tired, and his thoughts seemed to fly in all directions. He just could not stop worrying about everything today. With a deep frown creasing his forehead, he remembered the conversation he had had with his doctor and friend just a few weeks ago. Fred Ranf had warned him what stress and worry were doing to his health. His heart had been beating irregularly for some time, and he suffered from occasional spells of weakness and dizziness. Fred had prescribed some little pills to help him when these episodes occurred. But he had ignored Fred's advice to slow down, to spend less time at the office, and more time walking in Marianne's rose garden. How could he do such a thing without alarming his family? They were all busy and happy in their own worlds and he aimed to keep it that way.

"If I had a son, I would be happy to turn things over to him," he thought. "As it is now, my place is here." Providing a good life for his family was uppermost on Wilhelm's mind. "What do my three girls know about my business?" Sure, they had visited the factory; he wanted them to know where he spent his days. As the girls were growing up, he had shown them the process of glass and mirror manufacturing, but they had other interests, and had no real concept of what was going on in the business world.

Two years ago, when his firm had received an extraordinary order to create three enormous chandeliers for the newly refurbished opera house in Buenos Aires, his daughters, as well as Marianne, had shown rare interest and enthusiasm to see the finished product. Johann had driven them down to the factory to see the magnificent chandeliers before they were crated and shipped across the ocean. But since then, they were content to pursue their own interests which was as it should be. Smiling, he remembered Margarete's recent recital and was immensely proud of her success. He had not realized or appreciated Margarete's great talent before the recital. He looked at her with totally new eyes today. There was a young woman with goals, along with determination, and willingness to work diligently to achieve her dream.

His Lisbeth, however, was a different matter. She had no idea what her goals might be, and he suspected that her decision to study Interior Design, was most likely made only to please him. Lisbeth was lively and energetic, and her father could only hope that she would find interest and enjoyment in her studies. He sensed a restlessness, a certain yearning in her, yet could not define exactly what it was. One thing was certain; she wanted a different, more exciting life than her sister, but she had no real plan for her future, as Margarete had.

At the moment, Wilhelm was happy to know that his girls were enjoying a few days at the shore. He hoped they would relax and have some fun. Margarete, especially, deserved that.

The shrill sound of the telephone roused Wilhelm from his musings. With ashen face and trembling hands, he listened as his wife delivered the news to him. Grabbing his jacket, he raced out of his office, almost colliding with Kurt, who was about to knock on Wilhelm's door.

"Get Johann," he croaked to his secretary. "I must go home immediately, there is an emergency. Quick! Quick!"

Kurt watched him running down the corridor as if the devil was chasing him.

"Wait, I'm coming with you," Kurt yelled after him, hoping that nothing had happened to Margarete. His long strides, overtaking Wilhelm, he opened the door, just as Johann drove the Daimler through the factory gate.

Arriving at home, Wilhelm and Kurt found the usually calm household in a state of excitement. Hearing the story of Lisbeth's almost tragedy and her rescue, a shocked Marianne had panicked and called her husband. Only he would know what to say and do.

As Margarete related the story for the second time, the whole episode began to take on glamorous proportions. By the time Wilhelm heard the story, Marianne had calmed down somewhat. Lisbeth was resting upstairs, and Wilhelm relaxed visibly, as everyone spoke at the same time. Kurt sat quietly, taking in every word, as he looked at Margarete with adoring eyes.

"But where is this Lorenzo? Where is our hero?" Wilhelm wanted to know. He looked around and saw a tall, dark-haired young man leaning against the French door leading to the terrace. With tears in his eyes, Wilhelm extended his hands, pulling him into a bear hug, thanking him over and over, from the bottom of his heart. As Marianne brought cool drinks and invited everyone to sit on the terrace, Kurt, seeing that everything was safe and under control, quietly left the house. Slowly he walked to the corner, where he hoped to catch a taxi home. Wilhelm and the women were too taken with the handsome stranger; there was no room for him at this time.

Lorenzo was feeling uneasy now. He intended to leave as soon as he had delivered the two sisters to their home, but Marianne insisted he stay. It was not difficult to persuade him, as he hoped to get another glimpse of Lisbeth. What a beautiful girl she was, even when she lay pale and shivering on Hans Peter's boat. How lucky for him to have been at the right place at the right time! Her family's overwhelming gratitude made him feel welcome in their midst and gave him a feeling of warmth and inclusion.

Soon, Lisbeth, rested and joyful again, came bouncing down the stairs and joined everyone on the terrace. She was greeted with cheers, hugs and kisses. They were all grateful for her lively presence. Margarete, too, was refreshed and her worried look gone.

Now Wilhelm wanted to know everything about Lorenzo, who formally introduced himself. "I am Lorenzo Alberto Moncrief, and I come from Argentina," he said as he bowed to Wilhelm. His distinct accent and demeanor cast a mysterious spell on his listeners, particularly on Lisbeth.

"And what brings you here into these northern waters?" Wilhelm inquired. Haltingly, with a charming smile, he began to tell the Lindemanns about himself. He had been raised on an *estancia* (estate) named *Bien Cielo*, near Buenos Aires, where his father and his father before him, raised cattle. About 20 years ago his father began raising race horses which were now their main product. Lorenzo was an only child, his brother having died in infancy. Along with his parents he lived on over 800 hectares approximately 60 kilometers from Buenos Aires. His grandmother, Nonna, lived on her own property nearby.

"You ask what brings me to your northern waters," Lorenzo continued in his careful if limited German. "My father is very good and generous man. After I finish my studies at university he give me this wonderful present—a trip to see something of the world before I settle down and help him with race-horse business. So here I am."

"And we are all glad that you are," Wilhelm exclaimed. And as his heart swelled with love and gratitude, he embraced Lisbeth again.

"And who is Hans Peter?" Margarete wanted to know. "He was part of the rescue too."

"I live at his mother's guest house, and he invites me go sailing with him sometimes. I'm glad we went sailing today!" Lorenzo replied.

He continued telling them about his travels, how he had crossed the ocean and visited Spain first. In the last few months he had visited Italy and France, and had now spent several weeks in Germany by special request of his grandmother. Later he would travel to England and return from there to Argentina at the end of the summer.

"Why did your grandmother want you to visit Germany

in particular?" Marianne asked eagerly.

"My Nonna is very special to me," Lorenzo replied. "She was born in Argentina but descended from German immigrants who settled the area in the 1860s. We do not know where her ancestors came from, but Nonna is still very proud her heritage. I wanted to see the country and tell her something about the land and people."

"Does your Nonna still speak German?" Marianne wanted to know. She was fascinated by the story.

"Yes, she can still speak a little. She grew up with the language. She even taught me a few words," he said with a wink at Marianne. "Whenever I stayed overnight at Nonna's, she always said, *"Schlaf' wohl, mein Schatz."* (Sleep well, my darling.)

"Wunderbar!" everyone replied, and Marianne smiled, wondering just where his ancestors had come from.

"Today everything is Spanish, and Nonna speaks only Spanish now," he continued. "But she still very proud of her roots. She will enjoy hearing all about my travels and meeting your family."

Despite his limited German, Lorenzo continued a lively conversation. Wilhelm was more animated than ever. The near tragedy was almost forgotten, and the group spent a happy and memorable evening together.

Lisbeth was unusually quiet, but her glowing eyes and radiant smile told everyone that she had eyes only for Lorenzo, her hero, her knight in shining armor.

Margarete and Marianne went into the kitchen to prepare an evening snack together while Lisbeth sat, mesmerized by Lorenzo's voice. The conversation between the two men embraced one topic after another as they seemed to have known each other forever.

Lorenzo finally said good night with the promise to return again soon. Shaking Lisbeth's hand, he told her, "Promise me to be careful. Do not swim so far from shore again."

"I promise. I'll be more careful," Lisbeth smiled back.

"I hope to see you again soon. I will come and check you are all right," Lorenzo promised, and Lisbeth, filled with new and strange emotions, could not utter another word. But her happy, beaming face did not escape notice by anyone.

That evening, as his daughters quietly retired to their rooms, Wilhelm reflected again on the day's events. How close had his family come to disaster today? Should he have let the girls go by themselves? Who was this young man who saved his daughter? Should he have taken time from his busy schedule to vacation with them as even his doctor had suggested a while ago? Wilhelm was more concerned then he cared to show Marianne.

Still, with a thankful heart, he smiled. What could have been a tragic day, turned into a day with a happy ending after all! Closing his eyes, he embraced his sleeping wife and thanked God.

THREE

Tired as Wilhelm was, he could not fall asleep. His thoughts were churning as the day's events replayed in his mind. Lisbeth's fascination with Lorenzo had not escaped his notice, and he smiled tenderly. "Worse things than falling in love could happen," he thought, remembering his own youth. He had fallen in love with Marianne at first sight. And what a wonderful marriage they had had! He turned to his wife who was sleeping peacefully beside him and touched her gently.

Still sleep eluded him. Not wanting to disturb her with his restless tossing, he decided to get up. Suddenly he felt very strange. A painful pressure in his chest almost immobilized him. Fierce pain traveled down his left arm. With a trembling voice he cried out for help, falling back down on the bed and waking a fearful Marianne.

"Margarete, Lisbeth, quick, call Dr. Ranf. Something is terribly wrong with Papa. Call quick!" Marianne cried in anguish as she cradled Wilhelm in her arms.

"Wilhelm is a very lucky man," Dr. Ranf explained. "A minor heart attack, for certain. But it could have been a major one."

The family had assembled in Wilhelm's hospital room while the doctor gave his prognosis as well as his instructions. Returning to the office was out of the question for the time being, and stress of any kind was to be avoided. However, with rest and moderation of activities Wilhelm would recover, the doctor reassured them.

With a great sigh of relief everyone, especially the patient, relaxed. How close they had come to losing their beloved Papa. But Marianne was chiding herself, "How could I not have known? All his worries and restless nights—why didn't I try to slow him down?"

The news of his bad heart had been a total shock to them all. Much as Wilhelm had tried to shield and protect his family from any unpleasantness, this time he had no control of the situation. Thankful to be alive, he promised himself to make some changes. Yesterday he could have lost his little Lisbeth; today he could have lost his own life.

"How life can change in an instant," he mused. "Enjoy every moment as long as you can," he promised himself as he drifted off to sleep.

When Wilhelm woke, he was happy to see his family. "Hello, Liesl; hello Gretl," he smiled as both girls hugged and greeted him.

"Papa, we are not little girls anymore. Why do you call us those silly baby names?" Lisbeth pouted. But bursting into another brilliant smile, she hugged her father again.

"Yes," Wilhelm thought, "they have grown up, but in my heart they will always remain my little darlings."

Reluctantly he had begun calling them by their full names as they had become teenagers, but inside he still thought of them by their endearing nicknames. As he looked at them, he realized with a shock that, yes, they had become young women. "I must cherish the time I have with them. Before long they will leave our nest; but not just yet. For now they're still ours."

FOUR

The next few weeks brought a different routine to the Lindemann household. Marianne devoted her total time to taking care of her husband. She made sure he spent his time resting on the terrace, napping, taking medications precisely on time, and following a special diet. She limited visits, made sure he was only surrounded by happy faces, discussing only good news.

However, there was one person whose visits she could not curtail. At least three times a week Kurt Walter would arrive at the house with a bulging briefcase to report the activity at the factory. Hard as she tried to keep Wilhelm from working, as she called it, he was adamant. He and Kurt would spend several hours together going over business matters. Wilhelm felt very confident that things were running smoothly.

"We just received a repeat order from Huber's for 1,000 dresser mirrors. It came just in time too, as we are finishing another large order. Things are going well. We are busy,"

Kurt relayed to Wilhelm. "And fortunately we have not lost any more employees in the last few weeks, so everything will continue smoothly."

Wilhelm immediately recalled a conversation they had had a few weeks earlier. They had been discussing the sudden resignation of Adam Heller, his chief designer. Wilhelm had been stunned. Since then, he realized anew that many more Jewish people were fleeing Germany every day. What was happening to his country? What other changes and upheavals were yet to come?

Kurt looked forward to his almost daily visits with his boss. For him, Wilhelm's heart attack had an unexpected plus. With each trip to the house, he hoped to catch a glimpse of Margarete. But he seldom did. He had sat all alone at the back of the theater at her recital. He didn't want the Lindemanns to see him, but he had wanted to hear Margarete sing and quietly share in her special evening. Her soaring voice and beautiful songs had touched him to the core and filled his heart with longing. He had very special feelings for her, but she was his employer's daughter, and he felt awkward about that. Besides, she had her young man, Peter, of whom Wilhelm spoke warmly. Kurt's heart was bursting with love and pride for her. He was happy for her success and yet sad for himself. He had stolen out of the theater, dreaming he could openly give her his love as well as his admiration. But for now, this secret would remain locked quietly in his heart.

Since her recital he had seen her only a few times. She always greeted him with detached courtesy and was usually on her way out, or nowhere near. Once Kurt saw her leaving the house with her friend Peter from the conservatory. "Margarete doesn't even know I exist," he thought sadly. "To her I'm only her father's employee." But he still held out hope of seeing her. For now he had to be content with that.

Lorenzo, too, had become a regular and welcome guest in the house. In fact, he was one of the few visitors Marianne allowed to spend time with her husband. Lorenzo's bright smile, his charm and easy-going nature seemed to have a therapeutic effect on Wilhelm, and he looked forward to each visit.

Lorenzo had his own reasons why he came so often—he could not wait to see the beautiful Lisbeth again. During the last weeks they had met many times, slowly and shyly becoming acquainted. One afternoon he found Lisbeth reading in the gazebo. Marianne was making lemonade for everyone, and he offered to take two glasses to join her. Lisbeth was overjoyed to see him.

"Here, sit on the swing with me. It's so nice and relaxing out here." And Lorenzo was only too happy to oblige. They spent the whole afternoon out there, talking about themselves. Before long Lorenzo's visits with Wilhelm became shorter and shorter as he and Lisbeth spent more time together. Soon they spent most of their days together, playing tennis, going sailing with Hans Peter, going to the movies, cycling and meeting Lisbeth's friends. Lorenzo was quickly accepted by them as he became a well-liked, fun-loving member of their group.

Wilhelm and Marianne both noticed Lisbeth's involvement with Lorenzo, and although Marianne was somewhat concerned, Wilhelm squashed her anxieties.

"They are young and happy," he said indulgently. "Of course she adores him. He saved her life. Don't forget, he is also different from anyone she has ever known. He is charming and handsome. Why shouldn't she enjoy his company?"

Marianne shook her head, but she did not want to alarm Wilhelm with her disturbing thoughts.

Wilhelm closed his eyes and thought about his daughters. He wanted them to be happy. "Here I am, being treated like an invalid. How I wish I had taken more time to do the things I like." Still, he was grateful for Marianne's tender care and his loving family around him.

Lisbeth was happy. As she was dressing for a date with Lorenzo and her friends, she was chattering non-stop with Margarete. Every other word was Lorenzo. Margarete smiled indulgently as Lisbeth continued with her stories.

"Are you in love with him?" Margarete teased.

"Ah, ah, I don't know," Lisbeth stammered, blushing a deep pink. But the truth was that being with Lorenzo made her happier than she had ever been. She also felt a very special bond with him as she truly knew that she owed her life to him. She knew that she loved being with him, listening to his stories of his life in Argentina, his travels and adventures. His charm, his good looks, his captivating voice, his obvious admiration for her filled her heart with joy. She knew that she had fallen deeply and hopelessly in love with him. She was totally confused and afraid, and exhilarated in his presence.

Lorenzo, too, had felt a strong attraction to her from the moment he had pulled her miserable, shaking body out of the water. She was beautiful; she was lively and energetic; she adored him; and he loved spending every moment with her. But he knew his time with her here in Germany would be coming to an end soon. He knew he did not want to leave her, but he did not know what to do. For the time being he would treasure every moment he had with her.

For Lisbeth, everything took on a new dimension. The walks in the park, swimming and sailing, movies and dancing were twice the fun. Lorenzo also loved having a beautiful woman on his arm and enjoyed the attention and admiring glances that often followed her. His heart skipped a beat each time her luminous blue eyes looked at him with admiration and what he hoped—love. Never before had he known a girl as lovely, as different, or as challenging as Lisbeth. Lorenzo did not realize that Lisbeth, too, dreaded the thought of his approaching departure.

After several weeks of excellent care and recuperation, Dr. Ranf permitted Wilhelm to return to his office for a few hours a day. Marianne had hoped to have him at home much longer, but Wilhelm felt wonderful and was ready to resume a normal life. Johann had kept the car polished, and was looking forward to driving Wilhelm around town again. Kurt and the employees had planned a small "Welcome Back" celebration for Wilhelm, and he was touched beyond words. Never had he known how much he was loved and respected. He was ecstatic to be back. His recovery period had given him time to reflect and appreciate every small thing in life. He had promised himself to worry less and try to accept and handle things as they came. Returning to work was a great milestone for him. How fortunate he had been to recover completely, his daughter had been spared, his older daughter had achieved her goal and had a bright future. All is well, Wilhelm thought as he settled into his office, enjoying the many bouquets and cards decorating the room. He smiled broadly as Kurt entered, prepared to get to work again.

The summer was going by quickly. Normalcy returned to the Lindemanns' household. Marianne was content, enjoying her gorgeous garden. The girls were involved in their own activities, and she had to admit she loved the quiet house. Margarete and Peter, as well as Lisbeth and Lorenzo were in and out, but most of the day belonged to her. Occasionally she met her friends for lunch or shopping, but she thrived in these last lazy days of summer. It had been quite a turbulent, busy time, and Marianne looked forward to calm, undisturbed days ahead.

FIVE

On this crisp, clear morning Lisbeth and Lorenzo were cycling along a rutted country path.

"How much farther?" Lorenzo puffed, riding up a slight incline.

"Just over to the woods—see over there on the left," Lisbeth turned and smiled mischievously. "It isn't far."

"Good, good. I'm getting tired and hungry too," Lorenzo called to her, blowing her a kiss.

A picnic basket was strapped to the back of his bike, and as Lisbeth had promised, it wasn't long before they reached the edge of the shadowy forest. They found a cozy, level spot underneath a majestic oak tree. After leaning their bikes against the tree, Lorenzo collapsed on the grass, laughing.

"What a great ride!" he exclaimed, gulping for air. Lisbeth laid out a small cloth and began to unpack their picnic. Both were quiet now, taking in the restful view of the valley below. They relaxed as they finished their simple meal in silence. Lisbeth seemed unusually quiet and introspective. Lorenzo wondered why his usual stories could not seem to cheer her up today.

"What is it, *Cara* (Darling), why the long face today?" he coaxed.

Lisbeth looked up at him, and with a deep sigh she answered, "Oh, Lorenzo, don't you know? It's so wonderful being with you, and in a few weeks you will be leaving. How can I stand not seeing you again!" She couldn't go on and began to cry softly.

Lorenzo lifted her tear-stained face to his. Kissing her gently, he whispered, "I do not want to be without you either," pulling her closer to him. Slowly he began kissing her eyes, nose, and finally her willing lips. "I don't know what to do. I want to stay with you. But I know I must go home soon. I have been away too long. All I know is that I want to be with you forever."

"So, what can we do?" Lisbeth whimpered through her tears.

"I know; I will not go to England," Lorenzo replied. "To be with you is a thousand times better than visiting castles and cathedrals."

"But then what?" Lisbeth cried. "What are a few more weeks? You will still leave, and I will never see you again."

"That is nonsense! You'll come and visit me in Argentina. You will love it there. I know my family will like you, especially my Nonna! You will see. She will love you just as I love you."

There! The words had popped out before he had planned to say them. Lorenzo had surprised himself. He knew that all his thoughts and dreams were wrapped up with Lisbeth, yet the words "I love you" had been difficult for him to say, especially in a foreign language. Still, it was true, and Lorenzo was overjoyed that he could honestly look into Lisbeth's eyes and simply repeat, "I love you, Lisbeth. I love you with all my heart! *Te quiero! Te quiero!*" (I adore you!)

Stunned, Lisbeth lifted her head as her face glowed with happiness. Excited, overwhelmed, she heard the words she had longed to hear all summer. "Love, that's it, love! I love you too, Lorenzo, that's what it is. I love you. *Ich liebe Dich!* and want to be with you forever."

Declaring their love for each other seemed so simple, so right, so natural. They looked deeply into each other's eyes and kissed with renewed desire.

Lorenzo pushed away from Lisbeth, now speaking seriously as if he had just come to a decision. "Better yet, Lisbeth. You know what we will do? We'll just get married and then we will never be apart."

"M-m-married?" Lisbeth stuttered. "But how can we when you have to leave?"

"We could get married now as soon as we can, and then you can go with me to England, to Argentina, to wherever because we will always be together!"

Once the words had been said, Lorenzo could not stop talking about his love for her, his newly changed plans, their future. Lisbeth thought her heart would burst with happiness as she listened to Lorenzo's words. "But how can we do that? We don't have much time. What will Papa and Mutti say about this? Will they even let me go so far from home?" Lisbeth added worriedly.

Lorenzo silenced her with another tender kiss. "Your Papa loves you, and he wants whatever makes you happy. Let's talk to him tonight. Everything will work out, you will see. I will send a telegram to my family," he declared with youthful confidence.

With that happy thought, the two young lovers kissed again, forgetting all cares, thinking only of their happiness.

For the first time in her life, Marianne was unhappy with something Wilhelm had done.

"Here he is, recovering from a heart attack. I try to keep any excitement from him, and tonight he makes a major decision without even consulting me!" she stormed. "He drinks champagne and is as excited as a little boy on Christmas Eve!"

If she had not been afraid of upsetting him, Marianne would have gotten into her first real argument with her husband in 26 years.

When Lorenzo and Lisbeth had come to them tonight, nervously asking permission to marry, Marianne had had to sit down to recover from the shock. Never had it entered her mind that her little girl might fall in love and want to leave her home and family. It was all too soon for her. And to top it off, for Lisbeth to want to go to such a far-away place as Argentina.... It was more than poor Marianne could take in at one time. She had been so busy caring for Wilhelm that she had not noticed what was happening around her.

But Wilhelm was not surprised at all. In fact he behaved

as if he had been expecting it.

Smiling, Margarete had put her arms around her mother's shoulders, saying, "Mutti, have you been blind all summer? They are so in love, the whole world can see it."

But Marianne could not shake her concern. "In love, in love! Of course they are in love! But has anyone thought what it all means? Our Lisbeth will be leaving us, not just to move across town, across the country, but across the ocean, half a world away!" Marianne began to cry again. How could she face losing her youngest, her baby?

But Wilhelm had agreed, giving his blessing happily and without any doubts in his mind. Marianne could not understand her husband. Still, she had to go along, even if it was against her wishes. No one had wanted to hear her worries and objections. The truth was, Marianne had to admit, she had never seen Lisbeth happier, beaming with love and longing for Lorenzo.

Flushed with excitement, Lorenzo had embraced his fiancée, then shaken Wilhelm's hand and thanked him again and again. As he was accustomed, he had hugged everyone in the room, almost lifting Marianne off her feet. "Thank you, *Gracias, Danke schön!*" he'd repeated as he made a round of hugs for everyone.

Wilhelm had called for champagne, and Marianne had to join everyone in a happy toast. She had embraced Lisbeth and Lorenzo and congratulated them both. Smiling bravely as she held back her tears, she had thought her heart would break. Everything was just moving too fast for her. Too much had taken place in such a short time. "But this is a happy event," she said to herself. "I will not spoil one of the happiest occasions in my daughter's life."

The atmosphere in the room changed and became more festive as the young couple, Wilhelm and Margarete noticed that Marianne was now smiling. She seemed to have accepted this turn of events after all. All Marianne wanted was her daughter's happiness, and there was no doubt in anyone's mind that Lisbeth and Lorenzo were indeed deliriously happy.

Kissing her good night at the front door, Lorenzo whispered into Lisbeth's ear: *"Schlaf' wohl, mein Schatz!"* as she giggled with happiness. For some reason, those four simple little words, spoken in her native tongue, meant more to her than any other declaration of love.

The next few weeks were a total blur for Lisbeth. An engagement ring with a brilliant sapphire appeared on her finger, and telegrams flew back and forth between Argentina and Hamburg. At first, Lorenzo's family questioned his impulsive decision, but soon that was followed by acceptance and finally congratulations. They too wanted to know everything about Lisbeth, his chosen bride.

Marianne and Margarete immersed themselves in wedding plans and preparations which Lisbeth cheerfully approved. Wilhelm was quietly enjoying all the excitement, yet sad at the same time. Never had he seen Lisbeth so blissfully happy, and never did he regret giving her his blessing. Still, the pain of separation loomed ahead for them all.

Lisbeth was totally engrossed in her love for Lorenzo and could not get enough of hearing every detail of his far-away home, his family, friends, and the new kind of life she would find waiting for her there.

SIX

The wedding took place in Marianne's garden. The warm September sun cast a golden glow over the terrace and the gazebo in the center of the rose garden. The roses had never bloomed more beautifully than this year, as if they were on exhibit for a very special occasion.

Marianne's wedding gown had been lifted from mothballs and cleaned and restored. It fit Lisbeth perfectly, and seeing her beautiful daughter in it brought happy memories as well as a few tears to Marianne's eyes. She had to admit that she was getting caught up in the excitement of the wedding festivities. The shopping, the invitations, the flowers, the music, the menu for the reception required all of Marianne's time. Wilhelm was pleased that she was so absorbed in the preparations that she no longed fussed about him and his health. In fact, on several occasions he had worked in his office all day, and his wife had not even noticed. He was feeling better every day, and his energy level was higher than before his heart attack.

"Happiness is what made me well," he thought. "I know I will miss my Liesl terribly, but I am very happy for her. She was always yearning for adventure. Yes, now in Lorenzo she has found it. She is so much like my sister, Anni. May Lisbeth be as blessed as Anni!" he prayed.

Margarete too was caught up in Lisbeth's joy. She was to be the only bridesmaid and had chosen a pale blue silk dress for her sister's wedding. "It will be easy to plan my own wedding after this," she mused. "For Lisbeth we must get everything done in a few short weeks." Someday, when she and Peter were ready, she would take her time and plan every last detail and enjoy every single moment. But that golden day was still several years into the future.

Margarete had prepared several special songs for the wedding. The finale would be a haunting love song, the aria from *Lohengrin*—*Non ti scordar di me* (Remember Me Forever). She was almost as nervous as she had been on the day of her recital. Two of Peter's friends from the Conservatory would play violin and cello, and one of Margarete's friends the harp. Everything was prepared and ready when the wedding day finally arrived.

The caterers were bustling in the dining room and kitchen, setting up for the champagne toast after the ceremony. The gazebo had been decorated with white streamers and fresh flowers. Chairs had been set up in the garden for the closest friends of the family. A school friend of Wilhelm's, Judge Hoffmann, would be officiating at the ceremony, and a fine reception and dinner had been planned at the Grand Hotel.

As Marianne and Wilhelm were dressing, Marianne was

reflecting on the past weeks. Everything had gone so quickly, it all seemed like a dream. "And here we are, our little Lisbeth getting married to someone we hardly know." True, Lorenzo was a very likeable, charming young man, devoted to Lisbeth, and obviously very much in love. She had no doubt that Lorenzo came from a fine family, and that they would welcome Lisbeth. She had seen the telegrams of approval, congratulating and welcoming her. Nonna, the grandmother, had written a very kind and loving letter to Lisbeth. The thought of having this grandmother nearby was, for some reason, very comforting to Marianne. Still, her little girl would leave her, and that was very difficult for her to accept. However, seeing Lisbeth's happiness as well as Wilhelm's enthusiasm, she banished all but pleasant thoughts from her mind.

Wilhelm embraced his wife and kissed her tenderly. "Are we ready to go downstairs and attend our little Liesl's wedding?" he asked, and Marianne replied, "Yes, I'm ready, and may God keep her safe and happy always." But she couldn't suppress a sigh as she smiled and took her husband's arm.

Meanwhile, Lisbeth and Margarete were putting the final touches on their wardrobe. They alternated between laughter and tears as they chatted about what was about to happen.

"Little sister, getting married before me," Margarete teased. "Aren't you just a wee bit nervous?"

But Lisbeth was so overcome with love and anticipation of being with Lorenzo forever that it overshadowed her nervousness. Still, she felt an unaccustomed flutter in her chest. Taking another last look in the full-length mirror, Lisbeth almost did not recognize herself. Her long blonde hair had been coiffed into a crown of curls from which cascaded the exquisite long lace veil. Her large blue eyes, sparkling like stars, her face radiant with excitement and her slightly blushing cheeks added a special glow to her flawless complexion. Her mother's silk wedding gown encased her slender body with elegance and grace. With another last hug for Margarete, Lisbeth, suddenly calm and serene, picked up her wedding bouquet of pink roses, ready to take the first step into her new life.

All was finally ready. To the soft sounds of the musical trio, Lisbeth, the radiant bride, on the arm of her smiling groom, stepped out onto the terrace. All eyes turned to the glowing couple as they slowly walked down the decorated path to the gazebo. Surrounded by family and friends, Lisbeth and Lorenzo solemnly pledged their lives and their love for each other forever.

After a short honeymoon, the young couple returned to the Lindemann home. Wilhelm and Margarete enjoyed teasing Lisbeth by calling her *Frau* (Mrs.) Moncrief.

"Who is that?" Lisbeth replied. "It will take a while for me to realize that you're speaking to me. But it's a wonderful new name to get used to." She laughed while turning her wedding band on her finger. To her, it was the most beautiful piece of jewelry she would ever own.

"Señora Moncrief," Lorenzo called as he entered the living room, embracing his bride and whispering, *"Te Amo"*

(I love you) into her ear. Smiling, she wriggled out of his arms.

Seeing Hans Peter standing behind her husband, Lisbeth greeted him warmly, inviting him to sit. "Thank you, Lisbeth, but I must be on my way. I only helped Lorenzo with his belongings. We'll miss him at the guest house—not that we have seen that much of him since he pulled you out of the North Sea," he teased.

Both Lisbeth and Lorenzo smiled, remembering that fateful day that brought them together. "We owe you a lot, Hans Peter—you, your sailboat, and Lorenzo all saved me. And now, look how wonderfully it all turned out."

Again the newlyweds kissed as Hans Peter waved goodbye and closed the door quietly behind him.

Lorenzo's luggage was sitting in the foyer ready for his imminent departure. There was no need to unpack; Lorenzo was leaving in two days, close to his original schedule, and according to his father's instructions. His journey had taken somewhat longer than was originally planned, and his father was now anxious for his return. The marriage had been accepted with joy and anticipation at *Bien Cielo*, but Lorenzo did not relish leaving his young bride so soon. Yet he knew it was time to return home, face his responsibilities and prepare for Lisbeth's arrival.

She had applied for her passport weeks ago, but the wheels of bureaurocracy turned very slowly. Her father, who she thought could accomplish anything, could not speed up the process. Lisbeth had been racing to the mailbox every day, looking for her documents in the desperate hope that she could still sail with Lorenzo. It was not to be.

The morning of Lorenzo's departure dawned. Everyone in the Lindemann household was quiet and subdued. Johann was waiting near the garage. Even he dreaded the drive to the harbor as he knew how sad Lorenzo's sailing would make his beloved Lisbeth.

After a tearful farewell with promises and declarations of love, Lorenzo boarded his ship with a heavy heart. He missed his young wife already, dreading the twelve lonely days until his ship docked in Buenos Aires.

Lisbeth returned to the car with tear-swollen eyes. Old Johann placed his arm around her shoulder, which he had not done since Lisbeth was a child. She seemed like a child to him again—afraid, alone and needing to be held. Once in the car, Johann hesitated briefly. Shyly he handed Lisbeth a small box. She looked at him questioningly.

"It is a little present for you," Johann said softly. "It belonged to Trudi, and I want you to have it from both of us."

Lisbeth opened the box with trembling fingers and found a beautiful gold medallion on a fine golden chain. On the medallion was a simple white seagull carved in ivory. Lisbeth was speechless. She remembered Trudi very well and as a child had often admired the unusual pendant. She was deeply touched by Johann's thoughtfulness.

Seeing the joy the gift had brought her, he continued, "Trudi loved this pendant. I gave it to her so long ago. We used to take walks along the pier before we were married, and she always enjoyed watching the seagulls. She wondered where the gulls had been, what they had seen. If they could speak, what would they tell us?" Johann wiped a tear from his eye. Remembering his Trudi and the life they had shared always affected him with deep emotion.

"Oh, Johann, it is beautiful! Thank you for wanting me to have it! I know how much this pendant must mean to you."

"You are so welcome, my dear Lisbeth. Soon you will be flying far away just like the seagulls. When you come back to visit us you can tell us all about where you have been and what you have seen. You will be my little seagull."

With that, Lisbeth fell into Johann's arms and cried with a strange mixture of happiness and sadness. It was a special moment that she would keep in her heart and remember his love and kindness forever.

On the drive home Lisbeth closed her eyes and tried to sort out her thoughts. She had just said goodbye to her husband. How long would it be before she would see him again? Her heart ached with sadness and longing. How much she loved him! Knowing how much he loved her, she smiled again. How happy she had been with her young husband in the last few weeks. In her wildest dreams she could not have imagined being as happy and fulfilled as she did at that moment. Remembering his touch sent pleasant shivers down her spine.

"Now I have to be strong," she told herself. "In a few weeks I too will be sailing, and Lorenzo will be waiting for me." Determined to be positive, she resolved to enjoy every moment she had left with her family. "I will not spoil the time I have with tears and sadness. Lorenzo is mine. I know he loves me. He will be waiting for me. And I have much to do here to get ready to be with him."

With that, Lisbeth sat up straighter, wiped her tears and looked out the window, noting the beauty of the landscape gliding by. Fondling the pendant Johann had placed around her neck, she tapped him gently on the shoulder. "No more tears. Let's hurry home. We have a lot work to do."

Johann nodded, marveling at her new maturity. They drove the rest of the way in silence, but without tears clouding their vision.

Hoping her separation from Lorenzo would be short, Lisbeth's thoughts now turned to the many chores and all the frenzied activity awaiting her.

Wilhelm and Marianne were quiet and subdued after the excitement of the wedding and Lorenzo's hurried departure. They were both thankful Wilhelm had survived the hustle and bustle well. He returned to work, no longer keeping the curtailed schedule. Kurt no longer needed to come by the house with paperwork. The last time he had come was two days after the wedding. Lisbeth's gown was still hanging in the hallway. How he longed to see Margarete in this dress by his side! He thought of her constantly. He had even hoped for a longer recuperation period for Wilhelm, just for the chance of seeing her again. Unknown to her, she had an ardent, secret admirer in Kurt. But he simply didn't have the courage to approach her. For now he kept his love hidden in his heart.

SEVEN

Lisbeth's days were filled with shopping and packing. Soon her room was filled with crates and trunks awaiting her imminent departure. Margarete presented her with a new address book in which she had noted all the names of her friends as well as Tante Anni's address in the United States.

"We have such a small family, and yet so distant from one another! Tante Anni is far enough away across the Atlantic, and now you are going even farther away from us to South America." Margarete lamented.

"But you'll stay here, won't you, always?" Lisbeth asked.

"Yes, I will stay here so that you can always come home to us." Margarete was sure of that.

"But look at it this way," Lisbeth cheerfully replied. "You and Mutti and Papa will have great destinations to travel to. First you can visit Tante Anni and then sail south and visit us in Argentina."

"Oh, you silly Lisbeth! We would be spending weeks and weeks on the water, traveling halfway around the world."

As their easy banter flew back and forth, each one knew how far, how difficult, how rare their visits would be from now on.

"I promise you, Lisbeth, as soon as I graduate from the Conservatory, the first thing I'll do is to come and visit you. I know Mutti and Papa will want to come too, and we will have a wonderful reunion in your new homeland." Both girls smiled and hugged each other.

Day after day the postman delivered everything except the passport. Eager as she was to join her husband, Lisbeth truly treasured these last days with her family. She could only imagine how difficult it was for her parents to let her go, how deeply they loved her. Her father came home early every day now, and the reason was not doctor's orders. He wanted to spend as much time as he could with his beloved Liesl. There were many last visits with friends and classmates.

Finally, early in October, Lisbeth's long-awaited documents arrived. Everything was ready. The trunks were packed. Only the last goodbyes were left to be said. In one week Lisbeth was scheduled to depart, sailing on the steamship *Neue Welt* (New World). How appropriate the name! Truly she would be leaving for a new world.

Wilhelm had been so quiet the last few days, as though the enormity of Lisbeth's marriage was finally dawning on him. He and Kurt had finalized all the travel arrangements for her, and he had given her his final instructions. In

Buenos Aires, Wilhelm had a business acquaintance, a banker who had handled the finances as well as the shipping of Lindemann's chandeliers several years ago. On the night before Lisbeth's departure, Wilhelm and Marianne had a last serious talk with their daughter.

"My dear child," he said to her. "You didn't give us much time to plan a grand wedding for you. And now you are going far, far away from us. We know that you have a husband who loves you and who will take care of you. But we wanted you also to have something of your own so that you can buy the things you will need to make your new home. Therefore, I have arranged with Señor Alvarez of the *Banco Internacionale* to set up an account for you. You have your travel money and all you need for now, but consider the rest a gift from your mother and me. Look at it as part of your wedding present."

Tears were stinging his eyes as he embraced his little Liesl once more. Lisbeth, touched deeply, sobbed in her father's arms. She was stunned by her parents' foresight and care of her, even in the distant future. Filled with gratitude and love, she embraced both her parents, thanking them for the wonderful life she had spent with them. With a final hug and kiss, Lisbeth said goodnight as both parents wished her sweet dreams for the last time in her homeland.

Lisbeth clutched the letter for Señor Alvarez in her shaking hands as well as another thick manila envelope she was to deliver to him at the bank in Buenos Aires. She stowed them carefully in her large carrying case.

That last night Lisbeth and Margarete sat up and talked into the wee hours of the morning. Marianne too had come into her bedroom one more time for another last *Gute Nacht*. Lisbeth was very excited about the upcoming journey and seeing Lorenzo. But she was also scared.

"What am I doing?" she lamented. "I'm leaving everything I know. I'm going into a totally unknown life." Yet the desire to be with Lorenzo overcame her doubts, her fears and uncertainties. She finally slept, dreaming of the future while around her everyone was quietly missing her already, wondering if they would ever see her again.

The last morning dawned too soon. Breakfast was a very quiet affair. Johann loaded Lisbeth's two bulging carrying cases into the Daimler. One was particularly heavy, containing the many books Lisbeth hoped to read while on board ship. Marianne had also packed an additional bag full of knitting yarn, needles and patterns. She was very proud that she had taught her daughters a variety of domestic skills. She could not interest Margarete in knitting, but strangely enough Lisbeth had become quite adept at it. Knitting while letting her mind wander was very relaxing for Marianne, and something she enjoyed doing on long winter evenings. She hoped it would be a pleasant way for Lisbeth to pass the time while on the long voyage.

Lisbeth's large trunks had been delivered to the *Neue Welt* two days ago. After a last check that nothing of importance had been forgotten, Lisbeth gave her handbag to Johann and returned quietly to the house. Everyone knew why. Slowly she walked through each room, remembering, saying goodbye. With a final look from the terrace at her mother's beloved rose garden and the gazebo where, not long ago, she had stood, a radiant bride, joining her life with

Lorenzo, she whispered, "A*uf Wiederseh'n, Auf Wiederseh'n.*" She locked in her mind forever this final mental photograph of all she had known and loved.

The *Neue Welt* was a large steamship that docked regularly in Hamburg harbor every few months. Although it was mainly a cargo ship, it also contained a number of private cabins accommodating a dozen passengers. Fortunately, it was in port when Kurt and Wilhelm made Lisbeth's arrangements. It was one of the newest and safest steamships to which Wilhelm would entrust his daughter's passage. As the family arrived at the harbor, the early morning fog lifted and the *Neue Welt* gleamed in the sunlight.

Walking toward the ship, Marianne bravely tried to talk. "Oh, Lisbeth, I almost forgot to tell you," she began nervously. "In your big trunk I also packed two rose bushes for you. Don't worry. Johann got all the instructions from the nursery for how to pack them, how to feed them, how to plant them."

Lisbeth and the others stared at her incredulously. "You packed rose bushes for me to take all the way to Argentina?" she stammered. Wilhelm and Margarete exchanged amused glances.

"Only you, Marianne, would do such a thing," he smiled.

"What is so wrong with that?" Marianne protested. "These are special roses; they are very hardy. Lisbeth can plant them in her own garden on the *estancia*. Then she will always have something special from home."

"Yes, yes," everyone mumbled, grateful for the momentary distraction at this very stressful time.

"You are right, Mutti, it will be springtime down there when I arrive," Lisbeth said. "And I'm sure they will grow. Thank you, thank you so much."

Now the time for the final farewell had come. Lisbeth tried to be strong and not make the goodbyes too long. A last hug, a last kiss, another "thank you," another, "Don't worry about me," a last smile as the tears were streaming down her pale cheeks. With a last wave she resolutely walked up the gangplank, looking forward, yet wanting to go back. By the time she reached the passenger deck, leaning against the railing and waving to her family below, her tears had dried. With a confident smile she waved once more as the ship's engines began to hum. A couple of street musicians standing on the pier began playing the soft strands of the Hamburg farewell song. This brought a new wave of tears to the small group of passengers huddled at the railing, as well as everyone waving goodbye on land. The words of the farewell song echoed in Lisbeth's mind long after the home shore disappeared into the horizon.

Wo die Nordseewellen schlagen an den Strand
Wo die gelben Blumen blueh'n in's grüne Land,
Wo die Möwen schreien, schrill im Sturmgebraus
Da ist meine Heimat, da bin ich zu Haus*

---

* The entire song with English translation can be found in the Appendix.

EIGHT

Overnight the weather changed. A cold October wind was blowing off the North Sea. Marianne's garden needed preparing for winter. Even the last chrysanthemums were turning brown and dry. Lacking her usual enthusiasm, Marianne forced herself to do her clean-up chores in the rose garden today. Year after year, Johann had offered to take care of this job for her, and sometimes she had let him do it. This year, however, she wanted to do it herself. The dreary atmosphere of the garden matched her own sadness.

Even Margarete's long-awaited acceptance into the Hamburg Opera Chorus had not been able to lift her spirits. It was not fair to Margarete, she knew that. She should be able to share her daughter's joy, her excitement at being able to sing on stage. But she could not. She missed Lisbeth so much that she actually felt a physical pain. The reality that Lisbeth was gone was almost impossible for her to accept. "Why did we let her leave? How happy I was in the spring," she thought to herself, "when my roses first came into bloom. How I loved to spend my time out here thinking about our good life! How quickly things have changed in just a matter of a few months! I could have lost my husband. How strange it is that he had a bad heart and I did not even know about it until his heart attack! I almost lost my daughter in that swimming accident. How fortunate we were to have her back, only to lose her once again. But Wilhelm felt positive; he was so sure it was a good match."

Lisbeth's departure had been the most difficult day in her whole life. How she missed her happy face, her winning smile! Gone now forever, she was sure of that. Gone to a faraway place she had never ever thought of until her daughters had pointed out the great distance on the world map. But—and she had to smile in spite of herself—the power of love! What it can do to you! Lisbeth was happy, of that she was sure. And in the end, that is what counts in life. She, Marianne, had chosen a more quiet, settled lifestyle, and been totally content with her life. Her Lisbeth had made a different choice. Wilhelm was right. In many ways she was very much like Wilhelm's sister Anni who had done almost the same thing. Still, Anni had not married a stranger but her childhood sweetheart, Josef, and together they had taken a chance on a new life in America. It had worked for them— why not for Lisbeth and Lorenzo?

Marianne was raking the leaves out of the flower bed, pulling off the last shreds of the dried-up roses. How sad her garden looked now, how dull and cold! She shivered and pulled her jacket a little tighter. "I must accept things as they are. That is all I can do," she mused. "That is what I must do. I still have my Wilhelm, and I still have my Margarete. She has been my pillar, my strength all summer, through all the turbulent times. I am so glad she has her music, and I am so proud of her newest accomplishment. And I am so glad she has her Peter; they will make a perfect couple one day, and they will always stay here," she resolved.

With a deep sigh she looked around her garden, deciding to let Johann finish the job after all. Carefully she replaced the rake in the garage and rubbed her cold fingers. Her head held high, she walked briskly toward her warm and inviting house. After all, she still had a family. They still needed her and deserved more than her gloomy, morose disposition. With a little prayer for Lisbeth's safety and calm voyage, she entered her kitchen, ready to prepare dinner for her family, determined to show a happy face to all.

PART TWO

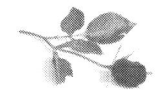

Journey South

NINE

The *Neue Welt* was steadily steaming southward. After the coastline had disappeared from view, Lisbeth walked slowly to her cabin, ready to settle in for the long voyage. Unpacking her suitcase, she spotted a box of her favorite hard candy her sister had stashed in a side pocket. Margarete's little surprise, which had meant to cheer her, unleashed a flood of tears instead. Lisbeth flung herself on her narrow bed, wracked by heaving sobs. The pain of separation hit her with a devastating force as a feeling of loneliness and heartache overtook her.

"How will I survive this journey, so far from my family and so far from my Lorenzo?" as a new wave of tears choked her. Finally, exhausted, she dozed off. When she woke, the ship was rocking through the choppy English Channel. Somewhat disoriented, she rose and took some uncertain steps around her cabin. It was a small room, but quite cheerful and comfortable. A soft armchair with a reading lamp sat in the corner near a small porthole. She lifted the curtain, but it was already dark. Seeing herself in the tiny bathroom mirror, she was aghast, her red, tear-swollen eyes staring back at her. It had been an emotionally draining, stressful, heart-breaking day, and she was very tired. Yet, despite it all, Lisbeth suddenly felt very hungry. With her old resolve, she forced herself to go on, to wash her face and dress for dinner.

That first lonely night aboard ship, Lisbeth was too wound up to sleep. Thoughts of home, her family, the past, as well as questions about the future churned in her head. She thought of Lorenzo and how much she loved him. As she slowly began to relax, she thought she heard his voice, crooning to her, "*Schlaf' wohl, mein Schatz,*" and only then did she drift off to a peaceful sleep.

The next morning she slowly began to adjust to her new surroundings. However, the constant pitching of the ship and the shifting of the horizon as the freighter plowed through enormous waves made her dizzy and nauseated. But after a day or two, the tiny blue pills Dr. Ranf had given her for seasickness began to take effect. As soon as she felt better she started to take interest in the new environment, going on deck for a breath of fresh air and getting acquainted with the other passengers. There were two German businessmen, dealing in beef and leather imports from South America. An Argentine antique dealer was returning to Buenos Aires. There was also an elderly couple who kept to themselves and appeared only at mealtimes. It was almost as if they were afraid to speak to anyone. There was also a father with his teenaged son who rarely participated in mealtime conversation. However, a young family, Roland and Sara Wolff, and their two children soon became Lisbeth's shipboard friends. Vera, the ten-year-old daughter, was lively and active. Before long she had charmed everyone on board, including the crew and the solemn captain. Aaron, her brother, quiet and studious, spent hours reading or playing chess with his father. They often met in the ship's lounge to listen to records, play games and visit. From Roland and Sara, Lisbeth learned that all three families were emigrating to Argentina to build a new life.

"That's just what I am doing," Lisbeth informed them. She had not thought of herself as an immigrant, but in fact she was.

"Why are you all leaving Germany?" she asked.

The couple exchanged glances. "You don't know? Well, perhaps it is better not to know," they replied.

"What do you mean?"

"What we mean, Lisbeth, is that we are all Jews, and as Jews we are no longer welcome in Germany. We are fortunate to have the means to leave and start over elsewhere. You are young. You are in love with your new husband. We are sure you have not followed the politics and the changes the Chancellor has brought to the country."

Lisbeth was shocked.

Roland sighed as his voice trailed off somberly. "Have you heard of the Nürnberg Laws that were passed last year? Jews have been deprived of their citizenship. Jews cannot attend university. It is a crime for a non-Jew to marry a Jew. And there are many more restrictions."

Lisbeth was speechless at hearing this news. Yes, she

had been too involved in her own life to pay much attention to events in the real world. She did remember overhearing a conversation between her parents regarding the departure of several of her father's employees who were Jews. Yet, when she asked, they seemed reluctant to talk about it. It seemed to have been of major concern to her father. Now she was beginning to see the bigger picture, could understand her Papa's anxiety and his fear of an uncertain future.

"Thank you, Roland. I am beginning to understand. How sad for all of you to be forced to leave, whereas I am going because my Lorenzo is waiting for me!"

Roland sighed and continued, "The reasons really don't matter. We are all leaving everything we know and love. We are all facing the unknown. We are strong, and we are going forward together to face whatever challenges lie ahead of us."

Nodding silently, they agreed, and this knowledge created a new and special bond between them. All of them knew they were not alone. As if by silent agreement, they never raised this subject again. It was as if they were ready to bury a painful past, not wanting it to cloud their future which was full of hope and anticipation.

The days began to pass quickly as Lisbeth found enough activities on board. On sunny days, if the wind was not too fierce, several of the passengers spent time walking the deck, back and forth, as that was the only physical activity possible on the *Neue Welt*.

She had found a photo book in the ship's tiny library showing the beauty of Argentina. She struggled through the English-language descriptions and learned many more facts about her new country than Lorenzo had informed her about. Of course, she knew all about his parents, José and Cecilia, his Nonna, his home, *Bien Cielo*, the small town Baradera nearby, but she knew of little else. Often she lay in bed imagining what everything might look like. She knew that the *estancia* was about 60 kilometers from Buenos Aires and that there was a train running from Baradera to the big city. Now she saw pictures of the mountains, the seashore, fertile farmlands and the large flat area called the Pampas where Lorenzo's home was located. There were photos of fields of grain and sunflowers. Lorenzo had told her about the great herds of cattle and sheep, and described a particular type of very tall Pampas grass. In her imagination she saw Lorenzo's home near the Paraná River. But mostly she tried picturing Lorenzo in the midst of the unfamiliar landscape. Suddenly she could not wait to reach her destination, to hold Lorenzo in her arms, to see her new home. She spent hours studying the book, wondering, imagining, dreaming and hoping for good fortune.

TEN

José Moncrief was one of the largest landowners in the *Pampas* (grasslands of Argentina). Surrounded by over 800 hectares of fertile farm and grazing land, his home stood on a rise near a curve of the Paraná River. José had inherited the *estancia* from his father Anselmo. When José was only 14 years old, his father had been killed in a riding accident. His mother Maria had continued to operate the ranch with the help of Manuel, the *estancia* manager, until José came of age. The raising of cattle and sheep, the sale of meat, wool and hides had always been the mainstay of the estate.

Over the years, José had turned his love of horses into a profitable business by raising and selling race horses. Nothing thrilled him more than attending the races, knowing that some of the contestants had been raised at *Bien Cielo*.

The *estancia* was a busy and bustling place. *Bien Cielo* consisted of many buildings: horse and storage barns, sheds, garages, bunkhouses and outbuildings of various kinds spread across the valley. Many of the *gauchos* (cowboys) lived on the property and performed the many daily tasks out on the range. Others lived in town or at outlying areas and rode in daily. Another group of ranch hands worked in the horse barns, raising and training the horses, preparing them for sale.

On a rise, somewhat removed from all the activity, stood the villa, overlooking the wide open spaces of the Pampas and the curve of the river. Surrounded by trees and a garden, the villa was an imposing two-story white structure with many large windows. The grand veranda, extending across the full length of the house, was supported by tall white pillars. Entering the courtyard, one was struck by the elegance and serenity of the house, surrounded by flowers and a gurgling fountain. When José's mother, Maria, had arrived at this house as a bride, there had been no veranda and no courtyard, only a large functional ranch house. The daughter of a wealthy landowner herself, Maria's ideas and dowry had made all the beautiful improvements possible. Maria had been very happy in this house with Anselmo and had been devastated to lose him at such a young age. José also loved this house, living with his mother and all the faithful employees who were like family to him.

When José married his wife Cecilia, he had hopes for a large family of his own, but it was not meant to be. Still he was very proud of his only surviving son, Lorenzo. Now it seemed Lorenzo had been gone forever. José was looking forward to his son's return from his European journey to help with the management of the vast family operation.

Today José sat on his shady veranda planning ahead for

the future and Lorenzo's homecoming. It seemed that he and Cecilia were always eagerly awaiting his return from somewhere. After attending grammar school in Baradera, Lorenzo moved to an academic *colegio* (boarding school) on the outskirts of Buenos Aires. His return for vacations and special holidays was always cause for celebration at *Bien Cielo*.

Then followed the university years when even some of Lorenzo's holidays were spent with friends at various locations. To José, he had always seemed somewhat restless as if confined, living on the *estancia*. For that reason José had come up with the grand scheme of sending his son on an extended trip to see the world. His hope was that Lorenzo would now see the *estancia* with new appreciation and would then be ready to settle down and assist with the management of the family business.

José took another sip of his cool drink, remembering the excitement of the last few weeks. He had been totally but pleasantly surprised when the telegrams began arriving, informing them of Lorenzo's marriage to a German girl, Lisbeth. Cecilia, however, had been shocked. She felt deprived of attending her only son's wedding. But now she too was looking forward to meeting her new daughter-in-law. José smiled. How impulsive his Lorenzo was, how charming and how headstrong! How quick to act and think later! Yet, this marriage might be exactly what Lorenzo needed to settle down and begin his adult life.

Although Cecilia was very curious about Lisbeth, she immediately could think of a number of things to worry about. How could Lorenzo bring home a young woman from a foreign country, from a different culture and language? Would she like living on a relatively secluded place, far from the convenience and excitement of a large city? The marriage also brought to an end the secret hope that Lorenzo might eventually wed Elena, a local girl whom he had known all his life and always sought out when he was home on holiday. At every dance or Fiesta, Lorenzo and Elena were seen together, and it was generally assumed that one day they would marry. The families knew each other, and José and Cecilia often stopped at Elena's father's cantina in Baradera.

"How would Elena accept such surprising news?" Cecilia wondered. She curbed her thoughts and said firmly to herself, "Lorenzo is old enough to know his own heart. I will be happy for him, and I will welcome Lisbeth with open arms." Cecilia adored her son, and in her eyes he was perfect.

Lorenzo's grandmother, Maria, now lived on her own property only two kilometers from *Bien Cielo*. When she had inherited her parents' homestead with its smaller, comfortable house, Maria decided to leave the villa and return to her childhood home. Her land had been leased to a neighboring *estanciero* (rancher) for many years, and Maria enjoyed living independently on that income. She continued to maintain two horses, one for her daily rides, the other for her two-seater carriage which she enjoyed using on her weekly trips to Baradera. José had suggested she buy a car and learn to drive, but Maria would not hear of it. Much as she enjoyed riding in José's car, she could not imagine giving up her horses or her carriage. She was grateful to her son when he invited her to ride along on visits to friends on other estates or to attend various events in the area. But she loved being independent and relying on her own wits and strength.

Today, however, Maria was getting ready for a very special ride. José and Cecilia were taking her to the train station in Baradera to welcome Lorenzo home. She was filled with happy anticipation. It had been a long time since Lorenzo had left on his journey. She was overjoyed at news of his marriage and could hardly wait until Lisbeth's arrival in a few weeks.

Lately she had tried to think in German again. During her childhood her parents and grandparents had spoken German at home, and her German roots were still there, but as Spanish became more prevalent in her daily life, the language of her childhood was almost forgotten.

"What a wonderful twist of fate," Nonna, as she was called, marveled that her only grandson would bring a girl from Germany into her life! With a last look in the mirror, a smiling Nonna went out to her porch, ready for the car trip to Baradera. Tonight would be like old times, the four of them having dinner together and hearing all about the new bride. "Life is good, even at my age," she thought, looking forward to a new chapter of life at *Bien Cielo*.

After his six-month absence, Lorenzo was looking forward to going home again. Sitting on the train chugging along to Baradera, his thoughts were of Lisbeth. He couldn't wait for her to join him and was anxious to show off his beautiful bride and to show her his spectacular country. Today even the treeless Pampas seemed striking to him with its vast rolling prairie and the variety of tall grasses. He saw massive herds of cattle with the occasional *gaucho* riding the range. Even the dry bushes growing along the creeks and river seemed greener and fuller than he remembered.

Soon the train pulled into the little station, and to his surprise and enjoyment, a small crowd awaited him. Along with his parents and his Nonna, several friends and townsfolk stood there to greet him.

"Ah, there he is. Our Lorenzo is back," they called.

"You are looking well. You are a married man now," they teased.

"We are so happy you are back, safe and sound," his mother cried, hugging him tightly.

"My congratulations too on your marriage, my son." José was shaking his hand and grinning broadly.

Many hugs and handshakes later the Moncriefs finally loaded Lorenzo and his luggage for the short ride home. Driving through the small town of Baradera, Lorenzo realized anew what a lovely, charming, old-fashioned place it was, and he immediately thought of Lisbeth again. She would love this place with the cobblestone streets and the well-preserved architecture of a time gone by. He couldn't wait to show it to her.

Arriving at the *estancia*, another welcome awaited him. Ranch hands and house staff waved and greeted him with enthusiasm. "Almost like the return of the prodigal son," Lorenzo couldn't help thinking. Nevertheless he was very touched by the show of love from everyone. News of his marriage had spread everywhere, and it seemed strange to be congratulated when his bride was not with him.

"You will meet her soon," he called cheerfully, wishing she were here right now.

That night the family enjoyed a wonderful meal together and stayed up very late. His parents were eager to hear all about his experiences, and Lorenzo loved telling them stories of his adventures along the way. The most important story was, of course, how he had literally fished Lisbeth out of the cold water of the North Sea. Nonna was very interested in all the details concerning Lisbeth's family and their way of life.

Cecilia asked, "How do you speak with each other? Does Lisbeth speak Spanish?"

"No, Mother," Lorenzo laughed. "I speak a little German, and we both speak our school English. So that is how we manage."

Cecilia shook her head. She could not understand how Lorenzo could fall in love with this girl when they couldn't even speak the same language.

"You are forgetting the language of love," Nonna said, and everyone nodded and agreed that there is such a thing.

"Lisbeth is a very smart girl," Lorenzo continued. "She will learn Spanish in no time. You'll see. I've taught her a few words already." He smiled at his mother as he put his arms around her. "Don't worry, Mother. You will love her, I know."

Cecilia smiled. It was hard to worry when she saw her son so happy.

After a few days of constant talking and telling stories, the excitement calmed and Lorenzo rested. He spent hours riding his horse and getting reacquainted with the routines of the *estancia*. Not much had changed in his absence as José and his managers ran a smooth operation. Wool and hides were prepared and shipped out routinely, cattle transported to auctions, grain loaded and sold. There were horses to be broken, trained and marketed. There was hardly ever a slow time at *Bien Cielo*, a busy and prosperous place. Fortunately, Baradera was only four kilometers away. It was the center of commerce as well as culture and entertainment in the area. The rail connection was invaluable to *Bien Cielo's* business success.

José was eager to show his son the books which he proudly kept himself. There was much to learn, Lorenzo realized as never before, but he was now ready to take on the challenge and make his father proud.

After settling in, Lorenzo knew he had one duty that could not be put off any longer. One morning after breakfast, he decided it was time. He saddled his horse and rode into Baradera. His destination was the cantina, hoping to find Elena there. He wanted to tell her himself about his recent marriage and hoped she had not heard the news from someone else. But in his heart he suspected that she already knew. The news had spread like wildfire, and Elena was anything but happy for him.

Before he even had a chance to greet her, she shouted at him, "You traitor! You liar!" She continued to yell at him, throwing the towel on the floor instead of wiping the glass in her hand. "Did you forget all about me on your famous trip? Have you forgotten what we've had together, how we just knew that we would be married one day? Were they all lies when you said you loved me?"

She was screaming and crying, not caring who else was in the cantina. "You go off on a trip to places I've never heard of and now you are bringing home a wife—someone you must have met only a few weeks ago." Elena was furious with Lorenzo, not allowing him to speak. Many eyes followed Elena as she pranced off in the direction of the kitchen, still yelling with a venomous voice, "I hate you. I hate you. I curse your marriage. I curse her. You will see—you will never be happy with her!"

With that she slammed the door, and Lorenzo stood stunned and speechless, the other patrons' astonished eyes upon him. He was dumbstruck by Elena's violent reaction. Sure, he did love Elena in a way. She was pretty and full of life. But he had totally forgotten her when he met and fell in love with Lisbeth. His bride would be arriving in Buenos Aires soon, and he could hardly wait to hold her in his arms again. But Elena's outburst bothered him a great deal. She had totally ruined all his anticipation and excitement.

"Everyone else is accepting my marriage and is happy for me. Why is Elena so furious with me?" he thought naïvely. "I have never, never promised her marriage! Perhaps in time she will accept things as they are." But realistically he knew that would never happen.

Lorenzo mounted his horse and rode slowly back to *Bien Cielo*. Many confusing and troubling thoughts crowded his brain. Never, never had anyone spoken to him in this way. Never, never had anyone shouted and cursed him as Elena had just done. He must keep Lisbeth away from her. He must explain to Lisbeth that Elena had assumed something that simply wasn't so.

As he approached his home, welcoming him as it glistened in the bright sunshine beneath a brilliant blue sky, he thought longingly of Lisbeth, knowing that she would be happy here. That, he had promised her. In a few more weeks he would hold her in his arms, and nothing, nothing, even Elena's fury, would stand in the way of their happiness.

ELEVEN

On the last night of the voyage, there was a festive feeling in the air. Excitement was gripping everyone on board. Tomorrow, tomorrow, what would tomorrow bring?

After the cheerful farewell dinner, Lisbeth was anxious to return to her cabin, finish packing and get a good night's sleep. Tomorrow she would see her beloved Lorenzo again, would hold him and never let him go. She could hardly breathe with love and longing for him. And yet sleep eluded her.

"Did Lorenzo receive my letter and telegram? Is he really going to be there waiting for me? What if he is not?" Questions of all kinds plagued her. Doubts and worries began to creep into her mind.

"Stop this, stop it!" Lisbeth admonished herself. "Everything will be fine. Lorenzo will be waiting for me tomorrow." She began to pray, "Please God, let tomorrow be a good day." With that, she fell asleep.

The alarm clock went off early the next morning.

Lisbeth could hear movement and activity as the crew, as well as the passengers, began their preparations for docking. She almost did not want to get out of bed. In some strange way the ship had become a new little world for her, her cabin a protecting cocoon. Today she would leave the *Neue Welt* to see her own real new world. She was ready and yet hesitant. But the moment of indecision passed quickly. There was no choice. Swiftly she rose and prepared herself for the day she had been dreaming about. Skipping breakfast, she hurried on deck to join the other passengers. Everyone was clustered at the railing, hoping to catch the first glimpse of the harbor and their new world.

With the aid of two tugboats, the *Neue Welt* docked with a few gentle bumps along Pier #207 in Buenos Aires. Few people, aside from the dock workers, were waiting on the pier. It was very easy for Lisbeth to spot Lorenzo immediately. Not only did he stand out by his height and good looks, but he was holding up a large hand-painted sign: "Welcome home, Lisbeth! *Te amo mucho!*" (I love you a lot!)

He was waving and calling her name, jumping up and down like a child. Lisbeth, too, feeling incredible relief and joy, waved wildly, calling out to him, while tears of happiness filled her eyes. Her Lorenzo had come, waiting for her with open arms! Lisbeth's fellow passengers on the *Neue Welt* cheered and applauded the happy couple. She was the only one of their group who had someone waiting for her. How lucky she was to be greeted with so much love! The other immigrant families looked nervous and apprehensive. But Lisbeth's radiant smile and obvious happiness spilled over on them, giving them also a measure of hope.

The next few hours were a blur to Lisbeth. Somehow she navigated through customs and immigration, had her baggage inspected, her passport stamped and stickered. She was finally able to leave the old red brick harbor building and set foot on a new land. All that was real to her was Lorenzo's presence. His smile, his kisses, his arms around her were all that mattered. She was so happy she thought she must be dreaming.

"It's all really happening. I'm here with my husband. I'm the luckiest girl in the world."

Lorenzo too, his heart beating with love and excitement, felt that he was the luckiest man in the world.

Lisbeth and Lorenzo spent the first week in Buenos Aires where Lorenzo had reserved a beautiful suite for them. "This will be our second honeymoon," he told her, "and it will be even better than our first."

"Yes, it's wonderful here," Lisbeth agreed. "The rooms at the Palacio are so elegant, the city is so beautiful, but most of all, we are here together and will never have to part again."

True, as much as they had enjoyed their short honeymoon, they both had known that separation was looming shortly. This time they would be together forever. They could not be happier as all their wishes had come true.

"What shall we do today, *Cara mia*," Lorenzo asked his bride, as they were finishing a lavish room-service breakfast a few days later. Lisbeth smiled contentedly. "You have shown me so much already, the elegant boulevards and parks, the museums, the shopping district, and tonight we are going to the opera. As you know, I must see Señor Alvarez at the *Banco Internacionale*. I promised Papa to bring him a letter and a business envelope. Can we do that this morning?"

"Of course, *Cara*, I have some business to attend to also, but I have put it off. It all seems so unimportant when I am with you. But you are right. Why don't we take care of those things this morning, and then we can relax and enjoy the rest of the day without any duties."

That decided, they dressed and left the Palacio. Lorenzo put Lisbeth in a cab with instructions to the driver, then sauntered down the street to visit his broker and discuss the upcoming racing season.

Lisbeth timidly entered the majestic old building of the *Banco Internacionale*. Looking around the huge marble-walled lobby, she saw mostly dark-suited businessmen carrying important-looking briefcases.

"Why didn't I ask Lorenzo to come with me and do the talking for me?" she thought nervously. But she had not, and now she was on her own. Bravely she stepped up to the nearest desk and asked to speak to Señor Emilio Alvarez. The young man looked up and asked her name, checking a list on his desk. He smiled pleasantly and waved for her to follow him. They walked down a long corridor until he knocked on the last door.

"Adelante" (come in), a deep voice called as her escort opened the door. He introduced Lisbeth to a kind-looking, graying man of medium stature. He smiled as he shook her hand firmly. His eyes sparkled as he exclaimed, "Lisbeth

Lindemann—pardon, Moncrief. I am so happy you have arrived in our beautiful city. I have been waiting to see you. Your father wrote to me some weeks ago about your coming. I am so glad you are here. Please, come in, come in."

Lisbeth was elated at such an unexpected welcome. Her dear Papa—he had thought of absolutely everything. "Señor Alvarez knows all about me. Why did I ever worry? I should have known Papa would pave the way for me." How thankful she was to him! Seeing Señor Alvarez' kind face, she knew that she had found a friend.

"Sit down, please," Señor Alvarez invited her, and called for coffee. "Tell me all about your voyage here," he continued in almost perfect German. This fact alone filled Lisbeth with a wonderful warm feeling. Trying to talk with Lorenzo was often difficult and cumbersome and took great effort on both sides. She knew the first thing she had to do was to learn Spanish. But for the time being, she loved just sitting and chatting with Señor Alvarez.

"Where is your husband? I was hoping to meet him too," he was now saying. "Is there a chance we could get together while you are still in the city?"

"Oh, yes, I think so. We will be here two more nights. Tonight we are going to the opera, but perhaps tomorrow you could meet him," Lisbeth answered happily.

"That's good. I will leave a message at the Palacio. Let's meet for dinner tomorrow night. I am sure my wife would also love to meet you. Let me see what we can arrange, and I will call you."

Lisbeth smiled and nodded agreeably.

"Now let's get to the business matters." Señor Alvarez

became serious. "Your father asked me to set up an account for you here at our bank. I have arranged everything according to his wishes. All you need to do is sign this paper, and I will hand you the account number and documents."

Lisbeth signed her new married name with a shaking hand, thinking lovingly of her father who had made this possible. The last piece of business was handing him the large plain manila envelope her parents had given her. Puzzled, Señor Alvarez asked, "And what is this?"

"Papa asked me to take good care of this and to give it to you personally. That is all I know about it. He said it was a business matter and you would understand."

Señor Alvarez took the bulky envelope in both hands and thanked Lisbeth for her personal delivery. Carefully he placed it in a desk drawer, locking it with finality.

Lisbeth gave a sigh of relief, having completed the business her Papa had entrusted to her. With another warm handshake, Alvarez repeated his earlier invitation and the promise to call.

"I am so looking forward to meeting your wife and you meeting my wonderful Lorenzo," Lisbeth smiled as she walked out with a spring in her step. Returning to the Palacio, Lisbeth felt proud of herself, her confidence and hopeful optimism soaring.

She wrote her first letter from Argentina:

Dear Mutti, Papa and Margarete!
Today I met your business friend, Señor Alvarez, and now I feel he will be my friend too. I turned the envelope over to him as you instructed. He told me all about my new

account, and I cannot believe your generosity. Thank you, thank you both. I know I will put the money to good use once I am established in our new home. Thank you.

Señor Alvarez invited us to dinner tomorrow, and we will also meet his wife. I am so happy that you introduced me to him, Papa. He is very kind and helpful.

Tonight Lorenzo is taking me to the opera, Rigoletto. I am very excited and look forward to seeing your chandeliers, Papa. Lorenzo and I have had a wonderful week here in the city. There is so much to see here, and Lorenzo is showing me everything. The streets are very wide and there are many boulevards with trees and flowers. Lorenzo says Buenos Aires looks very much like Paris. As you know, I haven't seen Paris, but I must say that this is a very beautiful place. Our hotel is just grand, and we enjoy room service and breakfast in bed almost every morning. Lorenzo is spoiling me and loving me very much. It has been a wonderful second honeymoon. But I am also looking forward to going to Bien Cielo soon.

The next day she wrote again to her family:

Rigoletto was wonderful! I kept thinking of you, Margarete. How I wish you were here! I can't wait to get some letters from you. Please write soon and write often. Papa, there are so many chandeliers in the opera house, but I remember yours. They are the most beautiful ones, hanging in the huge lobby. Just think, there is a part of you right here in Buenos Aires. I hope you will all come to visit me soon and can see for yourself. Mutti, you would love the parks with all the flowers. Write soon.

Love, Lisbeth

Lisbeth was packing again. She looked around the elegant room where she and her husband had been so happy this past week. As she waited for Lorenzo who was attending to last-minute arrangements, she sat in the club chair on the balcony, looking out on the bustling city. There had not been a dull moment, but despite all the activity, despite the joy of being united with Lorenzo, a little sadness and homesickness was creeping into her days. She tried to hide it from Lorenzo and overcome her anxieties. Seeing Papa's chandeliers made her so lonely for her family. After the long weeks on the ship, she realized for the first time just how far she was from home. The beautiful arias of the opera reminded her of her sister. Her thoughts had wandered back home instead of enjoying the splendid performance. Suddenly everything reminded her of home—the bustle in the streets, the buildings, the parks, the harbor—except it was not her home. All around, she heard a strange language, saw and experienced a new and different culture, ate strange and unfamiliar food.

 She remembered with a smile last night's dinner with Señor and Señora Alvarez. How kind and friendly they both were and how welcoming toward Lisbeth. Señor Alvarez, as well as Lorenzo, was very patient translating the conversation to Paulina and Lisbeth. And despite many trials and errors, they delighted in each other's company, laughing and promising to meet again and build a friendship. Yes, Lisbeth felt very confident that she had found true friends in Emilio and Paulina Alvarez.

 Soon Lorenzo returned to their suite, followed by the porter. "Are you ready, *Cara Mia?*" he smiled. "Ready to get on the train to Baradera and to meet my family? To see your new home?" Lorenzo embraced and kissed her.

"Yes, my darling. I am ready. I am ready to go." And Lisbeth truly felt ready to begin this new chapter in her life with Lorenzo.

TWELVE

The train ride to Baradera took an hour and a half with several stops along the way. Sitting on the wooden benches in the passenger compartment, Lisbeth thought it was the oldest little train she had ever seen. As it chugged along the ancient single track, smoke and soot were seeping through the leaky windows. However, this did not lessen Lisbeth's sense of anticipation. She looked around excitedly, taking in all the newness. Several passengers, obviously local farmers and townspeople, stared at Lisbeth curiously. She returned their stares with a friendly smile.

As the train rocked gently along, Lorenzo tried to explain the area and the scenery to her. In his eagerness, he slipped into speaking Spanish, and Lisbeth let him ramble on. She enjoyed looking at this new and interesting landscape rolling by. They traveled through vast grassy fields she knew were called the Pampas. Great herds of cattle and sheep were everywhere. It was springtime here, Lorenzo had explained to her, and the sun hung in a brilliant blue sky. They crossed several small streams and finally a large river.

"Look, Lisbeth! We are crossing the Paraná River. We are almost home. Remember I said I learned to swim in the Paraná? It runs through our *estancia, Bien Cielo*." Lorenzo exclaimed excitedly. "We are almost home."

Lorenzo's delight grew as they approached Baradera as Lisbeth became more apprehensive.

"Do not worry, *Cara mia*, everyone will love you; everything will be fine." Lorenzo, sensing her nervousness, placed his loving arms around her, kissing her gently.

Soon they pulled into Baradera station. The stationmaster, wearing an official cap and uniform, stood in front of a small group of people awaiting the train's arrival. Lisbeth scanned the small crowd, wondering if she could spot Lorenzo's parents. Lorenzo squeezed her tightly as he waved and called through the half-open window. "*Padre, Nonna*, here we are!" Lisbeth saw a tall, very handsome man waving back at Lorenzo.

"There's my father, Lisbeth, and my Nonna," Lorenzo exclaimed. With a final hiss of the steam engine, the train came to a stop. A few minutes later, Lisbeth was greeted by José and grandmother, Nonna. José formally shook Lisbeth's hand and spoke pleasantly. His eyes sparkled with pride and approval. Although Lisbeth did not understand one word he was saying, she felt a sincere welcome.

Nonna, a rather small, energetic woman, hugged Lisbeth and proudly repeated, *"Wilkommen, wilkommen"* (Welcome, welcome). She took Lisbeth by the arm and began walking toward the building. José patted Lorenzo on the shoulder, nodding his head, a happy smile on both their faces. There were a number of people milling around the station, and by their curious glances, Lisbeth could tell that they all knew who she was. Many nodded in her direction, smiling and waving at Lorenzo and his father.

Outside the station was parked the only car on the street. Proudly José opened the door for his new daughter-in-law. On the short drive home, everyone but Lisbeth was talking. She was quietly holding Lorenzo's hand, letting the Spanish conversation wash over her. "I must learn this language soon. I am missing too much," she promised herself as she looked out the window. What she saw was a charming, old-fashioned little town with cobblestone streets and simple stone buildings. There was a tree-lined town square boasting an elaborate fountain. A large white church, stores and cafés clustered around the square. Soon they crossed the Paraná River on a wide stone bridge. Lorenzo, pointing out various landmarks to her, held her close. Already Lisbeth liked what she saw and felt comfortable here. Nonna, turning her head, continued to smile at Lisbeth.

Lisbeth thought to herself, "I have never known my *Oma* (grandmother) and now I feel that I have found my *Oma* here."

They left Baradera for the short four-kilometer drive home. They crossed the Paraná once again and approached the *estancia*. As *Bien Cielo* came into view, Lisbeth was immediately taken by the majestic beauty of the large villa. The white building gleamed warmly in the afternoon sun as they drove up to the large veranda. Lorenzo's mother and several members of the staff were waiting at the top of the steps. Slowly Lisbeth stepped out of the car, waiting hesitantly. But Cecilia walked down the steps with open arms and hugged both Lisbeth and Lorenzo. Reserved and quiet, she looked into Lisbeth's eyes and smiled.

Soon everyone was talking and gesticulating, and Lisbeth walked as if in a dream. Lorenzo opened the massive door, inviting her into her new home. Nonna was right behind them, welcoming her once again with her limited but well-meant German words. Impulsively, Lisbeth turned and hugged Nonna, telling her in German, "Oma, I am so happy to be here, to meet all of you. Thank you for making me feel so welcome!" Oma's eyes misted with affection for the lovely young bride her grandson had brought home to them. From that moment on, Nonna became Oma-Maria to Lisbeth, and a special bond of love and understanding began to grow between them.

Lorenzo took Lisbeth by the hand, eager to show her all around the house. First he led her up a wide, elegant staircase with carved woodwork. The right wing upstairs, he explained, belonged to his parents, and also included several guest rooms. The other wing was to be their own apartment. With a flourish, Lorenzo opened the large carved door. "*Adelante, Cara mia,*" he announced proudly. Her heart pounding with excitement, Lisbeth entered the suite. There was a large master bedroom, an inviting sitting room, a bathroom, plus two smaller bedrooms. All were furnished with large heavy antiques. Dark velvet draperies framed the large windows. Colorful Persian rugs covered the wide plank wooden floors. Lisbeth was speechless. Their rooms were on a much grander scale than she had ever imagined. This was going to be her home from now on. This is where she would spend her years with Lorenzo.

"So, how do you like it?" Lorenzo was eager to hear her reaction. "What do you think, Lisbeth? Isn't it just perfect for us?" he prodded.

"Yes, darling, this is beautiful. I know I will be happy here as long as I have you by my side," Lisbeth replied, and was rewarded with kisses and hugs that lifted her off the floor.

"But, but..." Lisbeth stammered, pretending to be serious. "But where is my kitchen?" Lorenzo gave her a perplexed look. "A kitchen? You want a kitchen? The kitchen is downstairs, and so are the cook and housekeeper. You can cook there, if you want to, but really, why would you want to? Marta has cooked for us for years."

"I'm just teasing you, Lorenzo. You told me all about your Marta. Everything is perfect, Lorenzo. I was just joking." Visibly relieved, Lorenzo took her hand as they went downstairs to have dinner with the family.

The next week was a busy one for Lisbeth as she unpacked her trunks and began the process of settling in. Lorenzo could not believe that her mother had packed two rose bushes along with her books, pictures, and other memorabilia. "Roses!" he laughed. "Does your mother think we have no roses in Argentina?" he teased.

"I know. It seemed strange to me too, but she wanted me to have something special from her, something to remind me of home. They are very special roses, she told me, and we must find a spot to plant them very soon," Lisbeth replied.

"Of course, we will find a sunny spot for them," Lorenzo said indulgently. Lisbeth lifted the roses carefully, trying to read the planting instructions. But her eyes filled with tears as she read the roses' names. A beautiful pink one was called *"Heimatrose"* (rose from home) and a large yellow one was called *"Nordseerose"* (rose from the North Sea). Holding the rose bushes close to her chest, she began sobbing as a wave of homesickness washed over her. Wordlessly, Lorenzo held her close. Lisbeth looked up at him, smiling through her tears. "I'll be all right, Lorenzo. But seeing these roses and their names made me miss my family so much, so much!"

"Everything will be fine, *Cara*. I am here with you, and you will see your family again, I promise you."

Slowly Lisbeth calmed down, and holding her rose bushes tightly, she firmly resolved, "Let's go downstairs and find a spot in the garden. I want these roses to grow here in my new land. I want them to be as strong and beautiful as our love, Lorenzo." He didn't fully understand her long reply in German, but he was relieved she had stopped crying and become his sunny, lively and happy wife again.

The days flew by. Lorenzo spent every day with his bride, showing her around the *estancia*, introducing her to the people who worked around *Bien Cielo*. Lisbeth fell in love with the beautiful horses being raised and trained there. Lorenzo was happily surprised when she voiced her desire to learn to ride.

"That is good, Lisbeth. I was hoping to teach you. Around here, that is a must. Everyone rides, even my grandmother. She still keeps a riding horse."

Lorenzo was beginning to relax as he saw his wife slowly adjusting to a new way of life. She took great interest in all her surroundings and had already made friends with Marta, the cook, although they could not really communicate with each other. Cecilia and José also warmed immediately to Lisbeth's smiles and hugs.

Lorenzo was a patient translator at mealtimes and reassured everyone that Lisbeth was a very fast learner. He had already spoken to Alma, the town librarian, about teaching Lisbeth Spanish, and Lisbeth was very eager to learn. Life at *Bien Cielo* would not be boring at all. She looked forward to all the activities and challenges awaiting her.

The highlight of that first week was a visit with Oma-Maria at her home. Lorenzo gave her a ride on his magnificent stallion, gently trotting along the two short kilometers to Nonna's house. Lisbeth was breathless with excitement, holding on for dear life—never having been on a horse before—a new experience she was eager to make part of her daily routine.

Oma-Maria, as Lisbeth had started calling her on that very first day, was waiting on her wide front porch. Although she had seen Lisbeth several times since her arrival, today was filled with special anticipation as she prepared the tea table for Lisbeth's coming. She clapped her hands with joy as she saw Lorenzo's horse approaching her house and was thrilled to greet his young bride. Maria could not wait to become better acquainted with her. She hoped today was the beginning of many such visits and friendly talks.

"Come in, come," Oma-Maria called excitedly. She hugged her grandson and kissed Lisbeth, ushering them into the house. The old farmhouse exuded warmth and welcome, and Lisbeth felt totally at home. Photographs of Maria's husband Anselmo and of her son and grandson decorated walls and tables in the living room. Her wedding portrait hung in a prominent place, and Lisbeth admired the handsome young bridal pair of long ago. The table had been set with Oma-Maria's best china, and a delicious-looking cake was in the center. As Oma-Maria busied herself preparing the coffee, Lisbeth snuggled up to her husband, feeling welcomed and loved. The conversation became an experiment in creativity as Lorenzo tried to translate for Lisbeth, Oma-Maria attempted to use some of her almost-forgotten German, and Lisbeth tried using the few Spanish words she had learned so far. In the end the three shared many laughs and knew that they would always be able to communicate even without words. This happy "trial and error" afternoon remained one of Lisbeth's favorite memories of her early days in Argentina.

Returning to *Bien Cielo*, Lisbeth had a wonderful surprise waiting for her—three letters from home, one from her parents and two from Margarete. "The end of a perfect day," she thought, as she tore them open.

THIRTEEN

*D*ear Daughter Lisbeth!
We know you are still on the Neue Welt as we write this letter. But we look at the calendar daily and cross off the days until your arrival. We hope you have had a calm voyage and that you are well. We think and talk of you daily and know that you and Lorenzo must be happy being together at last. We can't wait to hear from you and are anxious to know all about your new home and Lorenzo's family.

We are all well here, but we will not deny that we miss you very much. It is quiet without you, but we will feel close to you when your letters come. Johann asks about you almost every day. He worries about you as if he were your grandfather.

The weather turned cold right after you left, and the winds are blowing off the sea. Otherwise there is nothing much to report. We are eagerly awaiting your mail. Take care of yourself and stay well and happy. We love you very much; you are in our hearts forever.

Your loving parents,
Mutti and Papa

Lisbeth's hands were shaking. She felt so connected with her family despite the many miles separating them. She hoped that her parents had received one or more of the many letters she had written on board ship and since her arrival in Argentina. Eagerly she reached for her sister's letters. The first one was very short, but it made Lisbeth extremely happy and elated for Margarete.

Dear Lisbeth!
I know it will be some time before you receive this letter, but I had to write you at once to tell you the most wonderful news. Right after you left, I finally heard from Mr. Kühnle from the Hamburg Opera. You remember he came to my recital last summer? I thought he must have forgotten all about me or that he did not like my performance. Well, guess what? Next week I will have a private audition with him and the music director, but he assures me that is only a formality. Then I will be in the chorus for the spring season. In the meantime, there will be much work to do. But I am so excited, I hardly know what to do. I wanted you to be the first to know, but this letter will have to do.
Enough about me, now. I am really looking forward to hearing from you with all your news. I know you are the one who has many exciting things to tell me. Hope you are well and happy with Lorenzo. I just know you will have a wonderful life, but I do miss you. Write soon.
Greetings to all,
Love, Margarete

"Lorenzo, Lorenzo, where are you?" Lisbeth was running down the stairs, waving her sister's letter. Lorenzo was just stepping out of his father's office, wondering what the excitement was all about and hoping it was good news.

"Good news," Lisbeth called to him. "Margarete will be singing in the opera!" With that she fell into his arms. "Isn't it just fantastic?" she asked.

"That is indeed great news," he replied, smiling at her. Whatever the news, whatever made his Lisbeth happy, made him happy too. Anything but tears. Tears made him very nervous.

> My dear sister Lisbeth!
> Today we received your long letters which you wrote on the ship. We are so relieved that it was a good and safe voyage and that the time passed quickly. Mutti and Papa are reading your letters again and again. They also shared them with Johann. He sends his greetings and is glad you arrived safely. Papa also wrote to Tante Anni and hopes that you and she will begin a correspondence. Somehow Mutti feels that Anni is closer to you than we are. I think it is a comfort to her, thinking South America and North America are closer because they are connected. We all miss you so much, but Mutti also worries about everything. I think once you write about every little detail to her, she will relax. Right now it is difficult to picture just where you are. Papa is fine, going to the plant every day, and also playing Skat (German card game) with his friends every week. Peter and I rarely have time to see each other. We are both busy with our classes, and rehearsals will start in a few weeks. But we are both happy and try to get together on the weekends. Now my dear sister, I wish I could be with you and see your new home. But as I promised you, as soon as I finish at the Conservatory, I will come to see you. We are all well. Do not worry about us. Just write soon and write often. The weather is cold and foggy. I wish it were spring already, and winter has not even begun. Take care. Love,
> Your big sister, Margarete

Late into the evening Lisbeth read and reread the letters, feeling sad and happy at the same time. Tomorrow she would answer her mail, but tonight Lorenzo was waiting.

My dear family!
Yesterday I received three letters from you. What a happy day! Thank you, thank you! Lorenzo and I are fine and we are so happy. I hope by now you have my letters telling you all about the house at Bien Cielo and the estancia. Everyone is very nice to me. Even if we cannot speak easily to each other yet, people are friendly. Did I tell you that Lorenzo's mother calls me Lissabetta? I have new names for them too. I call his father Señor José and his mother Señora Cecilia. Lorenzo's grandmother I call Oma-Maria, and she likes that. She is like a grandmother to me. She is so sweet and good and tries very hard to speak some German. She will help me with Spanish, and I will teach her German again. She lives in the house she was born in, not very far from here. It is a very simple but warm and comfortable house and has a large porch in front. From there you can see the whole valley and the road coming from Bien Cielo. She keeps two horses, one for riding and one for her little carriage. She goes to Baradera twice a week and has promised to give me a ride into town whenever I want. So far Lorenzo has been taking me around, introducing me everywhere. He says he is going to choose the perfect horse for me and will teach me to ride. Isn't that wonderful? Then I can ride to Baradera whenever I want and pick up my own mail. But don't worry. I'll be very careful, and Lorenzo will watch out for me.
I am getting used to the routine here. Usually I have breakfast with Marta in the kitchen. The men leave early to go about their business, and Señora Cecilia takes breakfast in bed. Marta is very nice, and I like watching her and learning, I hope. But I don't think I will have to do

much cooking here. There are servants cooking and cleaning for us. But I told Lorenzo that I would like our wing of the house to be private, except for one cleaning a week. I will tell you about our apartment in my next letter. I am still trying to get settled and arrange it the way I like. But all the linens and my beautiful pillow cases are perfect and make me feel at home.

Your roses, Mutti, arrived safely. They were so well packed that I am sure they will grow here. We followed the instructions and planted them on the side of the house in a sunny spot. I check on them every day and water them as your instructions told me. Lorenzo couldn't believe that you had done that. Oma-Maria thinks that was such an original idea, and she loves their names. They made me cry a little at first, but now they make me smile and think of you. Thank you again.

Papa, I took care of all the business with Señor Alvarez in Buenos Aires. He said he would write to you soon. Thank you again for your wonderful care of me and your generosity. I know there will be times and special things that I will need, and having this account gives me a feeling of security and confidence. Thank you again from both of us. Señor Alvarez and his wife Paulina are very kind and warm people. They have invited me to come and visit them when I am in the city. I feel that I have two friends there already. I hope they will come to Bien Cielo as they have promised us.

Now my dear parents and my dear sister, I see Lorenzo coming across the yard. It is time for lunch. The whole family meets for a large meal in the dining room around one o'clock, and after that it is siesta time. That means everyone takes a little nap. That is the warmest time of the day and everyone rests. Later in the day they all resume their work, and dinner is usually quite late. But I am getting used to it.

I hope you are all well and keeping busy. I miss all of you very much, but at the same time I am happy here. The *days pass quickly. There is always something to do. My knitting and my books are still in the trunks. I am busy learning new ways and the new language. Lorenzo is the most wonderful husband, and he has so much patience with me. He is teaching me Spanish, and Oma-Maria helps too. Soon I will start my lessons with Alma who runs the library in Baradera.*

Now enough about me. I want to know everything about home. Please write and tell me everything about everybody. I am so excited about Margarete's work at the opera. I wish I could hug and congratulate you this minute. I am always looking at the clock and calculating the time back home. When I am awake, you are asleep. I can't wait for your next letter. Hope you are well and take care of yourselves. Don't worry about me. We are doing fine. I miss you all so very much, but your letters keep me close to you. I have written to Tante Anni in New Jersey. I remember her well from when she came to visit although I was only around nine years old then. I can see already that I'll always be busy just writing letters. But then I will receive many letters too, I hope. I love you all and will write again soon.

Your grateful daughter, Your little sister,
With love to all, Lisbeth

Lisbeth finished her letters and sat back looking out her window. She had moved the large desk to the window so that she could see the front drive up to the house and the flowers around the fountain in the courtyard. In the distance she could see the curve of the river and the vast meadows beyond. The landscape, so totally foreign to her, was beginning to grow on her, and she was slowly learning to appreciate its vast beauty. Yes, she missed the city with all its attractions, but she knew that with Lorenzo she could be happy anywhere. Her little jaunts into Baradera and an occasional trip to Buenos Aires would surely suffice. She looked around her sitting room—the massive chairs, the heavy dark draperies, the colorful wool carpet on the dark wooden floor planks.

"Soon I will have to think about making some changes in this room to make it more cheerful and more up-to-date," she thought. But for now Lisbeth was satisfied. It was more important to make the changes in their bedroom. Already the room had taken on a different character just by using the beautiful white linens she and her mother had chosen for her dowry. The lace pillows on the chairs, the down-filled comforters, the framed family photographs everywhere had given the room a fresh, European look. Soon she would choose new fabric and replace the heavy velvet drapes darkening the room. Lorenzo liked the changes, but at Lisbeth's insistence no one else had been allowed to see them yet. She wanted to finish everything and then surprise Cecilia and José with her home-decorating talents.

Now she rose, and with a quick look in the mirror, lightly skipped down the stairs to join the family for dinner.

Before long the days fell into a pattern. Every morning Lorenzo took Lisbeth out for a riding lesson. The horse he had chosen for her was a chestnut mare, aged and calm, a perfect animal for a beginner. Lisbeth named her Fritzi and gave her sugar cubes every day. Lorenzo showed great patience in teaching his wife to ride. Although somewhat apprehensive in the beginning, Lisbeth showed some natural ability and fitness. When she came to the barn every morning, the stable boys usually stopped what they were doing and watched her mounting the horse and riding off with Lorenzo. "They are all laughing at me," Lisbeth joked. "But just wait and see. I'll show them I can learn to ride!"

"Of course you will," Lorenzo replied proudly. "You can do anything you want, and you will do it well."

Yes, there were many things Lisbeth had to learn here. She applied herself and was determined to learn not only the new language, but riding as well. Oma-Maria sometimes accompanied Lisbeth on short rides and was always full of praise. Twice weekly, when Oma-Maria took her little carriage into Baradera, Lisbeth got into the habit of going with her. While the older woman visited her friends, Lisbeth took her Spanish lesson with Alma at the library. Alma was very kind and chose easy children's picture books to teach Lisbeth. Even after a few short weeks, Alma was amazed at the number of words Lisbeth had already learned.

On the second trip into town they did a little shopping, stopped for a restful coffee break at a sidewalk café, and most importantly stopped by the post office. It was located inside a small general store and was run by Juliana, the young wife of the owner. Only a few years older than Lisbeth, she was the mother of a beautiful dark-haired baby girl. The baby's bed stood in the corner of the tiny post office as Juliana watched her child as well as tending to her duties as postmistress. The two young women became friends quickly despite halting conversation. Admiration for the infant with smiles and coos was a universal language understood by all. Oma-Maria's presence was very helpful, of course, and the joy the women felt at the arrival of each letter was obvious. Sometimes there were only the books and newspapers that Oma-Maria had ordered; other times, letters from Germany and the United States. Juliana became very excited about the international mail that her little post office suddenly handled. She was also intrigued by the various stamps which Lisbeth gladly shared with her. Soon the trips to the post office became highlights for Lisbeth. Even if there was no mail, Lisbeth looked forward to seeing her new friend Juliana and her baby girl.

Slowly Lisbeth became known to the townspeople and the merchants. More and more she realized that Baradera was more than a little hick town. Small and quaint as it was, it boasted a courthouse, several schools, stores and restaurants, a large church, a park with playgrounds, and even a movie theater. The Paraná River snaked through the town providing a swimming beach at the park. Situated along the main railroad line to Buenos Aires, Baradera had become a busy, bustling commercial connection to the outlying areas. Lisbeth was well aware of the prosperity and wellbeing this community represented. It was very fortunate that *Bien Cielo* was only four kilometers from town and therefore was accessible to all that Baradera had to offer and for the daily necessities of life.

Riding home with Oma-Maria today, Lisbeth felt very content. In her bag were letters from home. She had spent an afternoon with people she had begun to care about, and now she was going home to her loving husband. Lorenzo had recently mentioned having to go to Buenos Aires on business and had invited her to come along. She was now looking forward to that trip and was hoping to visit with Paulina and Emilio. Life was good and she was happy.

Dear Margarete!

It is hard to believe that I have been here for six weeks already. I am beginning to feel at home, and the days pass quickly. I really like my horse Fritzi and ride her every day. Lorenzo still rides with me, but soon I will try it on my own. Oma-Maria often rides over to see me, and we go out together. She has become a very good friend, and we manage to speak quite well to each other. I have also made another friend, Juliana, who runs the post office. I see her twice a week, always looking for mail from home. She has a very sweet baby girl, Teresa. I hope to find time to knit something for her for Christmas.

Tomorrow I will travel to Buenos Aires with Lorenzo and Señor José. They have business in the city, and I am looking forward to Christmas shopping and visiting with Paulina and Emilio Alvarez. I am so glad Mutti thought of sending some gifts along for the family here. I know that Señora Cecilia will love the scarf, as well as Oma-Maria her cologne. The photo book of Hamburg will be perfect for Señor José, but I have to find something very special for Lorenzo and for all of you. We will pack and mail presents from the city, and I hope everything will arrive on time. When we return, Lorenzo tells me, there will be a holiday Fiesta in Baradera, and he says it is always great fun. I will write and tell you all about it. I wonder how Christmas is celebrated here. It will be strange to have it in mid-summer. I think of you all the time, and you know I will remember you all especially at Christmas, wishing we could be together. Please write and tell me how Papa and Mutti really are. Their letters always tell me they are just fine, but I really want to know. I still worry about Papa's heart and hope he doesn't work too hard. How are you doing at school? Have you begun your rehearsals at the opera yet, or will you start after the holidays? Please write me all the details. I wish I could see for myself how everyone is doing. That is all for now.

I love you all, Lisbeth

Dear Lisbeth,

We love reading all your wonderful long letters, telling us the details of your new life. Johann always asks about you. He really misses you as we do. There is not one day that we do not speak of you and pray for you. It helps knowing that you and Lorenzo are so happy, and that is as it should be. I have been very busy at school and have had my audition with Herr Kühnle. Peter was right; it was only a formality, and I am happy to report that I did very well. Rehearsals will begin December 5.

Last night Papa and Mutti invited Peter and me to dinner at the Krone to celebrate. Peter is so happy for me! He was always sure that I would get the audition. He is my best friend and is always positive. I am really fortunate to have him in my life and I care so much for him. He sends his best regards to you both.

Yesterday we also received a letter from Tante Anni. They are doing well, keeping busy with their family and the garden center. Their daughter Monika is already eight years old and the boys Willy and Little Joe are six and five. She says they are outgrowing their little house next to the greenhouse and hope to move to a larger place soon. But I shouldn't tell you all that as she said that she wrote you a letter too. Everything is the same here.

Papa feels fine and goes to work every day. I'm glad he is back playing Skat with his friends once a week. Next week they will meet here, and you know how Mutti always fusses to have the best refreshments for them. Mutti is lonely for you, as we all are, but she is brave and keeping very busy. Her monthly lunches with her friends are always something she enjoys, and some of her friends also have grown children who have moved away.

As you know, many of the young men are being drafted into the military service. So far, I am so happy to say, Peter, being a student, is exempt. Papa says he is very relieved that Kurt Walter is "too old" for the draft. Isn't that silly? I never think of Kurt as being old; I believe he is

30. The weather is cold and foggy, and we always think of you and the wonderful sunshine you enjoy at Bien Cielo.

Mutti is knitting and shopping and baking for Christmas. It will be a different holiday for us as it will be for you. We are anxious to hear all about the different customs in your new country. I wonder if you will decorate a tree as we do here. Mutti said she will send you her Stollen (Christmas bread) recipe and hopes that you will be able to get all the ingredients. She also wants to send you some of her goodies but worries if they will taste good after weeks on a ship. You know she loves to worry. Now, my dear sister, we hope you are well and adjusting. Hope you are careful with your horseback riding. That is something else Mutti worries about. Papa thinks it's wonderful. Take care and give our best regards to all the Moncriefs. Write soon.

With love and best wishes,
Margarete

Lisbeth leaned back in the large comfortable chair by her window. She had read her sister's letter several times. She could just imagine the hustle and bustle in her mother's kitchen and all the activities in the weeks before Christmas. Delicious aromas of baking filled the air in anticipation of the holidays. Here at *Bien Cielo* the cooking and baking fragrances were strange and different, and most of the hustle and bustle around the *estancia* did not include her. A deep wave of homesickness washed over Lisbeth. As the initial excitement and newness of her life began to wear off, Lorenzo spent more and more time with his father, learning about the operation of *Bien Cielo*. Cecilia, always friendly toward Lisbeth, led a very quiet life, reading and embroidering. More and more, Lisbeth was left to her own devices. She kept busy preparing for her lessons with Alma. She read the Spanish children's books she provided. The best part of her days were her early morning rides with her husband. Lorenzo was quite proud of her efforts and her progress. Lisbeth had really no reason to be bored or lonely, but she had to admit that her moods and daily outlook greatly depended on her letters from home. When the letters arrived, she was jubilant and full of laughter. On other days she became sad and gloomy. But she knew that Lorenzo did not want to see her cry. On the few occasions when he had found her in tears, aching with homesickness, he had become distant and impatient.

"Why are you crying again? You knew that marrying me would mean leaving your family behind. Am I not enough for you?"

That was the first time Lisbeth had seen Lorenzo losing his temper, raising his voice to her and giving her a cold stare. "Oh, it isn't that, Lorenzo. I love you, and you only, and I'm happy to be here. I knew it would be hard not seeing my family, but I had no idea it would hurt so much. Don't you understand?" And Lorenzo would take her in his arms and hold her until the tears subsided.

Lisbeth promised herself to be strong and not let Lorenzo see her cry again. But still the tears would come at the most unexpected times, and she knew that she had to cry alone. Oma-Maria understood her feelings and would open her arms to her, letting her cry onto her chest, and no words were necessary. After Lorenzo's outbursts of anger and frustration, Lisbeth kept her ache, her homesickness, silently in her heart.

Even to Paulina and Emilio, whom she had come to love already, she showed no outward sign of her constant longing for home. To everyone who met Lisbeth, she was a smiling, happy, carefree young woman who adored her husband and her new life.

FOURTEEN

Lorenzo was excited to introduce his wife to the annual Fiesta being held two weeks before Christmas. He sprawled in the club chair watching Lisbeth put the finishing touches on her wardrobe. She was dressed in elegant black riding pants and the new embroidered sweater that Lorenzo had recently bought for her in Buenos Aires. She had wound her shoulder-length hair into a bun, and was now attempting to place the traditional black hat on her head at just the right angle. She tightened the chin strap and turned around to show her smiling face to Lorenzo.

"*Excellente! Tu es bonita!*" (Excellent! You are pretty!) Lorenzo exclaimed with fervor. He knew his Lisbeth was beautiful, even in the first moments of her wet rescue, but at this moment he found her even more stunning than she had been on her wedding day. His heart beat with love and pride as he rose and kissed her. "Careful, don't knock off my beautiful hat!" Lisbeth teased as she took his hand and they walked downstairs, ready to have a fun-filled day at the Fiesta.

The town of Baradera traditionally celebrated the holiday festival in the town plaza. It was a simple affair, but it brought all the people from the surrounding *estancias* and farms together to celebrate this special season. There was food and drink, music and dancing, pony rides and a carousel for the children. A variety of home-made sweets and local crafts were for sale. Cecilia always donated her beautiful embroidered linens, pillows and shawls, as others brought carvings, weavings, dolls, toys and paintings, fruit and preserves, wine and cakes. A wonderful carnival atmosphere brought everyone from far and wide. New acquaintances were made, old friendships renewed.

In the evening a small band played romantic Argentine music, and young and old danced and enjoyed the fellowship. Lisbeth was totally captivated by the excitement and the colorful festivities. Lorenzo was very proud to show off his beautiful bride.

Lisbeth enjoyed being introduced to many more of his friends and the whole community. She already recognized some people and was especially happy to see Alma, Juliana and her husband as well as some of the merchants who all greeted her warmly. She enjoyed every moment and had already decided to contribute some of her own handiwork next year. She was thrilled to find some local handicrafts to mail home to her family. She bought a wood-carving of a *gaucho* for her Papa, an intricately embroidered tablecloth for her mother and a hand-woven wall hanging for her sister. For Johann she found a small but exquisite painting of the grassy pampas with soft rolling hills in the background. She was more excited about her purchases than she had been in the elegant department stores in Buenos Aires. Lorenzo could not be happier, feeling that Lisbeth really was beginning to love his country and all that was familiar to him.

Later in the afternoon, José and Cecilia, as well as Oma-Maria, joined the young couple for a simple meal of *chorizo* (sausage), steak, fresh bread and grilled corn, accompanied by great mugs of *cerveza* (beer) and sweet local wine.

"Como dis frutas la Fiesta?" (How are you enjoying the festival?) several people were asking Lisbeth, and proudly she answered, *"Bueno! Me gusto mucho!"* (Great! I like it very much.) as Lorenzo and his family applauded her attempts at speaking Spanish. Oma-Maria patted her on the shoulder, announcing in German, *"Du bist die Beste!"* (You are the best) as they all broke out in happy laughter. What a wonderful day it was for Lisbeth! A warm feeling of satisfaction and belonging filled her, aware of the welcome and goodwill of all around her.

Soon Oma-Maria, José and Cecilia decided to go home, but Lorenzo and Lisbeth joined a group of young people for an evening of dancing and fun.

As the beat of the music increased, the rhythmic sound of the tango invited more and more spectators to the dance floor. Lisbeth and Lorenzo joined in, gliding and dipping to the strains of Argentina's favorite dance. Breathless, Lisbeth returned to their table, eagerly reaching for her cool drink.

In their absence another young woman had joined their table. Lisbeth had seen her at a distance once or twice, but she did not know her. Ignoring Lisbeth, she smiled brilliantly at Lorenzo, saying, *"Oh, ella es tu esposa! Es tiempo de que tu me presenta a ella!"* (Well, so this is your wife. It's time you finally introduced her to me.)

Lorenzo paled and was momentarily speechless. He recovered enough to place his arm around Lisbeth's shoulders and reply politely, "Yes, Elena, this is my wife Lisbeth. Lisbeth, this is Elena Ruiz. We went to school together."

"Mucho gusto," Lisbeth replied, leaning forward to shake Elena's cold hand. Although Elena's mouth opened in the semblance of a smile, her eyes were cold as ice.

"Lissabetta," she hissed like a venomous snake. Abruptly she turned her back on Lisbeth and Lorenzo and began talking to others at the table. Lisbeth turned to her husband, her eyes asking volumes of questions, but Lorenzo only shrugged his shoulders and behaved as if nothing out of the ordinary had transpired. However, everyone around them seemed uncomfortable and silent, having witnessed a disquieting rude moment. Elena rose, and with a last hateful glance at the Moncriefs, pranced away and was lost in the dancing crowd.

"Look, here come the *gauchos!*" Lorenzo called out, diverting Lisbeth's attention. A group of dancers, dressed in colorful costumes of the countryside, began the traditional Gaucho Dance, and Lisbeth was once more caught up in the hypnotic rhythms of the tango. The unpleasant moment was forgotten as Lorenzo held his wife close, whispering *"Te amo"* into her ear. Finally the evening ended with one more wild and exhilarating tango as the Fiesta came to a close. Tired but happy, Lisbeth and Lorenzo drove home in silence, each lost in thought. Lorenzo was relieved that the meeting between Elena and his wife had passed without an even greater outburst of emotion; Lisbeth felt a sense of belonging and acceptance despite Elena's strange behavior.

That night, Lorenzo's love-making was particularly ardent, full of deep emotion and desire, proving his great passionate love for her. Lisbeth responded with equal affection and total surrender. For years to come, she would remember this night as one of the happiest times she had spent with Lorenzo. In fact, she could not remember ever being happier in her entire life.

The next few weeks flew by rapidly. Lisbeth had packed her gifts she had bought at the Fiesta, along with a book about Argentina for her family. Juliana made sure the package went out on the first train to Buenos Aires and reassured Lisbeth that all would arrive safely in time for Christmas.

One day a large box arrived from Hamburg, containing lovingly wrapped presents for Lisbeth and her new family. Her spirits lifted immeasurably as she actually began looking forward to the holiday.

She had asked Lorenzo about getting a Christmas tree, but he regretted that small fir trees were not available for decoration. Lisbeth was sad at first but improvised by decking out a fairly tall bush she had seen growing near the Paraná River below *Bien Cielo*. The German glass ornaments that her mother had carefully packed in newspaper looked rather strange hanging on dry, barren branches. But Lisbeth was excited and full of energy, preparing for the special day as Lorenzo's family smiled at her indulgently.

Oma-Maria alone really shared her joy, calling the

makeshift Christmas tree a very beautiful *Tannenbaum*. Everyone knew that this would be a very special and memorable first Argentinean Christmas for Lisbeth.

FIFTEEN

Meanwhile, an ocean away, Marianne too was preparing for the Christmas holiday. But her heart was not really in it. Her thoughts were with her child, Lisbeth, absent from them for the very first time. How could she present a happy face to her family when all her thoughts were with Lisbeth? "Is she really happy? How will she survive the holiday when memories of home must be replaying in her mind?" Marianne loved to worry about everything, and at this sentimental family time she could create new worries daily.

As in previous years, she had done the shopping, the baking, and tonight she was looking forward to decorating the Christmas tree with Wilhelm and Margarete. She thought of the exquisite ornaments she had packed for Lisbeth, wondering how they would fit into Lisbeth's new foreign household. It never occurred to her that there might not be a fresh green, fragrant *Tannenbaum* at *Bien Cielo*. Daily she waited for the postman to bring the long-awaited, cherished letters from Lisbeth. Johann was almost as eager as Marianne and often made a point of walking down the street under some pretext, keeping an eye out for the letter carrier. Even the postman knew when he saw the exotic stamps on letters that there would be great joy that day at Burgstrasse #47.

Wilhelm knew by Marianne's smile or the sadness in her eyes if some long-awaited mail had or had not arrived for them. He missed his little Liesl as much as the others did but, trying to shield his family from any pain, he kept his thoughts to himself. He did not regret giving Lisbeth his blessing to marry and leave them, knowing she was happy with her young husband. Still he missed her terribly, but concealed his sadness in his heart.

Finally Christmas came and went with the usual celebrations of gift giving, festive meals and solemn church services. Wilhelm, Marianne and Margarete managed to have a joyful holiday after all, but it remained memorable only by the fact that their beloved Lisbeth was not with them and might never be again. Bravely they smiled and remembered her with love.

December 28, 1936
Dear Papa, Mutti and Margarete!
Christmas is over, and I want to write and thank you for all the wonderful presents. The sweaters for Lorenzo and me fit perfectly; the jewelry is gorgeous, and the books are just wonderful. Best of all, dear Mutti, was the Stollen and the delicious cookies. Some were broken but they taste just like at home. I am rationing myself, eating just a little every day. I feel as if I am with you again. Thank you, thank you! I hope you received our package on time and

that you had a wonderful holiday. We had a big Christmas celebration with a huge dinner for everyone here at Bien Cielo. On Christmas Eve we exchanged gifts just like at home. Then we drove to Baradera for Midnight Mass. The little church was filled, and of course the Moncriefs know everybody. But even I feel that I know some of the people here, especially Juliana and Antonio and their baby Teresa, and Alma, my teacher. You would be surprised that I can already use a few Spanish words with confidence. Everyone here loved the presents I brought from Germany, and I also knitted José a scarf. He liked it very much, but perhaps I made a mistake. It is so warm here now—when will he wear it? Cecilia gave me an embroidered stole, and Lorenzo a beautiful gold chain for the antique pendant I received from Oma-Maria. I love the silk scarves and stockings you sent, Margarete. I will wear them the next time I go to the city. Lorenzo often has business there, and I can always stay with the Alvarez family. Someday they will go to the opera, and then I will tell them about you, the opera singer. You are wonderful. I will write again after my trip to the city. All is well here. My riding lessons are coming along well, and yesterday I rode all by myself to Oma-Maria's place. José is so proud of me when I try my new Spanish words, and Cecilia always smiles. But I can never figure out what she is thinking. Lorenzo says that she likes me and is proud of me too, but that she is just the quiet type.

I have written to Tante Anni and have received a very nice long letter from her. I always thought that she lived so far, far away from us in Hamburg, but when I look at the globe, it seems that I am now twice as far from all of you. Where Tante Anni lives in America also seems incredibly far away. Wouldn't it be wonderful if we could all meet again! In the meantime I am looking forward to your graduation, Margarete. I have not forgotten your promise that you would all come to Bien Cielo for a visit as soon as you are finished with your studies. Two years is a long time, but I'm looking forward to that happy day.

Did I tell you about my unusual Christmas tree? There are no trees to buy here for Christmas. Lorenzo says there are only fir trees way up in the mountains, but around here they are not available. I cut a tall bush growing near here and dragged it up to the house. Then I decorated it with the beautiful ornaments you sent with me. My tree was unusual but still very pretty. I know Cecilia shook her head at my foolishness, but everyone liked it. Oma-Maria clapped her hands and just loved my pretty Tannenbaum. I missed you all very much, but somehow I still had a nice first Christmas here with Lorenzo. He says that New Year is celebrated in grand style here with fireworks and parties. He says that it is even more fun than the Fiesta.

How was your Christmas? I thought of you all the time, and in my mind I was with you when you went to church, when you opened the gifts and when you all sat at the dining room table for the special Christmas goose. I was really there with all of you! Give Johann a big hug for me and tell him his little seagull is seeing and learning many new and exciting things. I'm sending my love to all of you. Happy New Year!

Love to all, Lisbeth

SIXTEEN

The year 1937 began with a pleasant surprise. A letter arrived from Paulina Alvarez, inviting the Moncrief family for a visit in Buenos Aires. She hoped they would be able to spend some time in the city, enjoying a change of pace. The highlight of the week would be an evening at the opera, attending the opening of *Aida*. This invitation filled Lisbeth with childlike excitement.

"We can go, can't we, Lorenzo?" she pleaded happily. "It will be so much fun, and I can tell Margarete all about it."

Lorenzo smiled, *"Si, si, Cara,* there is no reason why we couldn't go," he replied. Actually, Lorenzo was most agreeable to the plans as he had felt somewhat restless himself. "Actually, this trip will be perfect," he continued. "I have been wanting to visit the racing stables at San Carlos de Bolivar for some time and learn more about their operation. It isn't far from Buenos Aires, and after a few days with you in the city, I will go on my own way, and you and Paulina will have a good time without me."

"Are your parents coming too?" Lisbeth asked.

"I'll have to ask them," he replied absentmindedly as he was already making plans of his own, perhaps including a visit to his old school friend Geraldo who lived in that area.

José and Cecilia declined the invitation immediately, not citing a reason. Perhaps they wanted Lisbeth and Lorenzo to have a few days without them, and they knew how Lisbeth looked forward to this diversion. Already she could hardly wait to tell the Alvarezes about her sister's acceptance in the Hamburg Opera Chorus, and to visit "Papa's chandeliers" at the Teatro Colon. Proudly she thought of her family and felt a special closeness despite the great distance. Sometimes everything seemed totally unreal to her, the unusual way she had met her husband, her marriage, and her long journey to a strange and distant land. And now, here she was, riding this old-fashioned train, learning a new language, new ways, and meeting new people. "I'm looking forward to dressing up and going to the opera in Buenos Aires. Is this really me, Lisbeth?"

She sat up straighter and came back to reality. "Yes, this is me, Lisbeth Moncrief; my husband is sitting across from me, and I'm really here in Argentina! Isn't this what I always dreamed of—to see the world and have an exciting life? Yes, I have done it, and my future is here with my darling Lorenzo." She opened her eyes as the train bumped along its way. She looked across at her husband, and as if he felt her penetrating glance on him, he folded his newspaper and laid it down.

"Well, *Cara*, we are almost there! I am really looking forward to a few days in the city. Aren't you?"

"Oh, yes. It will be so wonderful, and there is so much to do there. Paulina wants to take me shopping and show me more of the city. And I'm going to meet their children. It will be fun, but I already know that I will miss you terribly."

Lorenzo laughed. "You will be so busy, you won't even have time to think of me," he teased. He was also looking forward to his own activities, after the first days in town. To please Lisbeth he would dress up and go to the opera with her. But he was thinking more about seeing Geraldo and visiting San Carlos with him. As the train was arriving, he reached across and, taking her hand, pulled her onto his lap, encircling her in a tight embrace. As he repeatedly kissed her, Lisbeth forgot all about her uncertainties, her troublesome questions, and gave in to the joy of being loved and fulfilled.

As Paulina had hoped, the performance of *Aida* was fabulous. The beautiful music, the elegance of the stage, and the drama of the love story touched everyone. Lisbeth was moved to tears although she understood not one word of Italian. The repeated standing ovations, the excitement of the audience caught up with all of them. Even Lorenzo was surprised and moved by the music. Lisbeth began to understand Margarete just a little better: how one could actually fall in love with music as her sister had done. Paulina and Emilio were truly pleased that the evening had turned into this huge success for all of them.

Tomorrow Lorenzo would leave town. Emilio would return to the mundane world of finance. Paulina and Lisbeth would go shopping. But tonight was a little bit of heaven for all of them, a special night to remember.

After a few hectic days, Lisbeth finally had an afternoon to relax. With her eyes closed, she was lounging comfortably on the Alvarez' veranda. Tiptoeing quietly, Paulina carefully placed a tray with two tall glasses of lemonade on the small table beside her. Lisbeth opened her eyes sleepily and smiled at her friend. "Thank you. What a refreshing drink!" she muttered, taking a long sip.

"I thought you were sleeping. I didn't want to wake you," Paulina replied.

"No, no. I was just relaxing and resting," Lisbeth said.

"Good, good. I'm glad you are feeling better now than this morning," Pauline continued.

"This morning I was just tired," Lisbeth replied. "I didn't want to get out of bed. I guess all the shopping and all the late nights finally were too much for me," she laughed. "At *Bien Cielo* I never have a problem getting up and going on my ride with Lorenzo."

"Well, tomorrow you will be going home again," Paulina smiled. "I'm sure you've missed Lorenzo this week."

"Yes, I have. But it's been such a wonderful time here with you! I can't thank you enough for all you have done for me. Now I'm thinking about starting to sew my new drapes for our bedroom. I just love the material we bought today. Thank you for helping me choose it. When are you and Emilio coming to *Bien Cielo*? There is lots of room. Please come."

"Yes, we will come soon," Paulina promised, "when you are all settled in and your decorating is finished," she laughed. "I'm sure you are feeling at home there now, and we are glad you are making friends with everyone there."

"Well, not everybody! Most people are very nice to me, but not everybody."

At that moment Emilio entered the veranda, greeting them both with a friendly hug. "My, you are having a serious conversation," he teased, having overheard Lisbeth's last words. Lisbeth was suddenly eager to tell them about her unpleasant experience at the Fiesta. Knowing Emilio could translate for her, Lisbeth spilled out the story to them in German.

"That must have been upsetting for you, I imagine, but I think Lorenzo is right. Do not waste time worrying about people who mean nothing to you. There are enough others in Baradera and at the *estancia* who love you and want to be your friends," Paulina reassured her as Emilio nodded. Paulina was very careful not to show her uneasiness, hearing about Elena's contemptuous snub and coarse manner. Who was this Elena? What reason did she have to behave so rudely towards Lisbeth in public and in front of Lorenzo? Whatever it may be, right now Paulina knew that what Lisbeth needed was her support, her understanding.

She could sense Lisbeth's concern and suspicion. In addition, Paulina knew how greatly Lisbeth suffered from homesickness despite the love and care of her husband. She was still so young and vulnerable. For the first time in her life she was far away from home, from her family, from everyone and everything she knew. Lisbeth had haltingly confided in Paulina that the only cloud on her horizon was Lorenzo's temper and his inability to understand her feelings of loneliness and her longing for home. In the short months since her arrival in Argentina, Lisbeth had already decided that Lorenzo would not see the many tears she shed in private.

After a good night's sleep, Lisbeth awoke refreshed and ready to go home. She was anxious to get back to *Bien Cielo*, her Lorenzo, her home. As she stood up, however, she felt lightheaded and a bit queasy. "I'm too excited to eat breakfast," she told Paulina, adding to herself: "I just want to get back to Lorenzo."

SEVENTEEN

Riding over to Oma-Maria's house, Lisbeth felt a new sense of serenity, a complete peace of mind. As Fritzi was trotting along gently, Lisbeth enjoyed the touch of the warming sun, the light breeze, the calm beauty of the morning. She was happy and invigorated, anxious to share with Oma-Maria her wonderful experiences in the city. She was eager to start making her new draperies and needed Oma-Maria's help.

Oma was always there for Lisbeth, and they truly enjoyed each other's company. This morning Oma-Maria was already waiting on the front porch, drinking her strong Brazilian coffee. *"Buenos Dias, Guten Morgen!"* she called out to her friend. She ran down the steps, embracing Lisbeth as soon as she was off the horse. Soon they were sitting together, talking and laughing, sharing their love.

"You should have seen the stationmaster's face when I came home last week! Lorenzo was waiting for me with such a large bouquet of flowers that I couldn't see his face."

Lisbeth said. "It was so funny. Lorenzo wanted to hug and kiss me, so he handed the flowers to the stationmaster! You know, that man never smiles, but on that day he almost did."

"*Si, si,* I know how he is. He thinks he looks official if he puts on a long face. I'm glad you and Lorenzo made him smile." Both women had a chuckle about this and continued their conversation partly in Spanish, partly in German and they understood each other perfectly.

Finally Oma-Maria clapped her hands saying, "Lisbeth, I have been wanting to show you something special. Would you like to drive over to my father's vineyard today? Raul can drive us if you want to go."

"Oh, yes, that would be wonderful. Let's go. We can work on my drapes next week. I'm glad I'm feeling well again today."

"What is wrong? Have you been sick?" Oma-Maria wanted to know.

"No, no, nothing like that," Lisbeth relied. "It's just that while I was in town on several mornings I didn't want to get up. I didn't feel sick exactly, but somehow just not right. Then, coming home on the train, I felt that way again. I must have eaten something or maybe I was just tired from all the shopping," Lisbeth laughed. "Now that I'm home with my Lorenzo and here with you I feel just perfect."

Oma-Maria looked at Lisbeth in a strange, questioning way but remained silent. Lisbeth linked arms with her and together they walked off in the direction of the stables. Raul had the carriage ready to go, waiting to assist the women step in. Off they went, down the hill in the opposite direction from *Bien Cielo,* where Lisbeth had not been before. Oma-Maria was very quiet, but suddenly she turned and without explanation hugged Lisbeth tightly. Surprised, Lisbeth looked at her. Oma-Maria, in her direct manner, simply asked, "Have you ever thought you might be having a baby?" She clapped her hands again and simply said she had been praying for that to happen.

Lisbeth was stunned. What was Oma-Maria saying? Could it really be so? Why could it not be so? Suddenly it became very clear to her. Yes, that could very well be the reason for her tiredness. She turned to Oma-Maria, exclaiming, "Wouldn't that be just wonderful? I never thought I would feel like that. You are a smart lady, Oma. I hope you are right, but let's wait and see and not say anything yet. If I am pregnant, I'll be so excited. But I'll wait, then see the doctor, and then tell Lorenzo." The two women hugged again, hoping that Oma's wishes would indeed come true. Raul saw them giggling and hugging in the carriage behind him, and, though not knowing why, he too felt lighthearted and happy.

As they approached the vineyard, Oma-Maria told Lisbeth a little of its history. Her father, Roberto, had been called a fool when he converted 15 acres of his land to raising grapes. His own father had planted this seed of an idea when Roberto was just a boy. Remembering vineyards back in Germany, he always felt the climate and soil conditions in this area would be perfect for grape growing. However, he never had the time or the money to invest in a new and risky venture. He continued to farm and raise cattle as all the other immigrants in the area were doing. But in his heart he kept his dream alive and passed that dream on to his son. Roberto, upon inheriting the land, took the bold step and began planting a vineyard. The neighbors in this valley called his vineyard *"Locuro de Roberto"* (Roberto's folly) but that did not deter him. By the time Oma-Maria was born, the vines had matured. To his delight and the surprise of his friends and neighbors, Roberto had managed several successful harvests. To this day the vines thrived and produced a profitable crop. Oma-Maria was very proud of her father's determination and hard work as others began to follow in his footsteps. Now there were several other vineyards in the area, and all found a market for their products. The grapes were sold to a winemaker whose own vineyard lay closer to the coast, just south of Buenos Aires. Since her father's death, the vineyard had belonged to Oma-Maria. She had been leasing the *Locuro de Roberto*, as it was still called, to another grape-grower who was most pleased with the arrangement. It was from this place that Oma-Maria now received her income and was able to live independently.

Lisbeth was fascinated by this story and also amazed at Oma-Maria's own farsightedness and good business sense. "What a beautiful place!" Lisbeth exclaimed as she saw the vineyard spread before her in the valley and up the gently sloping hills. "I have never seen anything like this in my whole life," she thought as she marveled at the rows and rows of vines, tied to supports and wires. "Like soldiers marching in a parade." She slid off the carriage seat and ran down to inspect the grape vines more closely. Huge grape clusters hung heavily from the vines. "Oh, how beautiful it is here! I am so happy you brought me here. I simply could not imagine your vineyard before."

Oma-Maria smiled with great satisfaction. For some strange reason it was very important to her that Lisbeth liked this special spot on earth. This vineyard meant more to her than the rest of the whole *estancia* which she had already turned over to her son José.

"Tell me, Oma, why do you lease it out to strangers? Wouldn't José or Lorenzo want to operate this beautiful place?" Lisbeth asked.

Sadly the old woman shook her head. "You know, José is more interested in his horses and is much happier in the horse business. And Lorenzo, well, he is still young. Maybe some day he will decide to continue in the wine business. For now, I am happy with the arrangements as they are, and I'm so glad that you like this place too. I was always very close to my father, and here in the vineyard I feel that he is still with me."

"I understand perfectly. When I'm in Buenos Aires and see the opera house, I think of my father too and feel that part of him is right there with his chandeliers. Also, remember my mother's roses? I planted them and take care of them. It is as if part of my Mutti were right here in our garden—although they are not doing as well as hers back home." The women embraced. No words were necessary. They understood each other perfectly.

The next few weeks passed quietly as Lisbeth kept her hope and secret to herself. She busied herself with sewing, writing endless letters to her family and Tante Anni, concentrating on her lessons and spending every moment she could with Lorenzo. She looked forward to going to the movies with him as she was beginning to understand more of the language, and did not begrudge his card games or occasional evenings out with his friends. Her rides into town with Oma-Maria and her visits with Juliana continued to be a very important part of her new life. Feelings of homesickness still washed over her, but instead of giving in to tears, she tried to think happy thoughts: her family's promised visit in a few years and the probability of new life growing within her. "I have so much to be thankful for," she thought to herself as she walked into the garden for her daily visit with her mother's roses.

EIGHTEEN

It was February 1937 and Marianne felt restless. The holidays had been a subdued affair this year but had kept her busy. Now everything was quiet again, and she felt at loose ends. Margarete was seldom home, busy with her studies, voice lessons and rehearsals. Wilhelm spent full days at the office and even when at home, he seemed quiet and introspective. The weather was dreary and cold; even looking at her garden, she was sad. Everything looked bleak and barren, her rose bushes nothing but sticks. Not only did she miss her Lisbeth, today she missed everyone; it seemed they were all detached from her. As she looked across the yard toward the garage, she saw the lights on in Johann's apartment. On impulse, Marianne slipped into her coat and walked across the garden. In all the years Johann and Trudi had lived there, Marianne had never visited. But today she needed someone, anyone, to talk to.

Johann came rushing down the stairs, an anxious look on his face. "Good day, Frau Lindemann. Is everything all right? What can I do for you?" he asked, concerned.

"Oh, Johann, nothing really. I just saw your light on and thought I would stop by for a few minutes," she muttered.

"Of course, come in," Johann invited her, wondering why or what he had done to receive such a visit. His living room was small but inviting. Apparently he had been reading the newspapers as they were spread on the floor as well as on his easy chair. Quickly he gathered up the papers, apologizing for the disarray. As Marianne settled on the sofa opposite him, Johann offered to make a cup of tea for them. He disappeared into his tiny but spotless kitchen as Marianne relaxed and looked around. Memories of Trudi were everywhere. The handmade pillows, the crocheted doilies on the tables, a photograph of a smiling young Trudi taken many years ago. As Johann brought a tray with two steaming cups of tea, Marianne sighed deeply and blurted out the question: "How are you doing so well all alone since Trudi's death? Here I am with my family all around me, and yet I was so lonely today, I just had to come over and talk with you."

Johann smiled sadly. "I miss her every day. But strange as it sounds, I know she is still here with me. I feel her all around me. I talk to her, and I know she answers me. I try to keep the apartment as she would like. I cook as she taught me, and as long as I can live here I am not really lonely. I have my work, and I am so grateful for that. I have your family nearby. You are my family now. I hope you don't mind," he added modestly.

"No, no, Johann. We feel the same about you. You belong to us, and we need each other. That is why I came today. I needed you to help me. I was so lonely for Lisbeth, and the others are so busy. Johann, I feel better already."

They sat in companionable silence for a while, then Johann rose and opened a small drawer in his old battered desk. "Here is the last letter I received from Lisbeth," he said, handing her the envelope. Marianne was surprised. She had no idea that Lisbeth had written to him. "Yes, she wrote me for Christmas," he said proudly. "Your girls have always been special to me, and I am happy Lisbeth has not forgotten me."

Marianne smiled and began reading the letter. She was proud of her daughter for including a lonely old man in her new world. They chatted on for a while, giving each other hope and courage. "I'll have to be patient for two more years," Marianne was saying. "We promised Lisbeth a visit as soon as Margarete graduates. I just wish she weren't so far away. Sometimes I wish we had never let her go."

"Oh, Frau Lindemann, the time will pass quickly. But you know how happy she is with her husband. You can't deny her that happiness, even if it is hard for us to let her go. And perhaps..." he waved his hand over the newspapers. "There is nothing but propaganda in the papers. Times are not going to get better. Perhaps Lisbeth is safer where she is." Johann bit his tongue. He should not have voiced his worrisome thoughts, but Marianne seemed not to have heard him anyway.

"Here comes the postman," she shouted excitedly. "Maybe there is a letter from our Lisbeth. Thank you for the tea and the kind words. Thank you for being there for me," she added, and forgetting her usual reserve, gave him an impulsive hug. Hurriedly she ran downstairs, full of anticipation.

"I just hope there is a letter," Johann prayed as he cleared away the tea things and got ready to pick up Wilhelm from the office.

Wilhelm meanwhile sat at his desk waiting for Kurt. The young man was seldom late for a meeting, but that did not disturb Wilhelm today. He had not really concentrated on his own work either; for some reason his thoughts scattered in all directions. A sizeable order had come in yesterday from a major contractor in Bavaria who was building a large hotel. Happy though he was that his business was still doing well, he was beginning to have some concerns. More and more of his young apprentices were being called to military training, and he saw that as a loss for the future. But at least he had not lost any more of his key personnel. Today his thoughts were more of a private nature, missing his Lisbeth and seeing Marianne quiet and lonesome. But there was nothing he could do except promise them both a visit to Argentina as soon as Margarete finished her course of study. How proud he was of Margarete! Nothing made him happier than seeing his daughter reach her goals in her singing career. He hardly saw her these days, but he knew she was happy, as busy as she was. Her free time was spent with Peter, and why not? She deserved her happiness.

A sharp knock on his door stirred him from his daydreams. Kurt entered, his face flushed as if he had been running. "I'm sorry I'm late," he apologized as he pulled a chair closer to Wilhelm's desk. "Ah, what a day! Nothing but problems!"

"What is going on today that has you so rattled?" Wilhelm asked, knitting his brows. "We just got a large order. That should make you happy and keep us going strong."

"Yes, yes, that is good news. I am always happy when orders come in," Kurt said. "The factory is running smoothly. That's not the problem."

"Then what is?" Wilhelm wanted to know, and Kurt, sighing deeply again, leaned back and told him the story. Earlier in the afternoon, when Kurt had stepped into the "silvering room" of the mirror division, he saw two of his men involved in a serious discussion, bending over some papers. Thinking there was some sort of problem with the work process, Kurt stepped up behind them to offer his help. In the noise of the workroom, the men did not hear Kurt. Suddenly seeing him, they jumped apart, startled and alarmed. One of the men quickly folded up the paper and shoved it into his pocket.

"Is there a problem? Can I help you?" Kurt inquired. But the men just shook their heads and looked uncomfortable.

As Kurt began to walk away, the older one, Gustav Reiner, touched Kurt's sleeve and called him back with his eyes. "We were just talking, we, we, ah, we were just talking about Max, you know, Max Vogelsang, our old plant manager..."

"Oh, yes, Max. Have you heard from him lately?" Kurt wanted to know.

"Oh no, no, we have not heard from him. We don't even

know where he is really. But we were just talking about him, how smart he was, and how lucky for him that he could move away."

Kurt looked at them stupidly, not understanding what they were talking about. Then slowly he realized that both men standing before him came from Jewish backgrounds, both Gustav and Erich Adler. Alarmed, Kurt asked, "What are you talking about? Are you planning on leaving too?"

Both men fell silent. Finally Gustav spoke. "Erich and I, we also feel we need to leave this country, but we just cannot do it."

"Why not? I do not understand any of this."

"Herr Walter, it is all very simple. Hard as we try, we simply do not have enough money to take our families and leave. We have sold all we had that was valuable, some jewelry, some gold coins, but it is not enough. There is nobody we can borrow from. There is just no way. Can you help us? Is there any way?" Reiner's eyes were pleading. Kurt stood motionless for several minutes. He knew what the men were saying: "Help us, or we will die here."

Kurt looked at the men's faces and saw their anguish. They had both been loyal workers at Lindemann's long before Kurt joined the firm. He didn't know what to say to them. He honestly did not know what he could do for them. Finally he found his voice and told them, "I will talk to Herr Lindemann himself. Maybe he will have some ideas. Maybe he can find a way." With that, he turned and walked away, his heart hammering in his chest.

There was silence in the room as Kurt finished his story. He looked at his boss inquiringly. Wilhelm tented his hands under his chin as if searching for an answer. Finally he said, "Kurt, is there a way the annual bonus could be paid out earlier? Is there a way our firm could pay these men their vacations earlier? That is all I can think of just now. See what you can do. Do some calculations, and let's see if those amounts would help Gustav and Erich. Find out who else in the plant is in the same situation. See what you can find out and do it quietly. We can't have everyone requesting early payouts. But this situation is serious, and I cannot ignore it. If I can, I will help them." Kurt had always respected and admired Wilhelm, but never more than at this moment. Quietly he rose with the promise to come up with some figures in the next few days.

Wilhelm remained in his chair motionless. His head was spinning. His heart was beating frantically. "What next, what next?" he thought. "If this continues, we will have to close the plant or parts of it." But the immediate problem was foremost in his mind, how to help the people on whom he had depended for so many years. He shook his head, his mind clearing. "We will find a way. There must be a way to do it, even if I have to take it out of my own pocket," he resolved. With that he walked out of the office, hoping Johann was waiting for him.

The day that had begun gloomy and stressful for both Marianne and Wilhelm had a happy ending. There had been a letter from Lisbeth in the postman's bag, Margarete had a rare night off, and Marianne was now happily cooking a special dinner for her family. Wilhelm had come to a simple decision while riding home with Johann. Whatever Kurt's calculations, he would provide the extra funds needed for his employees' daring step into an uncertain future. Wilhelm had worked hard all his life and had achieved great financial success. But he had not done it alone; he had done it with the help of loyal and dedicated people. Money was only important for what one could do with it, Wilhelm thought, and at this time he was prepared to use some of it to help his devoted workers. He knew it was simply the right thing to do. That decided, he relaxed and chatted easily with Johann. The chauffeur happily related that a letter had arrived from Lisbeth and that he had had an especially nice visit with Marianne that day. This news in particular cheered Wilhelm and he could not wait to get home to his family.

In the end, the little exodus from Lindemann's Glass Works went quickly and smoothly. A total of seven workers and their families were thrilled and grateful at Wilhelm's incredible solution. With the vacation and bonus payouts and the additional funds Wilhelm so generously provided, they were able to quit their jobs with dignity, pack up their belongings and buy train tickets to a new life. They were anxious and uncertain but hopeful and calmly elated. Thankfully and with tears in their eyes, they shook hands one more time, wishing each other the best and muttering *auf Wiedersehen*, although they knew that would never be. Wilhelm was touched by their courage and determination, and it was difficult to know who was happier or more grateful, the giver or the receivers.

NINTEEN

On their next weekly excursion to Baradera, Lisbeth turned to Oma-Maria and declared, "Guess what? You were right, Oma! Do you remember our conversation at the vineyard? I know I am pregnant! But this morning, let's go to Dr. Mesta's clinic to be sure." Oma-Maria dropped the horse's reins and hugged Lisbeth fiercely. She clapped her hands and laughed out loud. "Bravo, bravo. That is wonderful." She just couldn't contain herself with happiness. Fortunately, the horse knew his way and trotted along placidly.

In Baradera, Oma headed right to the clinic where she let Lisbeth off. Then she continued to the boarding stables and walked with a quick step and a smile on her face toward the library.

"Where is Lisbeth today?" Alma wanted to know, prepared to begin her lesson.

"Oh, she will be a little late. She went to see Dr. Mesta this morning first," Oma replied, winking and placing a finger on her lips. Alma smiled knowingly and invited Oma-Maria for a cup of *mate* (tea) in the back room. They had a lot of catching up to do.

As Lisbeth came out of the doctor's office, she practically collided with an older woman coming down the street. It was Fernanda, the town gossip. According to her friend Juliana, if you wanted any news spread about town, you told Fernanda. She had actually acquired the nickname "Radio Fernanda."

"Pardon, pardon," Lisbeth smiled as she quickly ran toward the library. She couldn't wait to tell Oma-Maria the great news. She knew it and yet she was too excited to really believe it. "Yes, yes! I'm really going to have a baby. We must go home and tell Lorenzo right away. September, September—it isn't really that far away." Arriving at the library, she was almost out of breath. Bursting in, she saw Oma-Maria with Alma in the back room. There was no one else in the little library. But even if there had been, Lisbeth did not care. "Oma, I have good news!" she proclaimed. "Let's go home right away. I must tell Lorenzo!" With that she pulled Oma-Maria up from her chair. There was no time for a lesson with Alma today. Alma smiled knowingly, sharing the joy of the young woman she had come to love.

Lorenzo was sitting in the small office behind the horse barns, working on the breeding records. His father kept meticulous notes on each individual horse from birth to sale. He chronicled every detail from genetics to weight gain and development, body measurements to temperament. Lorenzo found this process tedious and boring, but José was adamant. When he sold a filly to be trained as a race horse, he could tell the buyer everything he might need to know about that particular animal. He found it a most helpful selling and training tool. As José was trying to teach Lorenzo every aspect of the horse business, he insisted that Lorenzo actually do the work himself as part of his training and education. Lorenzo tended to trust the various jobs to his workers and was more interested in negotiating the ultimate sale. Of course, what he enjoyed most was going to the races with his father and his friends. Today Lorenzo was staring out the window, not in the mood to record what, to him, seemed like insignificant details. He had a good view of the road leading up to *Bien Cielo* and spotted his Nonna's carriage coming up the hill. "Why is she coming back so early?" he questioned. He knew that on the day she and his wife went into town, they usually spent most of the day there, missing the family's main mid-day meal. Curious, he stepped outside just as they were about to pass the stables. When Lisbeth saw him, she waved wildly, jumping off the carriage before it had even come to a complete halt.

"Lorenzo, Lorenzo, I have some exciting news to tell you," she called, running into his arms. "We're having a baby," she whispered in his ear, hugging him and jumping at the same time.

"Wait, slow down, really? We are having a baby?" he asked incredulously. Then a happy grin spread across his handsome face, and Lisbeth could swear she saw his eyes misting with happiness. "I love you. I love you!" is all he could say, kissing her and twirling her around as if she were a child herself. Oma-Maria still sat in the carriage, the reins slack in her hands, sharing in the happy moment. How blessed she felt for having lived long enough to see yet another generation!

That day the mid-day meal was particularly festive. Although Marta had only prepared the usual soup, bread and beef stew, Lorenzo brought out a special bottle of wine, *Locuro,* made from the grapes of Nonna's vineyard. José and Cecilia were beaming at the news, congratulating Lorenzo and kissing "Lissabetta." In the excitement, no one bothered to translate the rapid Spanish conversation to Lisbeth, but she knew they were all happy and excited. She heard the words *Bebe, Septembre,* Dr. Mesta, and other words she understood sprinkled throughout the meal, and comprehended the Number One topic. Exhilarated but tired, Lisbeth was finally able to leave the table and head upstairs with Lorenzo to their private quarters. Never had a siesta sounded so good to her before, and soon she closed her eyes and relaxed in the comforting arms of her husband.

He looked at his wife sleeping peacefully in his embrace and felt overwhelmed with tenderness and love for her. Soon they would have a child, become a real family. He hoped it would help Lisbeth overcome her feelings of loneliness and homesickness for her family. He began fantasizing about the child but he could not see himself as a father just yet. Perhaps they would have a son. What would they name him? Or a daughter? Slowly his eyes closed and with a smile he too drifted off to sleep.

The next day Lisbeth was busy writing letters. She could not wait to share her news with family and friends back home, as well as her Tante Anni in New Jersey. She called Paulina and Emilio Alvarez, excited that she could tell them in person.

When she and Oma-Maria drove into town the following week, Lisbeth stopped at the post office first to tell Juliana. Juliana giggled happily and congratulated Lisbeth, but did not seem very surprised. It seems that "Radio Fernanda" had already done her broadcasting. Just having seen Lisbeth leave Dr. Mesta's clinic was enough for Fernanda to break the news to everyone. Of course, Lorenzo and his parents as well as Oma-Maria had told their friends and neighbors. Lisbeth did not really mind that the whole town seemed to know about her pregnancy. Everyone she knew and met was happy for them and wished her well. It was the second time in less than a year that the Moncrief family was making news in the area. First Lorenzo's marriage in a far-away place, depriving them of a wedding celebration. Now the news of a baby was a topic everyone enjoyed talking about.

There was one person who was angry and upset about the events at *Bien Cielo*. Ever since Lorenzo had returned with his foreign bride, life had been miserable for Elena. She had been bitter and dissatisfied every single day. "Why did Lorenzo take that damn trip to Europe? Why did he marry a girl he had only known a few weeks? Why did he bring this blonde stranger here and expect me to accept her, or even like her? It should have been me, me! Lorenzo is mine! All I want is Lorenzo! I will never accept her, never! And now she is pregnant, and everyone in town is happy for them." Elena dwelled on the past, reliving the times she had spent with Lorenzo. She knew that he loved her, only her, and kisses do not lie! Her anger flared towards anyone who even mentioned Lisbeth's name. She became more withdrawn, was unkind and bad-tempered even toward the customers in the cantina.

Her father had tried to reason with her, telling her to let go. But Elena refused. She continued to scheme and plot revenge. The fact that Lorenzo was married did not deter her at all. Learning that Lisbeth was pregnant only presented a new challenge to her. She would bide her time, but she promised herself to get Lorenzo back one day, whatever it would take. She had loved him for as long as she could remember, and somehow she would succeed in regaining his love.

Unaware of the evil brewing nearby, Lisbeth basked in her happiness. Lorenzo became even more attentive to her, taking long walks with her and offering to drive her wherever she wanted to go. The horseback riding was put on hold for the time being, and even the rides in Oma-Maria's buggy were curtailed. But Lisbeth did not mind. She knew everyone was concerned with her welfare and that of the baby. She couldn't wait for September when she could hold her baby in her arms. But until then there was so much to do, and Lisbeth woke to each new day with excitement and happy anticipation.

TWENTY

It was early April and still cool in Hamburg. But today there was no wind, and a pale sun struggled through the thin clouds. Marianne was in her garden when Lisbeth's letter with the happy news arrived. Marianne needed to be outside; if nothing else, she had to begin her spring clean-up. Dry shriveled leaves from the old apple tree in the corner were embedded in the rose bushes. Johann had offered to help her, but Marianne was anxious to be outside and do the work herself. She had barely started when she saw the postman walking toward her neighbor's house. She dropped the rake and ran to the postbox. Sure enough, there were two letters from Lisbeth along with a mountain of papers and mail that held no interest for her. Running back to the veranda, she dropped everything but the letter addressed to her and sat down on the dusty bench. As she began reading, tears of happiness ran down her cheeks. She laughed and cried at the same time, reading and rereading the contents.

"A baby! Oh, I'm so happy! We are having a

grandchild!" she said out loud to herself. Excitedly she jumped up and ran into the house, ready to call Wilhelm at his office. But then she stopped. "No, this is much too important to tell him on the telephone," she thought. She wanted him to read the exciting news himself. With renewed vigor she went back to her rose garden, raking and trimming, while her mind was already on what she could make and buy to mail to Lisbeth and her precious baby. When a few hours later she saw Johann drive out of the garage to pick up Wilhelm, she went inside and took a relaxing bath. Then she dressed in the new spring dress she had just bought the week before, fluffed up her hair, and put on her good pearls. When *Opa* came home, he would meet a happy *Oma*.

> April 1937
> Dear Lisbeth:
> Thank you, thank you for your letter with your exciting news. I am just thrilled for you both and wish you the best. How are you feeling? I wish I could see you and watch you grow.
> Mutti and Papa cannot stop talking about their grandchild. They have told absolutely everyone they know. I know Mutti will start knitting and shopping tomorrow. She even talks about sending you a baby carriage. Papa said he hopes you have a good doctor. Please reassure them so they won't worry. I am sure Lorenzo and his whole family are all very happy for you, and I hope they all take good care of you.
> Everything is fine here. I keep very busy with rehearsals as well as my studies, and I love every minute of it. The new season will begin in the fall, and I hope I will be ready by then. Peter sends his congratulations and best wishes.

Please write again soon. We love and miss you.
Margarete

May 1937
Dear Margarete:
Your letter arrived yesterday and my friend Juliana brought it here to Bien Cielo. Thank you. I love hearing all the news, even if there is no news.

Soon you will finish your spring semester and I hope you will have a little free time between rehearsals and voice lessons. Will you have any vacation this summer?

Remember how much fun we had last summer? It is hard for me to believe that only last year I met Lorenzo and got married! Now we are expecting our baby and I am very happy. Lorenzo says he can hardly wait until his son is born. How does he know? Frankly, I am hoping for a girl. But we will love whatever we have.

It is fun thinking of names. There is still so much to do to get ready. One of the smaller rooms next to our bedroom will be the nursery. Oma-Maria will help me make new drapes, and next month I will join Lorenzo and his father on my last trip to Buenos Aires before the baby comes. Then we will buy the baby bed and whatever we still need to make the room pretty.

I know Paulina will help me, but I wish you were here as well. But I am counting the months until you graduate in two years and will come and visit us. I am feeling well and have gained some weight. I can feel the baby move now, and Dr. Mesta says I am healthy and will do just fine. I am a little nervous about the birth, but Juliana tells me not to worry. And really, I am too happy to be worrying. I will leave that to Mutti!

I am still busy with my Spanish lessons, and Alma says I do very well. It is true—I am beginning to feel much more confident and not embarrassed when I make mistakes. Everyone is very helpful.

Now my dear sister, please give my love to everyone

and write again soon. I will write again when I return from Buenos Aires. Then I will have more to write about. Greetings and love to all!
   Lisbeth and Baby

The week spent in Buenos Aires was uneventful but quite productive. With Paulina's help, everything needed to furnish the nursery was purchased. Lisbeth was overwhelmed with the number of things a baby required. Lorenzo left the shopping pretty much to the women and occupied himself with business matters. But it pleased him that Lisbeth was so happily involved in preparing for their child. She had blossomed in her present state and was more beautiful than ever. He couldn't keep his eyes off her, and it was obvious to all who knew him that Lorenzo was one happy and proud father-to-be. Lisbeth basked in his love and attention.

The days and weeks slipped one into another while Lisbeth lived in a state of pleasant anticipation. One day Lorenzo brought home a large box that had arrived at the station earlier that day. Paulina had found some German books and magazines in the city for her. She was glad of the new reading material, even though the magazines were outdated. She was also expecting the crate to arrive from her parents soon. What fun it would be to unpack all of her mother's treasures! She really missed her daily rides but walked down to the stables daily to bring Fritzi some sugar cubes. One of the ranch hands groomed Fritzi and rode her every day. She still went into Baradera once or twice a week for her lessons and her mail pick-up. But now Oma-Maria came to *Bien Cielo*, and Manuel drove the women into town.

Sometimes Lisbeth longed for more independence and had approached Lorenzo about teaching her to drive the car. Lorenzo had stared at her with uncomprehending eyes. "You want to drive the car? Why would you? You have me or José, or Manuel to drive you to town, to the doctor, shopping, your lessons or your post office stops. I don't understand—why do you want to drive?"

It was too difficult for Lisbeth to explain it to him. She simply did not have the words to describe her longing to be herself, to be free, to be independent and self-sufficient. From the tone of his voice she understood perfectly that whatever else he would give her, driving lessons were not on the list. For the moment she could accept that, but she continued to nurse the hope that one day he would change his mind. Today she would have loved to visit Juliana on the spur of the moment. She couldn't walk that far in her condition; she had no bicycle even if she were allowed to ride it. Oma-Maria and her little carriage were taboo at the moment. Of course, she could ask someone to drive her into town, but today it seemed too much bother.

One day after writing four long letters, Lisbeth did ask Juan to drive her to the post office. There was no urgency in mailing her letters, but she felt the need to have a visit with Juliana and baby Teresa. She hoped Juliana was not busy and would have time for a cup of tea and a chat. Quite often she practiced new words with Juliana and learned new phrases with her. Sure enough, Juliana was overjoyed to see her. Teresa was sleeping soundly in her crib, and things were quiet. Juliana poured a steaming cup of herbal tea for

Lisbeth, and they settled down to talk. Juliana gently touched Lisbeth's belly and felt the baby move. Both women smiled and relished the miracle of the life within. This peaceful moment was shattered by the slamming of the general store door. Juliana rose and looked through the window from her office. The grocery clerk was nowhere to be seen, but the customer coming down the aisle was headed toward the post office anyway.

With a feeling of dread Juliana saw that it was Elena Ruiz. What a misfortune, just as Lisbeth was visiting her here! It was general knowledge that Elena was jealous of the new Señora Moncrief, a name she had assumed would be hers one day. People remembered how she had ranted and raved at the news of Lorenzo's marriage, how she claimed that he had told her he loved her. It was a delicate subject, and so far people had tried to shield Lisbeth from Elena's vicious tongue. Juliana did not know what to do at this moment. She tried to stand in front of Lisbeth, but Elena had already spotted her sitting near the baby's crib. She began yelling at Juliana, then looked at Lisbeth with venom in her eyes, screaming, *"Putta, Putta!"* (Whore). Then Elena turned abruptly and slammed the door on her way out. Juliana was stunned. She put her arm around Lisbeth and spoke soothingly, but Lisbeth was in shock. She understood very well that Elena hated her.

Lisbeth decided not to tell Lorenzo about her second bad encounter with Elena. Yet she could not get it out of her mind. Finally, days later, she discussed it with Oma-Maria. At first Oma tried to appease her by telling her Elena's outburst had nothing to do with her. But Lisbeth did not believe her.

"She looked directly at me as she was yelling that word. *Putta!* I am sure it is a bad word. I asked Cecilia, and she told me never to use it." Lisbeth was near tears. "Why is she so mean to me? Is she Lorenzo's old girlfriend? What does she want from me? My husband?" Lisbeth had finally put her fears into words.

Oma-Maria sadly shook her head. "Didn't Lorenzo tell you about her? What a temper she has? They grew up together, went to school in Baradera together, but later when he went away to school he hardly saw her. Perhaps they liked each other, but that is all. There never was anything serious between them. I know that for certain. Maybe Elena was hoping for more, but I know Lorenzo had no serious intentions toward her. I know that he loves only you. There is nothing for you to worry about."

Somehow that did not sound convincing to Lisbeth, but she did not know how to handle this situation. Baradera was a small town after all, and everyone knew everyone else and their business. She had never been treated like this in her life, and it hurt her a great deal. Tearfully she looked at Oma-Maria, hoping she could help. Oma put her arms around Lisbeth and murmured more consoling words, but in her heart she resolved to speak to her grandson about this matter. This should be the happiest time in their lives, waiting for their first baby. And nothing should mar this happiness, especially a troublemaker like Elena.

"Let's forget about it. It is not worth worrying about. Let's be happy and look forward to many more happy days until our baby comes."

Lisbeth smiled and promised to try, but her heart was

troubled. She needed a lift to put her back in a good mood. A small white envelope with a foreign stamp did the trick.

> *July 1937*
> *Dear Lisbeth:*
> We hope the crate with all the baby things will arrive soon. Knowing how you love to read, I have also sent a few books and magazines. Before long you will be busy with your baby and not have much time. I also wanted to send some newspapers, but Papa says the papers only report bad news.
> How are you feeling? Have you gained much weight? Can you sleep well? Mutti wonders about these things every day. But Papa says you are young and healthy and that all is well. I have a few weeks vacation now and spend much of my time with Peter going to the beach and sailing. Every time we are out on the water, I remember how you and Lorenzo met last summer. How time does fly! So many things have happened to all of us since then!
> We are all fine and can hardly wait for news of your little one. Mutti's garden is beautiful again. It is a good year for roses, she says. How are your rose bushes doing? I keep forgetting to ask. Even Johann asked me about them last week. Be sure to tell us. Johann is well and sends his greetings. Tonight some of Papa's friends are here as well as Kurt, but all they discuss is business and politics. Mutti has gone to bed early, and I wanted to have a visit with you. Is Lorenzo still marking the days on the calendar? It will not be too long now. We love hearing from you and wish you all the best. Love to all of you, especially Oma-Maria who takes such good care of you. We are so glad you have a new Oma.
> *With love,*
> *Margarete*
> *P.S. The wicker baby carriage was shipped in a separate crate.*

Early August 1937
Dearest Margarete,
Yesterday two huge crates arrived at the station. Juan and another ranch hand took the horse and wagon to pick them up. We all had so much fun unpacking last night!

The baby carriage is perfect—no damage. It is so much nicer than the old perambulator Lorenzo and José had brought down from the attic last week. But Lorenzo's old wooden cradle is still beautiful, and we will use it for our little one. All the wonderful blankets and outfits Mutti knit and bought for us made me cry. How sweet of her to select all the right things! Our baby will not want for anything with loving grandparents and aunt as you. Thank you from our hearts.

The baby's room is finished; the angel picture is hanging on the wall and the teddy bear is sitting on the bed waiting. Last but not least, thank you for the great books, magazines and even picture books for the baby! Soon the great day will come.

I think of Mutti and Papa and what wonderful parents they have been to us. I wonder, and I hope that I will be a good mother too. Lorenzo is still marking the calendar, and before long it will be September. I am feeling just fine. I am getting rounder and rounder every day, and the baby is moving all the time, especially when I try to sleep.

Tell Mutti and Johann that we planted the roses according to their instructions. They are not blooming yet, but they have healthy-looking dark leaves. They are still small, but I am sure that by the time of your visit they will be blooming for you. Thank you again for all the precious gifts. Our baby thanks you too. Tell Papa not to worry about the newspapers and the bad news. I very seldom see a newspaper that contains anything about home, and the radio does not broadcast what is going on there. So please keep me informed. Danke schön for everything and for your love.

Auf Wiedersehen! Adios!
Your loving Lisbeth

TWENTY-ONE

One August evening brought more excitement to *Bien Cielo* than ever before. Lisbeth had been tired and sluggish all day, but that was not unusual in recent weeks. Suddenly a fierce pain shot through her abdomen, taking her breath away. Cecilia dropped her embroidery and ran to find her son and her husband. They were sitting in José's den smoking cigars and discussing the latest horse racing news.

"Lorenzo, come quick! Lisbeth is in great pain. We need the doctor!" She ran back to Lisbeth in the parlor and helped her get out of the chair. Just as Lorenzo entered the room, another wave of pain washed over her. "*Cara*, what is it? It's not time for the baby!" he cried, but Lisbeth smiled feebly. "This baby must have a mind of its own," she gasped. "Call the doctor quickly!" She stood unsteadily holding on to her belly. José just stood mesmerized by the scene, unable to move. It suddenly became real to him; the baby they had talked about for months was real. It was about to be born.

"José, help Lorenzo get Lisbeth up to bed. Come on,

move!" Cecilia was suddenly in charge, and the two men began moving as if in a daze. With four strong arms to support her, almost lifting her off the floor, Lisbeth was helped upstairs to her room. Gently Lorenzo and José laid her on the bed as Cecilia came upstairs right behind them. She shooed them out of the room. "Get Dr. Mesta, hurry! Hurry!" She settled Lisbeth comfortably in bed, and, pulling up a chair, sat down holding her hand. "Don't worry, Lissabetta, the doctor will be here soon, and soon you will have your baby," she tried to comfort Lisbeth. But Lisbeth's only thought was, "It's too early. We need two more weeks." Another wave of pain pierced through her as she held on tight to Cecilia.

Meanwhile Lorenzo had sent Juan to pick up Dr. Mesta and the midwife. Usually Dr. Mesta's presence was not required at the local deliveries, but Lorenzo had insisted that he be present at the birth of his child. "*Si, si*, Lorenzo, you are like all first–time fathers. Do not worry. I will be there if that is what you want," Dr. Mesta promised. Lorenzo now ran up the stairs two at a time. "*Bueno*, the doctor is coming!"

Cecilia smiled and kissed Lisbeth's brow. "Everything will be fine. Good luck to you. *Hasta la vista!*" With that she closed the door quietly and went to join José in the parlor. They smiled at each other; soon there would be a grandchild, another Moncrief, an heir to *Bien Cielo*. They sat down in nervous anticipation, prepared for a long night.

Lorenzo's heart was beating so fast he thought it would jump out of his chest. He pulled the chair closer to the bed, then thought better of it and sat on the bed next to Lisbeth.

She clenched her teeth as pain after pain ripped through her body. Lorenzo gently stroked her face, kissing her hair, her cheeks, holding her hand and whispering loving and consoling words. Lisbeth held on tightly, thankful for Lorenzo's presence. She thought without him at her side, she would simply die. She smiled bravely, knowing that with each pain she was getting closer to holding their baby in her arms. "Together we will get though this," she prayed, as another pain took her breath away.

Dr. Mesta was thankful he had promised Lorenzo to attend his child's birth. First babies were often difficult, and this one would have been too much for Frida, the old midwife, to handle alone. He finally persuaded Lorenzo to leave the room and get some rest. So he sat with his parents, drinking endless cups of strong coffee, anxiously listening to the sounds coming from upstairs. Finally, just as the sun rose over the hill behind the Paraná River, Dr. Mesta slowly descended the stairs with a wide smile on his face. "Congratulations," he beamed at Lorenzo, shaking his hand. "You have a beautiful daughter, a perfect little girl."

Amid tears of joy and happy laughter, they all congratulated and hugged each other. Lorenzo started running up the stairs impatiently to see Lisbeth and his baby, but Dr. Mesta held him back gently. "Just a moment, young man, as soon as Frida finishes bathing and dressing her patients she will let us know, and you can go up and see them."

Meanwhile José, the proud grandfather, poured *Pisco* (grape brandy) into four tiny crystal glasses, and despite the early hour, four happy toasts were raised in honor of the new little Moncrief who had joined their family.

When Lorenzo finally saw Lisbeth and the tiny bundle in her arms, he was too overcome to speak. Tenderly he kissed his wife and carefully touched the baby's cheek. "Congratulations, *Madre*," he finally said. Together they unwrapped the blanket and inspected their *bambina*—ten tiny pink fingers and toes, the sweet little body, the perfectly shaped little head with just a hint of blonde fuzz. Carefully they wrapped her up again, and Lorenzo gently placed her in the cradle that had been in the family for two generations. "You are just wonderful, Lisbeth," Lorenzo whispered. "*Gracias, gracias* for our baby. *Te amo.* I love you so much."

Exhausted but exhilarated, Lisbeth closed her eyes. The happiness and contentment she now felt in her own little family was indescribable. Her life was complete. Lorenzo too felt great satisfaction, a new sense of responsibility and a new feeling of self-worth and sheer elation. He was eager to jump on his horse and proclaim to everyone that he was a father.

"Telegrams! I must send telegrams to Germany and New Jersey!" he thought, remembering his promise to Lisbeth. Racing toward Baradera, it suddenly came to him that he didn't even know the name of his baby. "We will decide later," he thought, anxious to share the great news. Forgotten were his hopes for a son, forgotten the old speculations, he basked totally in the happiness his Lisbeth and his daughter had brought to him.

August 18, 1937 To the Lindemann Family
Burgstrasse 47, Hamburg, Germany:

Happy to announce birth of our daughter 5 o'clock this morning. Mother and baby are fine. Much love, Lisbeth and Lorenzo

Being young and healthy, Lisbeth recovered quickly. She basked in the love and attention surrounding her and felt boundless energy in a short time. Nina, a young girl from Baradera, was hired to help her with laundry and bathing the baby. But Lisbeth was content to rock her little one herself and found other little jobs for Nina. "Later on," she thought, "when I resume my riding and my lessons, it will be wonderful having Nina around to help me."

Today as Lisbeth sat nursing her baby, she was struggling with a decision. She and Lorenzo had not decided on the baby's name before Lisbeth gave birth. Now that the baby girl was born, Lorenzo had left the decision solely to her. Although she had thought of a perfect name long ago, she wanted her husband to be part of the decision. But he stood firm. "Whatever you decide to call her will be fine with me."

Now Lisbeth heard Lorenzo's rapid steps on the way up to their rooms. A wide grin appeared on his face as he saw Lisbeth cuddling his tiny daughter. Kissing them both, he sprawled in the opposite chair. "And how are my girls today?" he inquired sweetly.

"Fine, very good, but I have decided that today we must finally give our little darling a name," Lisbeth replied.

"*Bueno!* Is it Maria, is it Manuela, is it Rosalia?" he joked.

"Not quite," Lisbeth smiled, "but you are close."

"Good." Lorenzo leaned forward, touching the baby's

tiny feet. "What will it be?"

"Her name will be Rosalinde. What do you think of that?

"I like it very much. Rosalinde—how did you decide?"

"I have been thinking so much about my parents, how far away they are and how they are missing knowing our baby. I thought about my own mother, now that I am a mother too, and about how much Mutti loves her roses, and about Papa, and our family name, Lindemann. Combining those two names, I came up with Rosalinde, in honor of my parents. What do you think, Lorenzo?"

"I told you, I love the name. It will be perfect for our little doll. Your parents will be so happy, and I think Rosalinde Moncrief sounds elegant and beautiful, just as she is—and her mother!" With that, Lorenzo rose and held his little family in a tight embrace.

Everyone in the family was happy with the name, particularly Oma-Maria, as her name was added as the second name on the birth certificate. All Lisbeth needed to complete her happiness was a letter from home. She was curious about their reaction. She had laughed out loud when the congratulatory telegram had arrived from her parents and sister, wondering if the child had a name. Lisbeth was sure they would be surprised and proud of her choice, showing them how much she loved and missed them. Her Rosalinde would always remind her of home.

TWENTY-TWO

The days flew by as Lisbeth and her baby developed a new routine. Rosalinde was a very calm and contented infant, nursing and sleeping peacefully for hours. Friends and neighbors stopped by almost daily to admire the child. Cecelia was most proud to show off her new granddaughter and could not get enough of holding her. Oma-Maria now came almost daily, eager to help. But with everyone hovering around, and the services of young Nina, there was not much left for her to do. She loved looking in on the baby, then telling Lisbeth she would ride into town to see if there were any letters from her other far-away grandparents.

Today she had brought two letters for Lisbeth who now sat happily reading and rereading the mail from her excited parents. They were overjoyed but sad at the same time, not being able to hold their first grandchild. The choice of name had been a great success. They could not believe how clever and thoughtful their daughter had been in naming her first child in their honor. Lisbeth smiled with happiness as she closed her eyes and tried to picture the scene back home in Hamburg. How proud and happy her parents were, and how they were planning to visit Lisbeth as soon as Margarete graduated!

Oma-Maria sat opposite Lisbeth, gently rocking the baby in her arms. She remembered her own contentment when her son José was born. It seemed only yesterday that her grandson Lorenzo was born. As she sat holding his first child, Oma-Maria felt blessed indeed. "Isn't it amazing," she remarked to Lisbeth, "how you just know what to do once you become a mother! You are such a good mother, Lisbeth. You take such good care of this little one."

"Oh, I am so happy with her. I could just sit and hold her all day. It will be hard not to spoil her," she smiled. "I told Lorenzo she is not breakable, and he is only now beginning to hold her once in a while."

Sometimes Lisbeth could not understand her husband. Although he had been ecstatic at the birth of his daughter, he was now more quiet and composed, leaving the care of Rosalinde to Lisbeth and Nina. When Lisbeth asked him why he was so reluctant to hold and play with the baby, he just said, "Wait until she gets a little older. Then I will teach her things, to ride her pony and things like that. For now, Rosalinde is your baby to play with," kissing the baby gently on the forehead.

Slowly Lisbeth resumed her former activities and her daily rides, sometimes with Lorenzo, but mostly alone. She and Oma-Maria went into Baradera once or twice a week. But each time Lisbeth remembered the wretched encounter with Elena and hoped and prayed not to run into her again.

Elena's nasty tongue was still wagging. She could not endure the thought that Lorenzo and his little family were happy together. When she heard from the local midwife the news of Rosalinde's birth, she hatefully commented to Frida, "So, it is only a girl!" Even seasoned old Frida, who had seen and heard many crude and heartless comments in her life, was shocked beyond words. Fortunately there were many more kind souls in Baradera who had come to love Lisbeth and who shielded her from Elena's attacks. When nagging doubts and worries attempted to crawl into her thoughts, Lisbeth resolutely pushed them aside, concentrating on her love for her husband and child.

One day two months later Lisbeth sat contentedly rocking Rosalinde. Full of wonder she gazed on the beautiful baby in her arms. Rosalinde had the fairest complexion with just a hint of blonde hair. Her cheeks had filled out and glowed a rosy pink. The baby was sleeping peacefully as Lisbeth adored the tender soft eyelids with long curved lashes hiding her big blue eyes.

"What a beauty she will be," Cecilia often said to her son, and Lorenzo smiled proudly and agreed. His little daughter was indeed becoming more beautiful every day.

Tonight the house was very quiet. Lorenzo had left right after dinner to visit friends in town. He promised not to be late, and Lisbeth had even urged him to go. He had been working so hard, and she wanted him to have a little diversion.

Next week, Señor and Señora Alvarez were coming for a short visit, and Lisbeth was sure that it would be a refreshing change for them both. She looked around the living room which was bathed in total silence. José sat reading the newspaper, and Cecilia was working on her embroidery again. Lisbeth often wondered about Cecilia's hobby; there were embroidered pillows everywhere, embroidered blouses, shawls, table linens and napkins. In the beginning, Lisbeth had wondered how Cecilia could continue embroidering day after day without getting bored. Certainly she was in charge of the household, the smooth running of a large complex. At the same time, there were helping hands all around.

Now after living on the *estancia* for a whole year, she realized in some ways her life had been paralleling Cecilia's. In the early days of her life at *Bien Cielo*, Lisbeth had found the leisurely pace appealing, giving her time to sleep late, go riding with Lorenzo, visit in town and take her lessons. But if it were not for the baby and the care she required, Lisbeth suspected that the quiet life in the country could become boring. She was beginning to understand why Cecilia immersed herself in her handiwork. She derived much satisfaction from her accomplishments and thrived on everyone's admiration and praise.

As Lisbeth gathered up her baby and proceeded up stairs, she looked almost enviously at the quiet companionship José and Cecilia shared. Suddenly she missed Lorenzo. "Why can't he spend more quiet evenings at home with us, his family? He is either working or off playing cards with his friends." Before long the horse races would start again, and this year she knew that she would not be going with him. "We'll have to talk about this sometime," she thought as she placed the baby in her crib.

Rosalinde stretched contentedly. As Lisbeth looked down on her, she realized perhaps for the first time the true sense of loss her parents must have experienced at her leaving. Their great love for her had let her go—to Lorenzo, and now to this, her own child. With longing thoughts of home, she finally fell asleep.

When Lisbeth woke the next morning, all was right with her world again. Lorenzo was by her side. "Are you in the mood for a little ride with me this morning?" he asked. Lisbeth, of course, was eager to spend some time with him. "I have to drive into town later. Would you like to come with me, visit with Juliana while I take care of business?"

"Oh, yes, I would love to do that." Yes, it was going to be a wonderful day. Everything was fine, and perhaps there was even a letter waiting for her.

TWENTY-THREE

Another summer is gone, Marianne thought sadly as she raked the leaves under the apple tree. The roses were beautiful again this year. Everyone was well, and August had even brought them a new grandchild. As thrilled as they had been at the news of Rosalinde's birth, there was also great sadness with the realization that they could not really be a part of her life. More and more the ramifications of Lisbeth's marriage and move to a foreign land became clear to Marianne. "When will I see them again? Will this new grandchild ever know us, her mother's family, her homeland, her history?"

Marianne raked harder, pulling at the grass beneath. Every fall as the garden faded and went dormant, Marianne became melancholy and sad. This year was no different. In fact she felt sadder than ever before. There were times she felt useless. "Who needs me anymore?" she thought sadly. "Wilhelm is busy with work and not thinking of retirement." She had to admit she had never really taken an interest in the business. It was just something Wilhelm did. It dawned on her now that she really did not know anything about it, and Wilhelm did not share his problems with her. Margarete was out more than she was home, totally occupied with her own work at the Conservatory as well as at the opera. "If Lisbeth were here with her baby, I would be so happy to spend time with her, take the baby for a walk, see her grow and develop. As it is, I might as well not have a grandchild!" Bitter tears welled up in her eyes as she let herself be drawn in by her sadness.

Johann saw Marianne in the garden and remembered a recent conversation he had had with Wilhelm, who had confided that he was worried about his wife's sadness and loneliness and her inability to accept life as it was. Even the happiness Lisbeth was experiencing did not seem to comfort or cheer Marianne. He had even suggested booking a voyage to Buenos Aires in the spring. But Marianne insisted they wait until Margarete finished her education. "We cannot go now. We cannot leave Margarete. We will not break up the family again. I want to see my whole family together. If we wait, it's only a little over a year, then we can all go together," Marianne had cried, so Wilhelm had agreed that they would wait.

At the same time he had his own worries, his own thoughts about the uncertainty of the times. More and more military personnel were visible in the streets, more and more young men drafted into the armed forces. What was behind all the military buildup? He and Kurt had discussed this on several occasions as the number of his apprentices dwindled. Lately, when he and his Skat buddies gathered to play cards, there was more talking and speculating than card playing. But Wilhelm could not discuss these things with his wife. In fact, he tried to shield her from any more anguish. He too missed Lisbeth greatly and wished he could see her holding his granddaughter in her arms. But he was able to accept the facts as they were, hoping and wishing for the day they would be together again. Margarete was scheduled to finish in the spring of 1939. That was only slightly over a year from now. Wilhelm was willing to wait and pray that Marianne would be able to do the same. In the meantime, he loved looking at Rosalinde's photo which stood prominently on the piano. She reminded him of his own little Liesl, so fair, so blonde, so sweet. His little sister, Anni, had been just as fair. He even thought he saw a resemblance.

As Wilhelm drove home with Johann discussing these things, he resolved to spend more time with Marianne and to find new ways to entertain her. He knew she enjoyed her luncheon meetings with her lady friends, and he resolved to speak to some of them, hoping they too would help him cheer up his wife. Even Johann promised to find a way to help.

Lisbeth was unaware of the disquieting atmosphere back home, just as her parents were unaware of her homesickness and sadness. The letters crossing the ocean in both directions were always cheerful, full of light-hearted words and insignificant details of daily life. Each tried to shield the other from worry or pain.

Christmas was approaching again, and on both sides of the ocean, people were preparing for the feast of peace and good will. Anni's letters were the only sincerely open and happy ones as her life with her husband and three children, their days filled with work and activities, proceeded smoothly and without complication. Anni's light-hearted nature, as well as her great optimism, assumed that everyone in her family, whether in Germany or Argentina, was also well and happy.

For Lisbeth, any letter was a ray of sunshine in her day, but for some reason Tante Anni's letters were always particularly uplifting. She wrote about the simple details of her life, what the children were doing at school, what they liked or did not like, how the plants were doing in the greenhouse, when their busy or quiet season began, who was working for them, and even about their new partner in the nursery operation. After reading Tante Anni's letters, Lisbeth could almost picture their life and their surroundings. How she hoped to meet them all one day as she felt that she knew them already!

New Year's greetings flew across the Atlantic again as everyone looked forward to the future. As Margarete had written, "Now we can honestly say NEXT YEAR! NEXT YEAR we are coming to see you, my dear sister. Next year, when I graduate, we will finally meet our sweet Rosalinde and see you again. It doesn't seem so long now, does it? This year will fly by, and next year we will be together. What a happy thought! In the meantime, what will this year, 1938, bring to all of us?" Everyone was filled with hope and anticipation.

TWENTY-FOUR

The year 1938 began uneventfully for the Lindemanns in Hamburg. After a brief cold spell in January, it became unseasonably warm. Although everyone enjoyed the pleasant temperatures, one knew it was only a matter of time before another violent storm would blow in from the North Sea. But the major storm brewing in the country was of a different nature. When on March 13, German forces annexed Austria, Wilhelm began to understand the *Führer's* preoccupation and campaign for *Lebensraum* (living space). Slowly the reasons for the compulsory military service, for the rearmament of the nation and the emerging political power became clear to him. "What will come next?" he wondered, dropping the newspaper. Still his life was not affected by this news, and all he could do was continue to be aware and alert.

Happy letters continued to arrive from Lisbeth, informing them of her life and the ever-changing news of Rosalinde's growth and the happiness she brought to *Bien*

Cielo. More and more everyone realized that she was a carbon copy of her mother, a sweet and contented child. As Wilhelm was reading the disquieting political news in Germany, Rosalinde was delighting her family by crawling around the house with her happy shrieks of joy. Lisbeth blossomed with motherhood and her new purpose in life. Lorenzo too, no longer afraid to hold his infant daughter, enjoyed her antics and found time to play with her every day. She responded with unbridled love for her Papa and raised her chubby little arms to him, wanting to be held. It was a quiet, peaceful and fulfilling time for the young family. Lisbeth's dreams looked to the future when she could share her happiness with her parents and Margarete.

For Margarete, too, the summer of 1938 was a happy time. Peter had graduated from the Conservatory with every conceivable honor. It was a day they had both eagerly looked forward to. Margarete and his parents were bursting with pride as Peter received his Master Degree. He had already been promised a prestigious job teaching and conducting a student orchestra at an exclusive private *Gymnasium* (high school). He still held fast to his dream of conducting a symphony some day, but at the moment he was eagerly looking forward to the teaching experience and the pleasure of earning a salary. The first step in his and Margarete's plans for the future had been reached. The following year Margarete would be receiving her degree, and it was an unspoken promise between them that they would begin building a life together. The endless hours of work and study, rehearsals and commitments, would finally culminate in joining their lives and dreams forever. Both young people glowed with pride and happiness as Wilhelm and Marianne congratulated Peter who was as dear to them as their own. The future glowed brightly, and the young people felt they were invincible.

In September, Wilhelm read with great interest every detail about the Munich Conference that Britain and France had arranged with Germany and Italy's leaders. In the end, when a peaceful occupation of the Sudentenland, part of Czechoslovakia, was approved, Wilhelm sighed with relief. At least there was hope of maintaining peace. Long discussions with his friends only reaffirmed his hope for a peaceful coexistence with their European neighbors. Any lingering doubts were overcome by the cheerful letter which arrived from Lisbeth a short time later. A new portrait of a smiling Rosalinde was the greatest gift to Wilhelm and Marianne. She carried the photograph with her for weeks, making certain that all her friends, neighbors, the grocer and the postman, had seen her beautiful granddaughter. Lisbeth and Lorenzo, along with Nina and the baby, were planning a vacation to a famous beach resort, Mar del Plata, in the next few weeks. Wilhelm and Margarete immediately began searching on their new and enlarged map of Argentina and found it about 80 kilometers south of Buenos Aires in a secluded bay.

"Today is one of the best days of the whole year," Wilhelm said to his wife as she sat totally relaxed in the chair opposite him. For once there seemed nothing for Marianne to worry about. Both her children were happy. Margarete was walking on clouds these days. Lisbeth sounded perfectly satisfied with her life and family. Wilhelm sat smiling, and totally absorbed in finding La Plata on the map. She herself was now counting the months and the weeks when, next year, they would be planning their reunion trip to Buenos Aires and the long and happy stay ahead. "Call Johann over, Wilhelm! Call Peter, Margarete! Let's all go out and celebrate together. We have so much to be happy about and so much to be thankful for." It was an evening to remember.

> *September 1938*
> *Dear Parents, dear Sister:*
> *Just a short letter this time...we are here at La Plata and it is heavenly! The weather is perfect, blue skies and white sandy beaches. It reminds me of home, but different. The town is pretty too with old buildings, shops and restaurants. Today Lorenzo went out on a fishing expedition. We are having a wonderful time and Rosalinde is a good little traveler. Nina is a great help as Rosalinde is now walking everywhere. This is the first time Nina has been away from home, staying in a hotel. It is a great adventure for her. She loved the train ride as much as our little Rosalinde did. Nina loves Rosalinde a lot and is very good with her. We are so lucky to have her. Hope all is well at home. I have sent our congratulations to Peter. I can just imagine how happy you both must be. Write soon and tell me all the news.*
> *Give our love to everyone.*
> *Your Liesl, Lorenzo & Rosalinde*

TWENTY-FIVE

October was coming to an end and everyone on both sides of the Atlantic began their early holiday preparations once again. Two important events were taking place in the family. The first one, although a surprise, put a spring into everyone's step. After keeping the news to herself for a while, Lisbeth informed the family that she and Lorenzo would once again become parents in the coming spring. She was elated at the news, knowing that Lorenzo and his family in particular, were hoping for a large family. In motherhood, Lisbeth seemed to have found her perfect niche. With Lorenzo at her side, life was perfect!

For the Lindemanns, already excited about their planned trip in the coming year, this news added another bonus. Not only would they be reunited with their daughter and meet Rosalinde, but they would have a chance to hold a new baby in their arms. A telegram was dispatched immediately. When Lorenzo returned from town that afternoon, he grinned happily, throwing Rosalinde in the air and catching her giggling and smiling. "Soon you will have a brother, or a sister, one for Mama, one for me!" he sang exuberantly. Lisbeth smiled quietly. What a wonderful year was ahead of them! A new baby in the spring, Margarete's graduation in the summer, and finally, after all the waiting, her family was coming. She could hardly contain herself.

The second piece of news came closer to Christmas and cast a sad spell over the end-of-year preparations and festivities. In the second week of December 1938, Peter received his draft notice. He had begun teaching on the first of September. He found great satisfaction in his students' progress and performance. At this moment he was busily preparing the student orchestra for the Christmas program. He was well liked by his colleagues and students. He had replaced an elderly, strict professor who was retiring. The students were ready for a young teacher with new ideas and a more contemporary approach to education and music. Getting ready for the Christmas concert was more satisfying to him than his musical debut recital at the Conservatory had been. He was anxious to show off his pupils to the parents, the administration, but especially to his love, Margarete, as well as their families.

At the moment, conducting a major orchestra was the farthest thing from his mind. Working with his young and promising students was the greatest reward Peter could ever have imagined. Everything was falling into place.

The draft notice, requiring him to appear by mid-January, hit Peter like a bolt of lightning. Having been exempt by age and student status, he had given it no thought. Now, having to tell his students after a most successful performance, and having to tell Margarete and their parents were the most difficult things Peter had ever had to do. He knew that his military duty was only for two years, yet it seemed like a lifetime to him. Great joy and great sadness—all in one year! But Peter knew he had no choice. He would do what was required of him, and then life with his beloved Margarete could finally begin.

TWENTY-SIX

In the week following New Year's Day 1939, Lisbeth received a long letter from her sister. Usually happy and upbeat, Margarete wrote for the first time the way she truly felt. She was sad, upset and angry. Peter's draft notice had surprised and shaken her. Not her Peter, not now, when everything was so perfect for them! She had felt so happy for him, excited by his new position. After only a few months, teaching had become more than just a job for him. It was just not fair to tear him away from his students at the very beginning of his career. Peter's looming two-year absence was the most difficult for Margarete to accept. Peter was trying his best to console her, but Lisbeth could tell that her sister was inconsolable. She had so looked forward to when they could finally have time for each other and could plan their future together. Everything was in suspension now; two years without him seemed like an eternity.

Peter was equally perturbed at this turn of events, but he knew he had no choice but to perform his duty. He was not alone; everyone in his age group was being called or had already left. All Peter and Margarete could do was to enjoy the last precious days together, pray for his safety and hope for a furlough.

Feeling Margarete's pain, Lisbeth cried as she read her sister's letter. She looked at the calendar. Peter would be leaving in a few days. How she wished she could hold her sister in her arms and comfort her! She could well imagine their feelings of uncertainty, loss and fear. She remembered her own longing for Lorenzo when he had sailed ahead of her and she was left behind waiting for her passport to arrive. The days had seemed endless, and recalling her own ache and loneliness brought tears to her eyes for Margarete and Peter. When would they see each other again?

Determined to cheer her sister up, she sat down to answer the letter. But what could she really say that would help? All she could do was to write about Rosalinde's antics, about her daily life. She stressed all that was positive in Margarete's life, her own upcoming graduation, and ultimately the trip to Argentina later in the year. Mostly she reminded her sister of the great love between Peter and her and that this love could overcome all the obstacles and help survive this delay in the fulfillment of their dreams. After all, Lisbeth had gone through a similar painful, although much shorter, separation. Now all her dreams had come true, and she wished the same for her sister. Lisbeth leaned back in her chair. Yes, everything had worked out well for her. She had her loving husband and sweet daughter, and now she was happily waiting for her second child. She began dreaming about all the wondrous events that would take place in her life this year. She hoped that Margarete would remember that she too had good things to look forward to, despite Peter's absence.

Sealing the letter, she kissed her sleeping Rosalinde and went off in search of Lorenzo or Manuel to drive her to Baradera. Once more she wished she could learn to drive. But she knew from her previous request that this topic was not up for discussion with Lorenzo.

"I'm so glad there is no military service here in Argentina!" she suddenly thought as she saw Lorenzo coming out of the stable office. "I would die without him!" she said to herself running into his arms.

After Peter's departure the days dragged for Margarete. She thought of him constantly and could not focus on her studies. The rehearsals and singing in the opera chorus had suddenly lost all the luster and excitement she had felt before. She spent her free time reading or just brooding in her room. When Peter's first letter finally arrived after four weeks of unrelenting basic training, Margarete cried with joy. Finally she knew where her Peter was, at a remote military base in the eastern part of Germany. He wrote about the hardships of learning to become a soldier, but also about the many friendships developing among his comrades. Most of all, he wrote of his love for her and the hope of seeing her again. When that might happen was uncertain, but it was enough for Margarete at least to be able to communicate with him by post.

She wrote him daily, and as the letters started arriving from him on a more regular basis, her mood and attitude improved greatly. She finally understood her mother's preoccupation with the mail after Lisbeth had moved away two and a half years ago. It seemed to Wilhelm that his household revolved around the daily arrival of the postman. The atmosphere was either gloomy or bright, depending on the contents of the postman's large leather bag. Wilhelm was becoming more anxious, more interested than ever in the daily news reports of national and world events.

Margarete's next letter to Lisbeth was much more cheerful. She was adjusting to Peter's absence and seemed more confident about the future. She was looking forward to the birth of Lisbeth's new baby and wrote with her former enthusiasm about her studies and the graduation coming up in July. She even mentioned a possible travel date for the long-awaited visit with Lisbeth and her family. It appeared that the early part of September would suit everybody, and Papa and Kurt were looking into the scheduling and possibility of traveling on the *Neue Welt*, the same ship that had taken Lisbeth to Buenos Aires almost three years ago. Lisbeth's heart jumped with joy. Finally! It was really going to happen.

Instead of putting Rosalinde into her crib for an afternoon nap, Lisbeth dressed her and placed her in her German baby carriage for a walk to Oma-Maria's house. She needed to share her good news with someone who would genuinely join in her happiness. She would tell Lorenzo and his parents at dinnertime. For now it was more important to see Lorenzo's grandmother who had become like her own.

She tucked Rosalinde securely into the carriage and was thankful for its solid construction. The two-kilometer walk up to Oma-Maria's house was easy, winding up a gentle slope, but the road was rough and gravelly, and required a sturdy carriage. Whenever Lisbeth set out on a walk with her baby, she remembered her parents and thanked them for this well-made vehicle which provided Lisbeth and her baby a certain amount of independence. She trotted happily up the hill to share her good news.

In a few weeks there would be a new baby to love, and it would be Nina who would take Rosalinde for her walks. What she looked forward to today was a good chat with Oma-Maria, not to giving birth to her child later that night. But that is exactly what happened. Returning home later that afternoon, Lisbeth went into sudden, hard labor, filling *Bien Cielo* with nervous excitement. After only a few hours, shortly after the midwife had been summoned, Lisbeth gave birth to another beautiful, strong and healthy daughter.

The birth was so sudden that Lisbeth could hardly believe what was happening until she held her screaming, red-faced baby in her arms. She was relieved and thankful for the quick delivery, smiling as she waited for Lorenzo to come upstairs and meet his second child. Quietly, almost shyly, he opened the bedroom door and tiptoed over to the bed. Gently he embraced Lisbeth and looked wonderingly at his new daughter. The baby had stopped crying and was peacefully asleep next to Lisbeth. Lorenzo picked up the little bundle, gazing, full of wonderment, at the baby. "She looks like me!" he finally exclaimed as Lisbeth laughed softly. Indeed, this child was totally different from

Rosalinde. She had a mop of black hair on her large round head, full chubby cheeks, making her closed eyes appear as mere slits. She weighed almost one and a half kilograms more than Rosalinde had weighed and did not seem like the fragile infant that her older sister had been. Lisbeth was thrilled that Lorenzo was so taken with the new baby, his love and pride showing in his face as he said, "My darling, *cara mia,* you have done it again! What a beautiful baby. I love you. I love her. I did hope for a son, you know, but now seeing this little angel, I could not be happier." Tenderly he kissed Lisbeth who felt complete relief and joy. She too had wondered if Lorenzo would be disappointed or how he would feel, but seeing him now holding the infant with such tenderness and care, she knew all was as it should be. Two beautiful little girls, "one for him, and one for me," as Lorenzo was fond of saying when they had talked about this child. "I know what we should call her," Lorenzo burst out jubilantly. "I know the perfect name for her! Angelina! Our little angel."

"Yes," Lisbeth sighed happily, "our angel she is!"

TWENTY-SEVEN

"Telegram! Telegram!" Marianne yelled as she saw the Daimler coming up the drive toward the garage. Knowing Wilhelm's habit of always coming to the front door, she ran back into the house, tearing open the front door and, waving the yellow telegram in Wilhelm's astonished face. "Telegram from Lisbeth!" she cried as she hugged him.

"Is it the baby? What is it?" But Marianne simply handed the telegram to him, watching a happy grin spread over his tired face.

> March 19, 1939, To Lindemann Family
> Burgstrasse 47, Hamburg, Germany
> Happy to announce the birth of our second daughter, Angelina Josepha Moncrief, 9 o'clock this evening. Mother and baby are well. Sister Rosalinde very happy. Our love to all, Lisbeth, Lorenzo and daughters

Wilhelm dropped his briefcase and hugged his wife, twirling her around as in a dance. "Isn't that wonderful! Two little girls! Just like our two! Oh, I am so happy for them. They can grow up together and have fun like our Liesl and Gretl. I can't believe it—our little Lisbeth, now a mother of two!" he exclaimed in high spirits.

"And best of all, we will see our little Angelina very soon! Just think, we will be holding this baby and Rosalinde in our arms in a few months. Have you talked with Kurt yet about scheduling our voyage?" Marianne added.

"Yes, my dear, we are working on it. I would like to sail on the *Neue Welt*, and I think she will be in port in September. Before long we will hold our three little girls in our arms. When is Margarete coming home? She will be so happy too."

As spring turned into summer, the various members of the Lindemann family across the North and South Atlantic Oceans were happily pursuing their diverse lives. Margarete was in the final phase of her studies, preparing for her exams and graduation. In April Peter had come home for a two-week furlough. To Margarete he was more handsome than ever, wearing his new uniform and sporty cap. How proud she was to be seen with him everywhere! Peter could not wait to visit his school and former students, to encourage them and to promise that he would be back. The time passed too quickly as he spent his time with his family and Margarete. Amid tears, it was once again time for another farewell. But this time the goodbye was not filled with the same anguish and fear. Peter hoped for another pass in a few months, and Margarete had the accomplishment of her own goals in view. Before Peter left, he and Margarete had come to the conviction that they would not wait for everything to be perfect before they made important decisions about their life. At the next furlough, when Margarete had returned from her trip to see her sister, they would sit down with their parents, make plans and set a wedding date upon Peter's release from the service. That decided, they both relaxed and parted with hope in their hearts. Lisbeth was right, Margarete thought. Love overcomes all. Love heals all. Love is all we need.

Marianne was busy in her rose garden, enjoying even the menial work, dreaming of the long-awaited reunion with Lisbeth and her family. She wondered how Lisbeth's roses were doing, already planning to give them her expert care and attention. She couldn't wait to meet her two granddaughters, reliving her own happy days as a young mother. Time had passed too quickly, but here was a chance to relive those happy days with a new generation.

Wilhelm's days consisted of his usual routine, but there was lightness and a glow about him that even his employees could not miss. Word had leaked out that he was taking his family to South America for a visit. The magic date was September 10 when the *Neue Welt* was to sail from Hamburg. Inside, however, Wilhelm was not as light-hearted as he seemed. In March of this year, when German forces had occupied the rest of Czechoslovakia, Wilhelm had been quietly concerned. It was reported as an almost non-event in the newspapers. Margarete and Marianne were almost unaware of the news as they were totally involved in their own affairs, so busy planning for the future that they forgot to be aware of the present. Wilhelm was determined to continue planning ahead and making his family happy. In his heart he vowed to keep his eyes and ears open, to be informed and prepared. With Kurt's encouragement, and the happy faces of his wife and daughter greeting him nightly, Wilhelm was in his own way preparing for the trip of his lifetime.

Even Wilhelm's sister Anni felt the long-distance excitement, writing letter after letter, hoping to persuade Wilhelm to extend his visit to include her in the United States. But this would be just too much for him. "Some day, Anni, I promise, we will come to visit you in New Jersey. When I retire, we will come. I promise," he had written to Anni's urgent plea. Anni knew that hers was an unreasonable request and that seeing Lisbeth and her babies took priority. Still she felt left out of the exciting preparations at her brother's house. She could only blame herself for not visiting him in recent years. But her husband and three children, their hard work at the garden center, had kept her anchored in the United States. "Someday we will be together again," Anni vowed to herself, happy that Lisbeth at least would see her family again. With regret, Anni remembered her last visit to Hamburg. Both her parents had died without seeing her again. "Lucky Lisbeth!" she thought. "She will not have my regrets to deal with."

Lisbeth was living in a state of heightened anticipation. Little Angelina was growing and thriving. As different as she was in appearance from Rosalinde, she was also different in temperament. Whereas Lisbeth's first baby had been calm and quiet, Angelina was demanding and made her appearance in their world known. She had a strong voice and used it freely. If she was hungry, her impatient demands could be heard in the whole house. When fed and happy, she could be the sweetest baby you would ever hope to find. Her hair was growing into soft black curls. Her brown eyes were large and luminous, and when she smiled, displaying a soft dimple in her left cheek, she stole everyone's heart. Rosalinde loved her little sister, and Nina had to watch her carefully as she tried to hold and kiss the baby.

Cecilia and José showed their love and pride in their usual quiet and undemonstrative way. Lisbeth's days were filled with much activity and satisfaction. She thanked God for Nina's help every day. It did not seem as important to go to Baradera every week. Oma-Maria brought her the mail. Lisbeth basked in the joy of her little girls and spent every moment with them.

When in July Lorenzo suggested she join him on a trip to the city to attend a major horse race, she was tempted to decline. But seeing Lorenzo's face, she reconsidered. "Why can't you come along with me?" he asked. "The babies are fine. We have Nina to take care of them. Oma-Maria will come too and help. Don't you want to go with me?"

Lisbeth knew he was right. She needed to spend some special time with her husband, and seeing Emilio and Paulina would also be a wonderful treat. "Of course I'll go with you. It will be fun. I have never gone to a really important race like this one," she added, and Lorenzo smiled and kissed her.

The little train was packed with travelers going into the

city for the biggest horse race of the year. Of course she knew from Lorenzo that horse racing and soccer were the greatest pastimes in Argentina. But she had not realized how many people from outlying towns like Baradera made the annual trip to Buenos Aires, mostly to attend this particular race.

They spent the evening at the Alvarez' home, enjoying a wonderful dinner and conversation. Lisbeth was very proud to be able to hold her own and participate in the social talk around the table. After a while, Paulina led Lisbeth into the small parlor as the men continued their discussions at the table. The two women had much to talk about. Paulina was telling Lisbeth about her children who were going off to boarding school in a few weeks. The two girls were 11 and 12, and only the youngest child, Alberto, would remain at home for another semester. Then he too would take the first big step into the world. Lisbeth could not even imagine how she would feel if Lorenzo would insist on sending her girls to such a school. "I can't even think about that now. My babies are mine. I don't think I could bear to part with them," she thought to herself. This reminded her of her own first big step into the far-away world. Her parents had let her go. "How could they stand the pain?" she wondered as she thought of her own precious daughters safely asleep in their beds at *Bien Cielo*. Lisbeth told Paulina the news of her family's planned visit later in September. With hugs and laughter, Paulina promised to come and meet them. She would be lonely without her own children at that time. The two women had much to share, and the time passed quickly. "Are you excited about the race tomorrow?" Paulina asked.

"I have never been to this one," Lisbeth said. "It must really be something. The train was full of people coming just to see this race."

"Oh, you will be surprised. It is one of the biggest events here in Buenos Aires! And to think that two of *Bien Cielo's* horses are the favorites! It will be fun. You have never seen anything like it."

Paulina was right. Lisbeth had never seen such a spectacle before. First of all, the arena was gigantic, holding thousands of people. All the spectators were dressed in their Sunday best, the ladies wearing hats. She was glad that Lorenzo had suggested how to dress. Before the race began, bands were playing, and decorated horses and wagons were parading around the track. Hawkers selling trinkets and souvenirs reminded Lisbeth of a *Volksfest* (festival) back home. Food and drink of all kinds were for sale everywhere. When the starting shot rang out, the crowd rose, cheering and applauding wildly. Lisbeth had never seen so many people so excited and swept up in the event. When one of *Bien Cielo's* horses came in second place, Lorenzo and Emilio jumped for joy.

After the race, the owner of the horse, Señor Hernandez, spoke at length with Lorenzo, smiling and nodding, quite satisfied with the outcome. He then invited the Moncriefs and the Alvarezes to a special dinner at a private club. Lisbeth told everyone how much she had enjoyed this totally new experience. Tomorrow she and Lorenzo would go back home again, and for the first time since her arrival in Argentina, she thought of *Bien Cielo* as home.

Soon her parents and Margarete would join her there, and with pride she looked forward to showing them everything that had seemed so strange to her three years ago but now was beginning to feel like home. Only a few short months from now her dreams would come true.

Meanwhile, her family was dreaming the same dream.

> *August 5, 1939*
> *Dear Parents, dear Sister:*
> *This will be the last letter you will receive from me before you sail on September 10. We are all well and hope the same for you. I am counting the days until your arrival and telling Rosalinde and Angelina every day that soon they will meet their Oma and Opa and their Tante Margarete!*
> *Soon Rosalinde will celebrate her second birthday, and little Angelina is not so little anymore. She is a big baby already and will be six months old when you come. She is very lively and friendly. Rosalinde can make her laugh out loud and loves to play with her.*
> *I can't wait for you to see our two little darlings. It is amazing how much Angelina looks like Lorenzo and Rosalinde like me. Oma-Maria comes to see the girls every day. She never had a little girl, you know. She told me she had secretly hoped to have a baby girl, but on the estancia men want sons. I am so happy Lorenzo is different. He adores our little girls. I can see the love in his eyes. Now I wish you a safe and pleasant voyage. You will love the Neue Welt. Señor Alvarez will let us know in case the ship comes in early or late. And do not worry,*
> *Lorenzo and I will be at the harbor to meet you. I am so excited I can hardly wait! Please tell Johann a great big thank you for taking care of Mutti's garden and everything around the house. And thank Kurt for taking care of the business. I want you to come and not worry about*

anything. We love you and we are waiting for you. Bon voyage! Until we meet again in September,
  With all our love,
  Lisbeth, Lorenzo and Girls

The letter delivered to Juliana at the Baradera post office, Lisbeth rode back to *Bien Cielo* feeling on top of the world.

As part of the final preparations, Lisbeth and Lorenzo had persuaded Oma-Maria to accompany them to Buenos Aires later in August. She had so enjoyed the company of Paulina and Emilio on their last visit to *Bien Cielo* and looked forward to seeing the city again after many years. It had been a busy week, the highlight being Rosalinde's second birthday celebration. Although she was too young to understand the reason for the party, she was as always a happy and cheerful little girl, enjoying the sweet cake and her new doll and doll bed. Even baby Angelina seemed less demanding, as if she sensed that this was a happy time. The entire household had become infected with Lisbeth's excitement. She and Cecilia had done all they could to prepare for the Lindemann family's arrival. This last trip to the city was to make sure nothing was missing for their comfort and enjoyment while at *Bien Cielo*.

That evening, at dinner with the Alvarezes the subject was, of course, the upcoming visit of the family from Hamburg. Emilio was unusually quiet, trying not to express his surprise and concern. He had been following the political and economic developments in Europe through the newspapers as well as his international business connections. Just as Wilhelm had felt, Emilio was uneasy about the German Führer. He knew about the annexation of Austria, the takeover of Sudentenland and Czechoslovakia, and the new alliance with the Soviets, in opposition to the British and the French. Although Emilio was not sure what all this meant, it did not bode well. He was so far removed geographically and had no one to discuss it with. Still, Emilio, thinking as a family man, would never undertake a journey halfway around the world when everything around him seemed so uncertain. But surely Lisbeth's father knew more about this and must have felt secure in making his travel plans. It was obvious that Lisbeth was overjoyed at the prospect of the family reunion, and he did not want to worry her unnecessarily. Perhaps his worries were totally unfounded, he reprimanded himself. "Let's hope and pray Lisbeth's family arrives as planned," he thought. "Lisbeth has been through a lot these last few years. She deserves to see her family and reconnect with them and share her new life and her young family with them."

The Moncrief family lived a rather secluded life on the *estancia*, and Emilio was certain Lisbeth had had no time to read Spanish newspapers or listen to the radio news. However, after dinner when he and Lorenzo sat on the veranda smoking their cigars, Emilio attempted to voice some of his concerns. Lorenzo, however, was either unconcerned or uninformed, or possibly not even interested in events taking place so far away from his home and everyday life. Emilio decided it would be best not to speak of his troublesome thoughts and not spoil the wonderful anticipation of the upcoming visit. Lorenzo was more interested in the latest plays and movies in the city, and therefore Emilio kept silent. "Perhaps I worry too much about things that do not concern me," he thought. But he had come to love Lisbeth as much as his own children and did not want to see her ever hurt or disappointed. "It will be such a good tonic for her, spending time with her sister and her parents—perhaps the final remedy for her homesickness which she has tried so hard to keep to herself and overcome." With a soft smile, Emilio finished his cigar and wished everyone a peaceful good night.

TWENTY-EIGHT

As Lisbeth was making final preparations on the far side of the South Atlantic, Wilhelm watched his wife's packing with caution and unease. Dark clouds of uncertainty had been gathering over Europe all summer. Wilhelm was diligently observing the various moves in the great chess game among the nations. He was convinced the reports were slanted and designed not to disturb the general population. He kept his worries to himself, discussing them only with Kurt and his male friends. There was no reason to worry the girls yet. They were so absorbed in the travel preparation that he did not have the heart to voice his concerns.

In April, when Mussolini invaded Albania, the French and the British extended their guarantees to neighboring countries. In May negotiations began in Moscow but were later suspended. Yet discussions of a mutual assistance pact with the Soviets continued. What did all this mean? Wilhelm wondered and worried. Were all these moves a prelude to war? A war between which nations? He had lived through one major war already and hoped they were not headed into another one. He did not trust the *Führer*, did not believe in the policy of German expansionism. Deep inside him grew a gnawing fear, a realization that the winds of war were blowing across the land. In August, as Marianne and Margarete began to pack their trunks, Wilhelm read with great consternation that the German and Soviet dictatorships had become allies. Allies against whom? What were the rumblings under the surface that he and the rest of the country were hardly aware of? Was he just an old man who worried too much?

There was a definite change in his own business. His work force had continually diminished; a decrease in orders was obvious. What orders did come in were for industrial-type glass instead of the pricier luxury items such as mirrors and crystal.

From day to day Wilhelm became more worried and morose, but he kept up a brave front for the two women in his house. He watched them laugh and shop, pack and plan, and in his heart he just prayed that his concerns would prove to be unfounded. The happy atmosphere in his home glossed over his fears, and in the presence of his wife and daughter, Wilhelm was as happy about their upcoming voyage as they were.

In early August Wilhelm read with great interest about a meeting between Italian and German foreign ministers at which the *Führer* gave a long and rambling speech, stating his intention to move against Poland by the end of the month. That night Wilhelm could not sleep. "What next?

What next?" he wondered.

He did not have to wonder long. On the first of September, German forces invaded Poland. When the French and British demanded a recall of troops, the demand was refused. Therefore, two days later, on September 3, 1939, formal notice was given to Germany that a state of war existed. The long armistice and period of relative peace was over.

For Wilhelm and his family, all happiness and hope for a peaceful life, all hope of seeing their daughter and her children were dashed, all the dreams shattered and broken forever. Marianne collapsed from shock, Margarete's body shook with uncontrollable tears, not only for their own private disappointment, but for Peter, for her country, and for everyone in all the nations whose lives would be forever altered by the ravaging forces of a devastating war.

There was nothing for Wilhelm to do but cancel their passage and send a telegram to his beloved Liesl. He knew her heart would break as his was breaking now. He would not see his little granddaughters in a few weeks; perhaps he would never see his Lisbeth again. As if in a trance he sent the telegram, then sat quietly in total exhaustion, his head in his hands, crying, as he heard Marianne sobbing loudly nearby.

TWENTY-NINE

When Lorenzo entered the cool foyer of *Bien Cielo* early in September, everything was quiet. As he ran up the stairs to their rooms, he called out excitedly, "Lisbeth, where are you? I have a telegram for you!" Quickly she opened the door and met him halfway down the stairs, wondering out loud, "A telegram? From whom? My family is coming in a few weeks..."

Lorenzo handed her the yellow paper, wondering himself why her parents were sending a telegram. Perhaps just a quick greeting before boarding the ship, he thought. Lisbeth tore open the telegram and tried to read it quickly. Actually, she read it over and over again, not able to grasp its contents:

> Dear Lisbeth and family,
> We regret to cancel our trip. War has been declared. Times too uncertain to travel now. We must be strong and keep hope and pray for each other. More news later. Love to all, Sadly, Papa

"What does this mean, Lorenzo? What is going on? No, no, it just can't be! They are coming in a few weeks. I don't understand," she gasped, falling into Lorenzo's arms. He held her sobbing, shaking body, also unable to understand.

"Why can't they come? What are they talking about?" Lisbeth cried out in anguish and anger. "If they cannot come here I'll just have to go home. I'll just have to see them there!" She beat Lorenzo's chest with her tight little fists, crying hysterically.

Lorenzo was stunned himself. What was it Emilio had been trying to tell him last month? He really had not wanted to listen. He knew there was unrest in Germany, but it had not concerned him. He realized that lately he and Lisbeth did not really talk much anymore. She was busy with the two children and he was equally occupied with *estancia* business. Though Lisbeth was making strides with her Spanish, Lorenzo knew that she was not listening to the radio news, nor did she have time to read the newspapers. Since Angelina was born, he and Lisbeth had been leading almost parallel lives, and even with Nina's help Lisbeth was more involved with the children than with him. Now, as Lorenzo was holding his sobbing wife in his arms, he realized guiltily how little he had shared with her. He should have discussed Emilio's concerns with her. He should have prepared her. There was always that chance that they could not come after all. He had failed her, and all he could do now was to hold her and tell her not to worry.

"The war will be short," he whispered. "Nothing will happen to your parents. Just be patient. They will come another time."

But the comforting words had no effect on Lisbeth. She sobbed and cried out in her pain, and there was nothing, nothing he could do to change things. "I love you. You are here with me, with our little girls. You have a family here with me. Everything will be all right again," he tried to console her. But the disappointment, the uncertainty, and finally the great fear for her loved ones were too much for Lisbeth. She could only let herself cry and sob in her husband's arms. She could not think; she could not face the future. She felt as if they had all died and she was left alone in the world. After the great joy of anticipation, a raw pain filled her heart. Who were those people starting a war and why? Lisbeth really did not need the answers to these questions. All she wanted was to see her family and all she knew was that this wish had been denied her. All the love from Lorenzo, all the hugs from José and Cecilia, could not change things, could not grant her desperate hope.

Finally, all cried out, Lisbeth collapsed on her bed in exhaustion. But before long she was racked again by tears and sobs of anguish. "What have I done, leaving them? I should be with them now as they face the dangers and hardships of war." The old pain of homesickness which she thought she had overcome deeply pierced her heart, more painful than ever. Suddenly the joy of her little daughters, the love of her husband, the acceptance by her in-laws, and the great encouragement and love so freely given by Oma-Maria, became meaningless as she let herself wallow in panic and self-pity. She had no idea what war really meant, what would or could possibly happen. All she knew was that war was bad, and it scared her to death. She imagined her family suffering from fear, hunger, cold, homelessness, and everything that was cruel and bad.

As the days dragged on, Lorenzo tried his best to get information through newspapers and radio newscasts. He tried patiently to reassure her and to translate every tiny bit of news, but to no avail. Day in and day out, Lisbeth woke with the same dread. "What is happening at home? Are they still alive?" Her imagination flared with visions of horrible misfortunes. She lived for her almost daily trips to the post office hoping desperately for news.

Weeks went by and there was only silence. Frantically she continued to write her parents as well as to Tante Anni in the United States. Her only hope now was that perhaps Anni had received some communication from Germany. She became obsessed with worry. She withdrew within herself, not wanting to see anyone or talk to anyone. Even Oma-Maria, who had always been able to cheer her during her bouts of homesickness in the early days, was unable to rouse her out of her stupor, silence and tears. The only solace she found was in her babies. Rosalinde was now two years old, busy exploring her world. Nina spent most of her time with her, playing with her and taking her for walks to Oma-Maria's house. Angelina, still a big and cuddly baby, could occasionally coax a little smile out of Lisbeth who would sit and rock her for hours, silent tears flowing down her cheeks as she daydreamed of home. When Lorenzo came home, she was lethargic, her energies spent. To his credit, he tried his best to take her mind off the war in Europe. But he just could not seem to reach her. All his offers to go riding, to visit friends, to go to the cinema, were rebuffed. She no longer seemed interested in her weekly lessons with Alma. Her visits to Baradera which she had so enjoyed in the past now only consisted of trips to the post office. Lisbeth had allowed herself to fall into a state of depression, alternating with panic, wallowing in fear and regret.

José and Cecilia felt as helpless as Lorenzo and became more distant. Lorenzo was at a total loss as to how to help her. Where had his lively, smiling, happy and loving wife disappeared to? Where had the ecstasy of their married life gone? Why was Lisbeth now so cold and distant as if the war in Europe was his fault? Never in his young life had he experienced the sad and gloomy atmosphere such as this in his home. His parents had always been calm and contented individuals, and his Nonna had always been the sunshine in all their lives. Of course, he had always been the center of attention in the family as well as in the community. Now everyone's attention was on Lisbeth, but it was an unhealthy attention.

When he had met Lisbeth, he had been charmed and captivated by her beauty and her quick laughter, as well as her obvious admiration of him. Loving her with all his heart and soul had been easy then. His step quickened and his heart leaped with joy whenever he saw or even thought of his beautiful wife. Even after the girls were born and her days became filled with their care, Lorenzo had always felt he was number one in her life. What had suddenly changed? Her all-consuming worry and disappointment had suddenly shut him out. Did she blame him for taking her away from her family? Was she placing guilt on him as well as herself? Lorenzo was a loving, but in many ways a simple, uncomplicated man. All he wanted was to have his old Lisbeth back. He spoke to Oma-Maria about it and asked for help and advice. As she and Lisbeth had formed such a quick and loving bond, he felt she was his only ally. Oma-Maria was doing all she could, visiting often, taking her on a ride in her carriage, inviting her to tea, and sharing her books. But none of these things seemed to be of interest to Lisbeth. She declined Oma-Maria's offers of time and companionship, wallowing in her worry and sadness instead.

Weeks went by, and there was no word from home. Then, just as Lorenzo was reaching a state of despair of his own, Juliana came riding out to *Bien Cielo* with not one, but two letters. Joy and happiness radiated from Lisbeth's face as she jumped into Lorenzo's arms, laughing and crying and kissing him all at once.

"Thank you, God," Lorenzo sighed. "Let the news be good. Let me have my loving wife back in my arms forever."

With a shout of joy, she ripped open the first letter. It was dated early in August and was from Tante Anni. The envelope was dirty and tattered as if it had been lost in the bottom of a ship's hold. Where in the world had this letter been for all those weeks? Still Lisbeth was eagerly excited to read it:

> *Dear Lisbeth and family:*
> *As always we enjoyed your last letter. We can only imagine how happy you are awaiting your family's visit. How I wish I too could see your Papa, my dear brother, whom I have not seen in over twelve years. Perhaps you can convince your parents to come up north and visit us on*

their way home. We're all looking forward to hearing about your time together. We are fine and working hard. The garden center keeps us very busy, but we are thankful the business is steady. Monika is now twelve years old and a great help with Willy, ten, and Little Joe, eight. Write soon. Love to all,
    Tante Anni and family

Overcoming her disappointment at Anni's long-lost letter, she turned her attention to Juliana who was holding the second letter behind her back. This was what Lisbeth had been waiting for, for two months.

October 10, 1939
My dear sister Lisbeth:
One month ago today we were planning to board the Neue Welt. How we had waited for this moment to be with you again and meet your little girls! Did you receive Papa's long letter? He wrote you all the details and sent newspaper clippings. We do not know if you will be receiving any of our mail from now on, but we will keep writing. As you can imagine, everyone is in a state of shock since the war began. We are all afraid, not knowing what will be. Mutti and I had not realized that war was a possibility, but Papa says he had fears all along. He had gone along with our plans, hoping his fears were unfounded.

Now the German troops have invaded Poland, and who knows what will come next. The best hope is that the war will be short. Already changes are taking place. Not only Peter, but all young men under 30 are being called to service, which means a great portion of Papa's workforce. Now some retired people have to fill many positions as at Peter's school. His classes are being taught again by the professor who had retired when Peter took his position. Now Papa and Kurt are discussing closing the glass works for several reasons. Kurt is almost 32 years old, and his age group may be called up next. Also, there is no business. Who will buy mirrors and chandeliers? Who will be building homes and hotels when times are so uncertain? You know how long we have badgered Papa to retire or slow down, but this is not what he had in mind. He is very sad, and closing the factory will be very difficult for him.

Mutti has unpacked our bags and is very quiet. This is a difficult time for her. Cleaning up her garden in the fall always reminded her of your leaving. This year would have been an exception, but it was not to be. Johann is helping Mutti and thinks in the spring we should plant vegetables and potatoes in the garden. He remembers the First World War when we were babies. But Mutti will not hear of it. Her garden will not be disturbed!

I am very fortunate that the director of the opera chorus was able to find a spot for me at this late date. At least I have this job now which I always enjoy. So far the war has not impacted us in our daily living. Stores and cinemas are open; people go to restaurants and the theater, and everything is running smoothly as before.

Of course I am always worried about Peter. He is stationed somewhere in the East, and I hope his letters will continue to come through.

Dear sister, do not worry about us. We are fine and going to be brave, hoping for the best. How we wish we could be with you right now, but we will be sometime in the future. Please keep writing as we will. Keep writing to Tante Anni also, hoping to stay in touch somehow. We know that you and yours are safe, and that is a great comfort to us.

Until we meet again,
Your loving sister Margarete

Sitting in bed, reading her sister's letter for the tenth

time, Lisbeth was excited and relieved, knowing they were well. Yes, Papa's firm would be closing soon; the young men were going to war; but her home was still there, her family together. Good old Johann! He would look out for all of them. Life seemed almost normal despite the war and the uncertainty. As if a heavy weight had been lifted from her heart, she felt more like her old self. She smiled again and kissed Lorenzo. *"Schlaf wohl, mein Schatz,"* Lorenzo whispered and heaved a sigh of great relief.

Life continued in the old pattern at *Bien Cielo*. The mood in the house was, if not happy, calm and content. Lisbeth resumed her riding, her visits to town and to Oma-Maria's house. She played with the children and took them on long walks early in the morning. In November she spent four days in the city with the Alvarez family. Paulina was always happy to see her and had a calming influence on her. Emilio too, like her Papa, tried to get as much news as he could about the events in far-away Europe. The major shipping lines that dealt with Germany had curtailed their exports and were changing their shipping routes. He promised Lisbeth to keep her informed of any news. As the two women went shopping, Lisbeth could not help but wonder what kind of Christmas her family would be having this year. She had received another letter from Tante Anni, relaying the same information Margarete had. Still Lisbeth lived from day to day, waiting for news. Back at *Bien Cielo*, her trips to the post office became as frequent as in the early days of her life with Lorenzo. Juliana had promised to deliver any mail personally, but Lisbeth had the urge to be there physically, as if that would speed up the process.

The whole town knew about her family, and even people she hardly knew stopped her on the street, expressing their concern. Lisbeth was touched by the many kindnesses shown to her. She had not realized that so many townspeople truly cared for her. Juliana had told her that she was the first foreigner to come to Baradera for as long as anyone could remember. Now Lisbeth could feel this acceptance, and a warm sense of belonging came over her. The encouraging words and warm hugs were a good tonic for her, and she almost forgot about Elena's rudeness in the past.

Yet, as Christmas approached and there were no more letters from home, she became agitated and fearful again. Slowly her daily disappointment turned to despair. She couldn't eat, she couldn't sleep, and everything being done for her seemed useless and in vain. No one, not even Lorenzo could lift her spirits. The only pleasure she allowed herself was to play with her children. Slowly she slid into the same depressed state as prior to receiving her sister's letter.

Lorenzo was becoming impatient with her, again at a total loss to know how to handle this problem. More than once he raised his voice, lost his temper, storming out of the house. The holidays were coming, but there was no spirit of happy anticipation in the air. José and Cecilia became more and more distant, feeling that she was neglecting her husband, making their son unhappy. Oma-Maria seemed to be the only one who could reach Lisbeth and try to cheer her up. She came to *Bien Cielo* almost daily now, playing with the children, bringing special treats and trying to lift everyone's spirits. Yet they all knew the only thing that could bring about a change was a letter from across the sea. It was as if a black cloud were hanging over the whole *estancia*. Despite the clear blue sky and brilliant sunshine, everyone could feel a chill settling over *Bien Cielo*.

The Christmas Fiesta was coming, but unlike the previous years, Lisbeth showed no interest in going. "How could I laugh and enjoy the festival when maybe my family is in real danger," she thought bitterly. Lorenzo coaxed and cajoled her to go with him, but she was adamant.

"Why can't you go to please me?" Lorenzo shouted. "It would be good for you, see some people, have a diversion. Your friends will be there. Come along and forget your fears for just a little while," he begged her the evening before the Fiesta.

"If the silly Fiesta is so important to you, then just go. You don't need me. Just go. You have your friends," Lisbeth replied angrily, raising her voice.

"But I want *you* there. Doesn't that count?" After a stubborn silence, Lorenzo continued, "No, I must not count. You know, Lisbeth, you are suddenly a different person. I don't even know you anymore. Always the tears, always the sad face...can't you think of me and our children? Can't you see that you cannot change anything? Do you only care about your family in Germany and not your family here?"

Even Lorenzo's outburst of all that had been building up in him did not bring Lisbeth to her senses. Instead of an answer, she dissolved in tears and ran to their bedroom, slamming the door behind her. Lorenzo sat, holding his head in his hands, not knowing what to say or do. What was his life turning into? Why did a war halfway around the world have to ruin his life? Slowly he rose, his jaw set in a determined way. "I'm going into town," he told his father who was coming in from the veranda. He walked down the hill to the shed where the car was parked. As Lorenzo raced down the dusty road, José shook his head sadly.

Lisbeth woke from her troubled sleep when she heard Lorenzo stumbling up the stairs to their room. Throwing his clothes on the floor, he fell into bed, the odors of smoke and alcohol wafting from him into her face. She pretended to be asleep, but silent hot tears covered her cheeks. She felt abandoned and alone.

Lorenzo was still sleeping soundly when Lisbeth rose in the morning. Everyone had left the house early to attend the festival. The house was quiet. Deeply regretting the last night's outburst, Lisbeth began preparing breakfast for her children and for Lorenzo. "As soon as he comes down to the kitchen, I'll tell him how sorry I am for behaving so badly. I will tell him how much I love him, and that I will go to the Fiesta with him," Lisbeth resolved confidently. However, when she heard Lorenzo running downstairs an hour later without a word or a glance in her direction, he left the house, slamming the heavy door behind him.

Late that evening when Lorenzo and his parents returned from the Fiesta, Lisbeth and the children were in bed, the girls sleeping peacefully. Lisbeth lay exhausted from a day of crying, sadness, bitterness and regret. That night and the many nights that followed, there was no *"Schlaf wohl, mein Schatz"* from Lorenzo. The words she cherished so much were never said again.

Christmas came. No letters arrived from overseas. Everyone at *Bien Cielo* was walking on eggs. The young couple's argument and continued silence was affecting everyone. A pall had fallen over every activity in the house. Even Oma-Maria, with her happy and easy-going nature, could not affect a change. Christmas Eve dinner was a big affair as usual for everyone on the *estancia*, but there was great tension in the air. Even the *gauchos* and field hands felt something different and indefinable. When the time came to leave for Midnight Mass in Baradera, Lisbeth was not asked to come along. With reproachful glances José and Cecilia quietly followed their son down the hill where Juan was waiting with the car. Lisbeth thought her heart would break at this latest rejection. She was suddenly afraid, not for her parents or sister, but for herself and her children.

"What have I done? I am losing Lorenzo. I know I am, but I don't know what I can do about it. I am too tired to think. I just don't know what to do." Her feeble attempts at reconciliation had been rebuffed. Lisbeth knew it was not just the festival. There were many small things adding up to a big problem, and she was sure it was all her doing. She was paralyzed with fear and depression. How she wished she could just leave everything, pack up her girls and go home!

"Home? Where is my home now? I don't feel I have a home anywhere!" Sadly she knew that she had traded one home for another, and now she was losing this one. "Where can I go from here? Where do I belong now?" These questions churned in her head relentlessly. "I'll speak to Oma-Maria. Perhaps she can help us all somehow. I can depend on her. She is always there for me." With a firm resolve to speak to Lorenzo on Christmas Day, to reach out to him again, to get him back, she went to bed. "This is Christmas Eve. Peace on Earth, Goodwill to all Men. I will make peace!" And with prayers for all the people she loved, near and far, she feel into a dreamless sleep.

Christmas Day dawned bright and sunny. Lisbeth woke early and smiled, remembering her resolve of last night. She cuddled up to Lorenzo and kissed his sleeping face. He sighed in a contented way and opened his eyes. As Lisbeth smiled down on him, for a fleeting moment Lorenzo saw his loving wife as he had known her in the past. Before he could say anything, Lisbeth kissed him again, saying in a sweet voice, "Lorenzo, please don't say anything. I am so sorry for the way I have been behaving. I do love you more than anything, and I want things to be as they were."

She was laughing and crying and kissing him all at the same time. But Lorenzo, although returning her kisses, was holding himself back as if he were not sure he could believe her. "What a sudden change of mood! If only it were true!" he thought.

Oblivious to his reticence, Lisbeth continued to dream out loud. "If only I could go home for a while, Lorenzo, to see my family, to know they are safe, then I would be all right. What do you think, Lorenzo? Couldn't I go home, despite the war? Just a short stay, please, please?"

"Lisbeth," he replied seriously, "you are not thinking. There is no way anybody can travel to Germany now. Do you understand what war means? Even if your family is safe, who knows what upheaval is taking place in the country? You are not thinking straight. It is not that simple."

But Lisbeth continued to talk, to dream of things that could not be. "But Lorenzo," she begged, "let me go to Buenos Aires next week. Let me speak to Señor Alvarez. Surely he knows what is possible, which ships are still sailing to Europe. Please, please, let this be my Christmas present!" she begged.

But Lorenzo shook his head and slowly tried to extricate himself from her choking embrace. "Lisbeth, you speak like a child. It simply is not possible. You cannot take two small children on such a voyage and be caught in a war. Please use your head. It cannot be done."

Lisbeth knew that she had asked the impossible, but she could not let go of hope that such a trip would be the answer to all her problems. Sadly she looked at her husband, knowing he was right.

"Enough of this now," Lorenzo said with finality. "Let's get ready. Did you forget we are going to Nonna's house for dinner? Let's not talk about this anymore. Let's try to make peace. But don't ask me for the impossible." With that he walked into the bathroom and began his shaving ritual.

Lisbeth slowly rose from the bed and tried to control her rising tears. She had not really achieved the peace she dreamed of last night. But at least they were making some sort of peace. They were speaking to each other again. They had two young children whom they both loved deeply. For their sake she would try, try with all her might, to regain their former harmonious life. "There is nothing I can do about the war. I cannot let worry and fear destroy my life here. I must be strong and pray that all will be well, just as Papa said. It will be a merry Christmas after all," she decided, hearing the girls' happy babbling in the next room and seeing her husband's handsome face reflected in the mirror. She smiled her old optimistic smile and tried to face another day.

THIRTY

The new year began in a positive way. After a peaceful Christmas dinner at Oma-Maria's everyone heaved a sigh of relief as obviously Lorenzo and Lisbeth had come to some sort of understanding. Only they themselves knew that their relationship was not quite the same. Still, friendly chatter and loving glances were once again exchanged between them.

As the days passed, Lisbeth seemed more cheerful and less demanding of her husband who seemed more quiet and subdued. She did not complain when Lorenzo came home late after a card game with his friends or if he didn't come home in time to dine with his family. Even baby Angelina seemed to sense the new serenity as she smiled, lying contentedly in her carriage. Rosalinde loved to sit on Lorenzo's lap whenever she had the chance, and a pleasant atmosphere seemed once again to envelope the Moncrief family.

One week into the new year, Juliana arrived at the

estancia with a letter for Lisbeth. It was not from Hamburg as she had fervently hoped, but from Tante Anni in New Jersey. Her happy chatter about her family, her life, her belated Christmas wishes were a sweet balm to Lisbeth's soul. But the greatest joy was an enclosed small Christmas card and a short letter from her parents. Everything seemed to be the same. They were managing well. They were hoping this greeting would reach the western shores of the Atlantic. Apparently a similar greeting had been sent to *Bien Cielo*, but had never arrived. The latest news, of course, lifted everyone's spirits. Lisbeth felt almost as if the war were just a bad dream and not a reality. She began thinking of a trip home again, but she knew Lorenzo would not allow it, even if it were possible.

The letter from her aunt, however, gave Lisbeth a new idea. What if she convinced Lorenzo to let her travel to the U.S.A. to visit her relatives there? The last time she had spoken with Señor Alvarez about the war and how it affected so much of Europe, he had mentioned that steamships were still traveling north along the coast to the United States. They were not, however, crossing the Atlantic to Germany. Perhaps this was the way to go, wait a while, be patient, and if nothing else happened she could convince Lorenzo to let her go.

Still she did not have the courage to suggest such a thing, as their new-found understanding and truce was still tenuous. Although their relationship was still strained at times, it had improved immensely since the previous fall. To everyone who knew Lisbeth, it seemed that she had finally accepted the war and the constraints it had put on her and her family's lives. She relaxed to a degree and no longer pestered Juliana daily about her mail. She continued to write long letters, hoping they would reach their destination. Lisbeth felt confident that the crisis in her marriage was past. Her old lightheartedness was slowly returning, and everyone in the household was breathing easier.

Lorenzo did not mind when his wife decided to take Rosalinde on the train to Buenos Aires, leaving baby Angelina in Nina's care. It was February and summer was coming to an end. The sun still shone brightly and the air was warm. At two-and-a-half, Rosalinde was a very mature little girl and already had a remarkable vocabulary in Spanish and in German. Paulina was thrilled to welcome the *muchacha* (little girl) in her home as she missed doting on her own daughters away at school. That evening the talk turned once again to the war in Europe. Señor Alvarez told Lisbeth that according to his sources there were no serious new incidents or invasions since Poland's capitulation in October. Of course, the world was sitting on pins and needles, waiting and watching. Lisbeth felt confident at this time that her family was in no danger.

After dinner that evening, Emilio casually mentioned that he and Paulina were going to travel to New York during the month of April. This piece of news made Lisbeth sit bolt upright. "What? You two are actually going to New York? Is it a vacation or business?" she asked excitedly.

"Well, actually it is business, but we will combine it with a vacation," he smiled. "The children are away at school, and there is no reason Paulina can't go with me for a few weeks." He went on to explain that every few years it was necessary for him to handle financial arrangements in person for several exporters. Establishing letters of credit and renewing import licenses in the United States was an important and integral part of his job. For Paulina it would be her first trip out of the country, and he thought she would enjoy it.

Lisbeth's mind was racing, her heart beating wildly. "I wish I could travel with you and visit my aunt," she blurted. Paulina looked at Emilio as they spoke at almost the same time.

"Oh, of course we wouldn't mind at all having you along. But that is a matter you will have to discuss with your husband first. I don't even know if there is space for another passenger on the ship, but I can find out. Also, there is the matter of required documents. I would have to investigate whether it is too late for such arrangements."

"I know. It's probably impossible," Lisbeth sighed, remembering a certain conversation with Lorenzo when she had been told in no uncertain terms not to dream of impossible things. Nevertheless, another seed had been planted, and her mind would not let go of the idea. She became so excited even at the possibility, that she could not fall asleep that night. She would need to look at the map. Springbrook, New Jersey. Was it anywhere near New York City?

The next morning Lisbeth rose early to catch Señor Alvarez before he left for the office. "Please, please find out if there is a cabin available, and all the other things I need to know and do. Please, please. I will speak with Lorenzo as soon as I get home."

Emilio smiled. "I will inquire, but that is all I can do. You speak with him, and then we will see!" He did not want to get involved in the Moncriefs' affairs, and certainly did not want to cause any problems. He almost wished he had not mentioned the trip at all. But he had, and now there was no stopping Lisbeth's excitement as she picked up Roselinde, twirling around and telling her, "Guess what, little girl? We just might be going on a nice long trip, you and Angelina and I! It will be so wonderful. You have cousins in America. Wouldn't you like to meet your cousins?"

"Please, Lisbeth, slow down. Don't get your hopes up. I don't know if any of this is possible, and you must discuss it with Lorenzo. He may not want you to leave and take the children on such a trip. Please wait and see, and don't count on it yet. There is too much to arrange and discuss," he pleaded.

But Emilio might as well have been talking to the moon. Lisbeth was already making plans. "And I have the money. It wouldn't cost Lorenzo anything to let me go with you," she continued.

Emilio shook his head. "Lisbeth, it is not about the money. You need to talk with Lorenzo. He will know what is best."

"Yes, yes, you are right, of course," she said. "I just got so excited thinking about it. I will talk to Lorenzo, but I know already what the answer will be. I know this trip will never come to be, but it is so good just to think about it!" Lisbeth answered sadly as Emilio picked up his briefcase and quietly closed the door behind him.

Paulina silently put her arms around Lisbeth. "Lisbeth, Lisbeth, I know how homesick you have been, how worried about your family, and how wonderful it would be to see your aunt. But please, wait and see. Don't set yourself up for disappointment. Talk to Lorenzo first and then we'll see."

Lisbeth nodded. She knew Paulina was right. Traveling with two children would not be easy; on the other hand, what a great opportunity to have Emilio and Paulina nearby to lend a helping hand! "Are you sure you would even want me along on your trip? Even if there is a cabin, and even if Lorenzo would let me go?"

Paulina smiled. "Of course, Lisbeth. It would be wonderful having you and the children on board. But that is not the question here. There are other things you must work out if you can."

Lisbeth nodded. It was time to get ready to return to *Bien Cielo* and find a way to convince Lorenzo of her plan.

On the train home, Lisbeth's mind was filled with all kinds of ideas. How should she broach the subject with Lorenzo? How could she convince him that such an opportunity might never come along again? Would Lorenzo want to go with them? April—isn't that a time when some of the work on the *estancia* is finished? What would his parents have to say? Would Oma-Maria help her to convince Lorenzo? Her heart was beating with excitement as the train pulled into the station. She was met by José, not Lorenzo, which dampened her spirits somewhat. But perhaps it would be better to approach her husband later when they were alone. She had decided to begin gently, telling him about the Alvarez' plans, and slowly easing into her own wishful thoughts. In her mind she already saw her children playing with their American cousins.

In the end, the whole process had been remarkably easy. Strangely enough, Lorenzo did not need to be persuaded at all. When she told him what Emilio and Paulina were planning, Lorenzo turned sharply, at first frowning. Then a strange little smile crept into his face. He said the most amazing thing: "Why don't you go with them?" he asked casually as if it were the most natural thing in the world.

"Go with them? Do you mean it? Really? Are you saying the girls and I should travel to New York with them?" Lisbeth could not believe what she was hearing.

"Well, actually, I think the girls are too young to make such a trip. They are perfectly fine here with me and my parents, and Nina. But you can go. Maybe it will help you with your sadness, your worries. I think such a trip would be good for you." Lorenzo smiled his charming smile.

"Oh, no, Lorenzo. You don't understand. I am not going anywhere alone. What is so wonderful about this trip is that I would have Paulina and Emilio on the ship to help me with the children. If I go, I am taking the girls. It would only be for a few weeks, and you could come too if you want to! Wouldn't it be great to travel all together?"

"I can't leave now. I can't go anywhere. But I will think about it. I'll have to talk to Emilio first. I think the girls are too small, but I will think about it. Let's talk about it after we know more from Emilio."

Lisbeth couldn't believe that Lorenzo was even willing to discuss or think about it. She had been prepared with reasons, arguments, pleading and tears but did not have to use any of them.

Actually Lorenzo seemed pleased with himself, to have come up with this suggestion. Lisbeth had not expected him to be so accommodating, even anxious to let her go. "Are you trying to get rid of me for a while?" Lisbeth joked, hugging and kissing him.

"Of course not, *Cara*, but it just came to me that if this is what would make you happy again, then that is what you need to do. Of course, we don't even know if it will work out. There is a lot to consider. Let's wait and see what Emilio has found out. I would miss you and the girls terribly, but perhaps it's the best solution for everyone."

"What do you mean, for everyone? It's our decision, and I would be so happy, so happy, if I could visit Tante Anni and her family. I would never complain or be homesick again, I promise! It's only for a few weeks, and I won't be alone on the voyage, and when we get there, my family will take care of us. Oh, Lorenzo, you are wonderful."

Lying in Lorenzo's embrace, Lisbeth felt lighter and happier than she had in a very long time. She felt sure that Emilio would find a way for her to join them, and she was convinced at this moment that Lorenzo, in his great love for her, would allow her and the girls to undertake this journey. How she loved her Lorenzo, how good he was, how generous! Lisbeth buried her face in his chest, happy and joyful once again.

The next morning as Lisbeth was descending the stairs, she heard raised voices in the parlor. She knew that Lorenzo was telling his parents about her plans and that they were obviously disapproving. Cecilia's voice especially could be heard above the rest. It reminded Lisbeth of another such discussion that had taken place shortly after her arrival. At that time she had not understood anything, but she knew that it had something to do with her. When she confronted Lorenzo about it later, he was reluctant to talk.

In the end it came out that Cecilia was upset and disappointed that Lorenzo had not been married in a church. To Cecilia, a ceremony performed by a judge meant nothing. At the time, she had insisted that Lorenzo and Lisbeth marry a second time in her church. Lorenzo refused, and Lisbeth was very proud of him. She was married once by Judge Hoffman. She had the certificate in hand, and a second marriage ceremony was not necessary. Still Cecilia pouted about it for some time, and Lisbeth was never sure that she had been forgiven or fully accepted for that.

Today, as she heard Cecilia's shrill voice rise above that of her son and husband, Lisbeth knew instinctively what the argument was about. Cecilia did not approve of Lisbeth's independence, and certainly not of taking the girls to New York with her. Lisbeth quietly retraced her steps and returned to her rooms. "I must be patient and just wait and see. We have not even heard from Emilio. Perhaps it will not work out after all, and Cecilia will be happy. But please, God, help me, let it work out for me, and I will never ask for anything again!" she prayed. After a while, Lisbeth dressed the girls for a walk to see Oma-Maria. She was the one person she could share everything with, the good and the bad. Oma-Maria would understand; she would stand by her always. Of that Lisbeth was sure.

Oma-Maria had not seen Lisbeth so happy in many months. "What is it?" she asked as they hugged each other.

"You will never believe it. If everything works out, the girls and I will be traveling to America to visit my aunt. Don't look so worried. We are not going alone. We'll be sailing with Paulina and Emilio. They will take care of us on the trip, and then we will be with my aunt. Isn't it wonderful? Lorenzo is making me so happy. He is the best!" Lisbeth beamed as she chattered away.

Oma-Maria had to sit down. This surprising news was almost too much for her. She was happy for Lisbeth. She knew how difficult the last years had been for her, and she wanted Lisbeth to have some peace and be happy. "Oh Lisbeth, what news you have brought me! I am missing you already. How long will you be gone?"

"I hope to spend a month with Tante Anni, but I am leaving everything to Lorenzo and Emilio to decide. I just hope it all works out. We should know quite soon. There is a lot of paperwork to do. But I'll leave all that to them. I just hope it all comes to pass. I wish Lorenzo could go with us, but he says that he can't leave right now. Are you happy for me, Oma-Maria?"

"Yes, child, I am very happy for you. But I must tell you, I will be counting the days until your return."

"Oh, my dear Oma, don't worry. The time will go fast, and before long we will all be together again. But seeing my family in America will be almost as good as seeing my family in Germany. Anni seems to get letters despite the war, and I know I will be happy if I can at least visit one branch of the family. Isn't it just wonderful? Isn't Lorenzo just the best, the best husband in the world?"

"Yes," Oma-Maria smiled wistfully, "Lorenzo is the best."

PART THREE

Journey North

THIRTY-ONE

It was amazing how quickly and easily everything fell into place. The freighter *La Paloma* which they were to sail on, belonged to the concern whose financial interests Emilio would be negotiating in New York. There were six private cabins and they could handle up to 14 passengers. The largest of the cabins was miraculously still available and could accommodate Lisbeth and her two children. The sailing date was set for April 12, and the duration of the voyage about 12 days. Emilio and Paulina were planning to stay in New York six days while the ship was unloaded and reloaded for the return voyage. Emilio suggested that Lisbeth and Lorenzo book an open return date for her, as the *La Paloma* left New York at the end of each month on its routine round trips.

Lisbeth had hoped for a four-week stay, but again Lorenzo surprised her by suggesting a two- or three-month stay instead. Lisbeth could hardly believe her good luck. She would miss Lorenzo terribly, yet this was an opportunity of a lifetime for her.

A telegram was sent to Anni advising her of the arrival date. A very happy reply from Anni arrived shortly thereafter, welcoming her niece and children with open arms. The time until departure seemed to fly by as Lisbeth was caught up in preparations. Lorenzo seemed more relaxed and spent much more time at home with them. Looking back, Lisbeth felt that this was one of the happiest times in her marriage. She knew that José would miss the girls. Cecilia said little, often shaking her head. Obviously she did not approve of her son's decision to let his family travel so far without him. She also disapproved of Lisbeth for her independence, her courage and her determination. But nothing could deter Lisbeth. She felt she was doing the right thing, and Lorenzo, her wonderful husband, had approved this decision completely.

The day of departure for Buenos Aires was coming closer. All paperwork was in order. Lisbeth's German passport was still valid. No special visas were required, and Lorenzo had signed a document giving his permission for the children to visit a foreign country with their mother. The suitcases were packed, the gifts wrapped, and the children's favorite toys and blankets would travel in a special take-along case. Lisbeth's documents, her tickets, the girls' birth certificates, her money were all safely tucked in the leather bag she had carried with her on her first ocean voyage. How far she had come in the last four years!

Today, all that was left to do, was to ride into Baradera to bid her friends goodbye. First Alma at the library who gave her two special children's books for the journey. Next to see Antonio at the general store, who also gave her special treats for the girls. She saved a visit with Juliana for last. They were sitting in the tiny post office, drinking a cup of tea and discussing the upcoming adventure. Juliana smiled, "You know, I am happy for you to go on this great voyage, but for me, I have never been farther than Buenos Aires, and I am perfectly content to live here the rest of my life. That must sound boring to you, Lisbeth, but I love my life here."

"Oh, but I do understand," Lisbeth replied. "I'm happy too, living with my husband and his family. But I don't have my own family here as you have. All your relatives are here—your brothers, all your sisters, your cousins. No one of my family is here, and I miss them all so terribly. I had so looked forward to their coming, but now, with the war, I don't even have their letters. I know nothing—if they are well or suffering or anything. Going home is impossible, but if I can see my aunt and cousins, that makes me as happy as going home. Can you understand that?"

"*Si, si*, I understand. I can only imagine how hard it has been for you. How you must have loved Lorenzo to leave everything you knew and follow him here! He is a very lucky man to have you."

"I am lucky too," Lisbeth went on. "He loves me enough to let me go on this visit. I know I will miss him so much, and yet I want to go. But I'm not going forever, just a few weeks or months and we will be back. Maybe the war will end soon, and we can all live in peace and see each other again."

"Let's hope for that. Let's pray for that," Juliana replied, filling Lisbeth's mug with more tea.

"Lorenzo will be busy at *Bien Cielo*, the time will fly, and don't forget, Juliana, he will be getting so many letters from me, he will have to ride into town every day and visit you here," Lisbeth joked.

Juliana laughed nervously. "Why haven't you come in with Lorenzo more often in the last few months?" she dared ask.

"Oh, I was so miserable and depressed, so worried about everything. I was not a pleasure to be with," she laughed. "But everything will be much better now. And when I return you will see me with Lorenzo all the time again."

Juliana looked into Lisbeth's eyes without answering. "Something is wrong here," she thought, but she would be the last person to hurt her friend. She had seen Lorenzo around the cantina many times, and local gossip had it he was seeing Elena again. Juliana had never liked Elena or trusted her. In fact she had tried to stay away from her. Lately Elena was walking around with a smug expression on her face like a woman with a secret. At one time everyone had assumed Lorenzo would marry Elena, but after he brought his bride home, that speculation had died down.

Still, in the past few months, Lisbeth had become quite the recluse, and Lorenzo had been seen at the cantina, drinking and enjoying himself quite regularly. Juliana had more than a suspicion that Lorenzo and Elena were spending time together, but she was not one to think out loud.

She was not the only one who had noticed the goings-on since the Christmas Fiesta. Was it was wise for Lisbeth to leave town for an extended stay? Probably not, she thought. "But Lisbeth knows nothing of the gossip, and I hope she never will. Whatever it is, I hope it plays itself out before Lisbeth returns."

The two young women hugged and kissed each other goodbye. "*Adios*, have a wonderful trip and write to me, please," Juliana called after her. "I work with other people's letters, but never have I received a letter of my own!"

"I will, I promise," Lisbeth called over her shoulder as she mounted Fritzi for the ride back to *Bien Cielo*.

The day had come to say *adios* to Oma-Maria. Saying goodbye to her was particularly hard. Lisbeth had not realized how much she loved and depended on the old lady, and would miss her terribly. "But it is only for a short time. In a few months I will be back."

"*Auf Wiederseh'n,*" Oma called from her front porch. "*Adios*! I'll see you again soon. *Adios!*"

Angelina did not understand what all the commotion and excitement was about, but Rosalinde remembered her earlier train ride and was anxious to do it again. After a quiet family meal, Lisbeth and the children went to bed early. Lorenzo sat and talked with his parents, and once again Lisbeth could hear their raised voices. Whatever they were discussing did not concern Lisbeth now as she settled down for a good night's sleep before the long-awaited trip north.

Lorenzo had been allowed to board *La Paloma* with his wife and daughters. The cabin was spacious and well appointed. The large bed could certainly accommodate an adult and two small children. There were closets, a small table and chairs, a mirror and dressing table, as well as a tiny bathroom. "There certainly would have been room for Lorenzo too," Lisbeth thought sadly. But she was thankful that he had given her permission to travel without him. Looking around, Lisbeth knew that spending twelve days in a confined space would not be easy at times, but she was willing to make the sacrifice. There was also a spacious enclosed walking deck where she could stroll with Angelina's baby carriage.

"You want to take that bulky carriage along?" Lorenzo had teased her. "There will hardly be room in your cabin to turn around." But Lisbeth had insisted. Angelina was used to her carriage, and Lisbeth wanted her to feel comfortable with familiar surroundings.

Now Lorenzo wanted to take a look at the rest of the ship, and together they set off to see the dining room and the small lounge, equipped with a phonograph, books and games. Lisbeth was confident the time would pass quickly. She knew that Emilio and Paulina loved her children, and the little girls knew and loved them as well. But now, as the sailing time approached, Lisbeth began to wonder if she had done the right thing, insisting on this trip and leaving Lorenzo behind. However, she was careful not to show him her doubts and worries. "Everything will go well," she assured herself, "and when we arrive, my family will be waiting for us."

A last hug and kiss, and Lorenzo had to leave the ship. Lisbeth took a deep breath and held tightly onto her children. A sudden panic seized her. "What if I never see my Lorenzo again? What if something happens to us?" A cold shiver ran down her back, but seeing a smiling Lorenzo waving his last greetings, she shook it off. With Emilio and Paulina at her side, she smiled bravely, waving a last goodbye to her husband on the pier.

As the ship eased out of the harbor, Lisbeth remembered her first voyage, the painful farewell with her family, the tears and uncertainty. Yet that loss was equaled by a great high, a sense of elation, knowing she would soon be reunited with her beloved Lorenzo. This time, however, Lisbeth experienced contrasting feelings. Yes, she felt sadness at leaving her husband behind. Yet that was overshadowed by something else, something totally new to her—something almost like relief, or a freedom, coupled with the hope that this separation would somehow clear things between them and rekindle a dying flame.

As *La Paloma* gathered speed, Lorenzo disappeared from sight. She took her children to their stateroom to settle in for the long journey. She felt sad and happy at the same time. On the one hand she had wanted this trip at all costs; on the other, it had been almost too easy to get Lorenzo to agree. It seemed as though he was almost happy to see her go. "But no, that is just my imagination. He let us go because he knew he was making me happy. That's the only reason, I know. He just wants me to be happier again because he loves me."

Gently Lisbeth put her children down onto the bed for a nap. It had been an unusual, busy day for them too, and within minutes they were both sound asleep. Lisbeth sat on the chair, putting her feet up on the bed. She closed her eyes and let her thoughts wander. "Here I am on a ship again. Who would have thought that I, little Liesl, as Papa often still calls me, would undertake two long ocean voyages within four short years? The first one south, across the Equator, to be with my new husband, and now north again to a new continent."

For Lorenzo, she had left all she knew; for his love she had left everything behind. Now a different urge propelled her. For the love of family bonds she had left her husband behind, if only temporarily. This time she was sailing north to meet relatives she hardly knew. But she needed to do it, hoping to find peace and contentment. Sailing north, so far north, as she had studied the globe before her departure—north, past Rio de Janeiro, north across the Equator again, north along the West Indies, north, all the way to New York City.

THIRTY-TWO

Wilhelm sat in his living room reading the daily war reports, while unbeknownst to him, his daughter and grandchildren were sailing north. Tired of the same government-approved propaganda, he dropped the paper, stood up and stretched. He stepped out on the veranda where he saw Marianne and Johann in the garden. Marianne was kneeling on a cushion, totally absorbed in cleaning up her rose bushes.

Behind the gazebo he could see Johann moving around with a bucket in his hand. With Johann's stubborn insistence and Wilhelm's gentle persuasion, Marianne had finally agreed to turn the grassy croquet court and lawn into a vegetable garden. One of Johann's friends had come with his tractor and plowed up the green expanse. Marianne could hardly look at it. But Johann was happy, tilling the soil, and today planting potatoes. He had plans to add cabbage, kohlrabi, beets, carrots and lettuce later on.

Wilhelm walked down the steps and nodded briefly to

his wife. He walked farther on to have a chat with his chauffeur, now turned gardener. "How is it going, Johann? You certainly have added a lot of extra work for yourself, haven't you?"

"Oh, yes, but it is nothing. You will be glad when we have our own potatoes in the fall, plus our own vegetables all summer," he beamed. "With the war on, you never know what might happen. And this way I know we will not go hungry."

Wilhelm smiled and hoped it would never come to that. But he knew this was Johann's way of contributing and taking care of the family just as Wilhelm was doing in his own way. He was always thinking of ways to secure his family's future. He was doubly glad now that he had made provisions for Lisbeth, not only her private account, but also the investment he had entrusted to Emilio Alvarez. He had heeded his father's advice as well, and invested in gold, securely hidden in his safe. His good friend, Lars Müller, head of the Hamburg International Bank, had managed to buy U.S. dollars for him. Wilhelm knew that he had done all he could to provide for his family in any eventuality. Despite these preparations, for the first time in his life he was actually afraid of the future and what this terrible war would do to all of them. With a deep sigh he reentered the house, turning the radio to a classical music station.

That evening Johann drove Wilhelm to the home of his friend Judge Roland Hoffman, who had married Lisbeth and Lorenzo only a few years ago. It seemed an eternity to Wilhelm since then. How he wished he could see her and his precious granddaughters! Wilhelm was looking forward to the monthly evening of Skat, cigars and conversation. But he had a feeling tonight it would be mostly a political discussion instead. When Wilhelm arrived, Lars Müller and Christian Wagner were already seated in the judge's library. Hearty greetings were exchanged as the doorbell rang again. They heard Hans Birkner's jovial voice greeting the judge's wife Ursula. Hans owned a shoe factory and was the perfect salesman. He knew everyone of importance in town and was happiest wheeling and dealing. He was a successful man who had worked hard to be who he was. His walking shoes for men and women were well known all over the country. Plain and simple, but of the best quality, perfect for walking the city pavements.

As the five men sipped their first cognac, the last Skat player arrived. A retired university professor, Albert Glaser, was a slight man with piercing, intelligent eyes. He had a worried look about him and sat down with a heavy sigh. "I almost did not come tonight," he declared abruptly. "But I wanted to say goodbye to you, my friends whom I have known most of my life."

Five astonished faces turned to Albert.

Before anyone could ask questions, he continued, "We all know what is happening here since the rise of the Party. We know that people like me are no longer welcome here. We all know people who were wise enough to have left the country years ago. But I did not want it to be true. I stayed, I hoped, I did not want to leave my country. But the time has come, and I hope it is not too late. Tonight, on the midnight train Lillie and I are leaving for Holland. I can't stay long, but I had to see you, my friends, one more time. Perhaps someday we will meet again. Until then, may God be with you."

With a quick handshake, Albert grabbed his hat and coat and disappeared. The men in the room were stunned. They all knew what Albert was talking about. Since Hitler's rise to power, the purge against the Jews had begun moderately as they were expelled from public posts and driven from professional life. Albert had already retired and did not fear for himself, but now conditions were almost intolerable and the time had come for him to take his wife and flee. The Skat group was helpless; they all knew that worse was still to come. There was nothing anyone could do but wish Albert and Lillie a safe haven in Holland. There would be no card game tonight, only subdued conversation.

Christian Wagner, one of the directors of the German Railway System, shared that he had been forced to choose between joining the National Socialist Party, or Nazis, or losing his position as well as his retirement benefits. He had chosen the latter. Lars, however, admitted that he had no other choice but to join the party. Hans, the shoe man as they called him, vowed never to join. He would rather close his factory than be forced to become a member.

Wilhelm sighed, remembering his own situation. When his manager Kurt Walter received his draft notice, they came to the decision to close the glass works. Business had been slow; the work force had diminished, and Wilhelm had suddenly lost his former energy and drive. Yet he told himself that it was only temporary, that the war would not last forever. Still it was a very painful decision for him. Two weeks after Kurt's departure, Wilhelm had closed out all accounts, paid the last bills, and shaken the hand of each of his trusted employees. His final, generous payout to each of them had not lessened the pain and sadness on both sides. "Till after the war," many of them told Wilhelm as they shook hands for the last time. Looking at the boarded-up windows, he locked the doors of the building and finally the huge entrance gate. He looked into the eyes of his old friend Johann, and no words were necessary. Both men knew it was a somber event, feeling uncertainty, futility, tragedy, and bottomless sadness.

Driving home in total silence, both remembered happier times. Aside from the death of his parents and Lisbeth's departure, this was the saddest day in Wilhelm's life. Sad as he was, at least he did not have to concern himself with having to join a political party against his will. He was also grateful not to have sons to be sacrificed in this war. But Peter and Kurt were as close as sons to him, and he feared for them.

He looked at his Skat friends. Hans' boys were still too young, but Lars had a son and a nephew on the Eastern front. Already war casualties were becoming a daily occurrence with more losses to follow. In every community sad words were being repeated: "Have you heard...Horst was killed...Markus is missing...Have you heard...Georg was injured...Have you heard?...killed...missing...injured..." and always bitter tears followed.

And worse was still to come. Several months after the closure of the glass works, on a quiet Sunday afternoon, there was an impatient ring at the Lindemanns' front door. When Marianne went to answer, there stood two uniformed officers of the *Reichspolizei* (National Police), requesting to see Herr Lindemann. Her heart racing, Marianne ran to get Wilhelm who was in his office. Without much fanfare, one of the officers handed Wilhelm an official-looking paper informing him that he was to relinquish his car, Johann's beloved Daimler, to the service of the *Vaterland* (fatherland). Wilhelm was stunned and speechless. His initial impulse to question or even to laugh was stifled by the stern look in the officers' eyes and the obvious impatience in their gestures. His head held high, Wilhelm led the men toward his garage. He called Johann and directed him to bring the car out of the garage. As Wilhelm handed the keys to the vultures in uniform, one of them gave him an official-looking receipt adorned with a seal, stamp and signature. Wilhelm handed the paper to Johann saying, "Frame this and hang it in the garage as a souvenir." He then turned slowly and walked, head down, back to his house. With tears in his eyes, Johann stared after his employer, holding the useless paper in his trembling hand.

THIRTY-THREE

In Springbrook, New Jersey, excitement was running high at the Bauer household. For the past twelve days the children had been marking the calendar until Tante Lisbeth's arrival. Finally that day had come.

After taking the children, Monika, Willy and Little Joe, to school early, Anni and Josef began their drive to New York City. *La Paloma* had docked early in the morning, but by the time the customs and immigration officials had come on board to inspect the cargo, it was near noon when the passengers were allowed to disembark. All during the drive, Anni had been checking her watch nervously, but Josef reassured her calmly that there was plenty of time. Still, it took a while to park the car and find the correct arrival hall.

As Anni expectantly scanned the crowd, it was easy to spot a rather anxious-looking young woman carrying a beautiful dark-haired baby girl in her arms. A middle-aged couple followed close behind, the man carrying a blonde three-year-old girl. As soon as Lisbeth heard her aunt's excited cry, "Lisbeth, Lisbeth, here we are!" her anxious look turned into one of pure joy. Before long they fell into each other's arms, laughing and crying with happiness. Josef stood quietly by, smiling at the happy family reunion. Then he too welcomed Lisbeth and her children with a comforting hug. Emilio and Paulina were introduced and thanked again for their assistance to Lisbeth during the voyage.

"You were just wonderful. I don't know how I could have managed without your help," Lisbeth exclaimed, hugging Paulina and Emilio.

"It was our pleasure," Emilio smiled, patting Lisbeth's shoulder. Indeed it had been a pleasant voyage for them all. Rosalinda and baby Angelina were the little stars among the small group of passengers on *La Paloma*. Everyone enjoyed the diversion the little girls' antics provided. There always seemed an adult available to play a game with Rosalinda or read a story. Even some crew members, when not on duty, volunteered to spend a little time babysitting Angelina, so that quite often Lisbeth was able to join the other passengers for a meal in the dining room. Other times she enjoyed quiet meals in her cabin. Having Paulina and Emilio on board gave Lisbeth a calming sense of security. She still basked in the unexpected love and understanding shown her by Lorenzo in letting her and the girls travel to see her relatives. Allowing her this trip was like a healing salve on her wounded heart. Despite the many misunderstandings, harsh words and continued tension in their marriage, Lisbeth now was filled with love and gratitude for her husband. Confident that this separation would be the bridge leading them to their former happiness, Lisbeth embraced her aunt with hope and contentment.

All too soon Lisbeth had to bid farewell to her great friends who were staying in New York. Once again, Emilio reminded Lisbeth of the information he had written down for her. "Remember, all you need to do is call the number I gave you. Mr. Jenkins will arrange your return trip. Everything has been paid for. All you need to do is inform him of your return date. You know that there is a ship returning to Buenos Aires at the end of each month."

Lisbeth hugged and kissed them both, thanking them over and over again for all they had done for her. Amid reassurances to remain in touch, they waved a final goodbye.

Rosalinde and Angelina were tired and totally perplexed at their new surroundings, but seeing their mother smile, they relaxed, still holding tight to her skirts. An hour later, their baggage stowed in the trunk, the baby carriage strapped to the roof, the little family crowded into the Bauers' car for the two-hour drive to Springbrook. The children snuggled into Lisbeth's arms and fell asleep instantly. Anni was full of questions, jumping from one subject to another. Lisbeth was too excited to speak and promised to tell them everything later as she could hardly keep her own eyes open. She had barely slept the previous night, partly from joy, partly from nervous expectation. The stress and anxiety of the day fell away from her as she lay back and dozed.

When she opened her eyes, the car was just coming to a

stop in front of the Bauer house. The brick home stood solid and comfortable, very homey and welcoming. Tulips were blooming along the sidewalk, and a purple lilac bush in full bloom was peeking over the white fence. A welcome banner, made by the three Bauer children, reached across the wide porch proclaiming "Welcome to America, Tante Liesl and Cousins!"

Once again Lisbeth was touched as she read the name her parents had called her when she was just a little girl herself. Being with her aunt and family was as close as she could be to her parents and sister, far away in a war-torn land. She was overwhelmed at the outpouring of love toward her and her babies. Monika, Willy and Little Joe were all waiting on the steps, greeting them with open arms and open hearts as if they had known each other forever. A wonderful feeling of belonging filled Lisbeth as she was enfolded into this warm and loving family. Without a doubt, she truly felt she had come home.

Lisbeth continued to marvel at the extent of the welcoming preparations that Anni had made for them. On the lower level of the house, a large guest room and bath were waiting for them. There was a large double bed for Lisbeth and Rosalinde. An old baby crib, freshly painted, was set up in the corner. A multi-colored handmade quilt covered the bed, and a new pink baby blanket was waiting for Angelina on her crib. A comfortable old rocker sat in the opposite corner, and soft decorative pillows added an inviting touch. The walls were graced with old family photographs which again brought tears to Lisbeth's eyes. But what touched her the most was the fact that Tante

Anni's children had lovingly assembled some of their old toys and placed them on the antique chest set against the wall. There was a well-loved doll, a teddy bear, a stack of picture books, building blocks and a wooden train set. Lisbeth held her children close, telling them how lucky they were to have a family such as this.

Guiltily she thought of Lorenzo, hoping he would understand and forgive her for feeling so totally contented. "How can this be? I love him so much, and I miss him already. And yet I am overjoyed to be here. He only let me go because he loves me so much. I know that. We will be happy again when I come home. This separation will be the best for both of us," Lisbeth told herself as she tried to banish these troublesome thoughts from her head. She was here now. She felt welcomed and accepted, and she would make this absence not only a pleasant holiday but a time of growth.

Even her worries about her family in Hamburg seemed less acute now. Here in the U.S., she felt closer to home. Although there were still thousands of miles separating them, the simple fact of traveling north relieved her anxiety. There was also hope for an occasional letter from Hamburg, as Anni had experienced. By contrast, Lisbeth had not had any communication after the very first letter at the beginning of the war. An optimistic smile spread over her tired face.

Lisbeth bathed and dressed her children for the festive dinner waiting for them. Monika was setting the table while the boys finished their homework. They were anxious to play with their little cousins as Lisbeth wandered into the kitchen to help her aunt. Wonderful aromas of baked chicken wafted from the oven as Anni finished the potato dumplings, like those her mother used to make.

"Tante Anni, I can't believe you are making all my favorite foods."

"Why not?" Anni laughed. "It isn't every day my niece comes to visit. Actually, you are the very first guests we have had from either side of the family. We are thrilled you are here, and if you think this is medicine for your homesickness, you are my medicine too."

Over Anni's shoulder Lisbeth spied a golden apple strudel sitting at the end of the kitchen table. "Oh Tante Anni, you even made strudel for me! Just like Mutti's! I love you!"

Anni smiled and blew her a kiss and Lisbeth truly felt at home. During dinner the conversation was very lively. The children wanted to know all about the ocean voyage. Josef was interested in the ship's cargo and the operation of the *estancia*. Anni wanted to hear about Lorenzo's family, especially Oma-Maria. There were so many questions. There was so much to tell.

"What kind of food do you eat there?" Little Joe wanted to know. "How do you get around? What does the house look like? What is your horse's name? Are you a good rider? How is your Spanish? How is your English?" The questions were endless, but Lisbeth was happy to oblige and answer them all. Long after the children had been put to bed, the adults sat up talking into the night, catching up, filling in all the empty spaces.

"Your Lorenzo must be a truly generous man, letting the three of you leave for months," said Josef. "I'm not sure I could handle such a long absence from my wife and children."

"Yes, Lorenzo is a wonderful man in every way. He has put up with my moods, my disappointments when Mutti and Papa could not come to visit me. I had so looked forward to seeing them, being with my sister and showing them my new life. I could not wait to show off my beautiful babies to them. And then the war came and took everything away from me. The worry about their safety and wellbeing completely overtook me. I just could not handle all that," Lisbeth told them sadly.

"We understand how hard these past several months have been. We are worried too, but you had hoped to see them. How difficult this time is for everybody!"

"Yes, it has been hard for me, and for Lorenzo too. I've been so depressed, crying and sad all the time. I didn't want to go anywhere with him, do anything. My homesickness was so all-consuming that I really was not a good wife to him. But Lorenzo is so understanding. He thought this trip would help me. I know already that I will be so much better after this visit with you."

Anni and Josef exchanged glances. They had had no idea of the tensions in Lisbeth's marriage or that she had been so affected by the war and her fear for her family. They too hoped this absence would benefit both sides, but they sensed that there was no simple answer to what sounded like a major problem.

"Yes," said Josef, "we are all concerned about your parents and Margarete. But we know that so far they are fine. Of course, the war is not being fought on German soil.

Just this week the German forces have seized Denmark and invaded Norway. I'm not sure I understand what is going on, but certainly there is no reason for us to panic. I'm still hoping that someone or something will stop this insane invasion all over Europe." Josef's calm voice and reasonable manner was a balm for Lisbeth's soul as they resolved to pray and hope. Everyone was quiet, letting their thoughts drift. But a somber mood prevailed about them.

"I have an open return ticket," Lisbeth said softly. "*La Paloma* continually makes round trips, returning to Buenos Aires at the end of each month. Lorenzo thought it might be good for me to stay until the end of the summer. Would that be all right with you if I stayed until the end of August?" she asked shyly.

"Of course, of course, stay as long as you like. We told you that before. In fact, it will a perfect time as the children have their long summer vacation then. This year we have promised them a trip to New York City. Willy is determined to see the Statue of Liberty which you saw in the harbor coming in. Do you remember?"

"Yes, I saw a tall statue on a small island, but I don't know anything about it," Lisbeth answered.

"Well, you will learn all about it from Willy. He is very enthusiastic about American history," Anni laughed. They continued making plans and telling Lisbeth about all the wonderful things they wanted to show her in America.

"Tomorrow we will take you all around Springbrook and, of course, to our garden center." With more hugs and kisses, they finally retired for the night.

"We hope you will be happy here," Anni said once again. "And maybe, with any luck at all, we might even get a letter from across the sea. Everything will be fine. I just know it will." Lisbeth nodded, hoping with all her heart that her aunt was right.

By the time Lisbeth and her children rose the next morning, the sun was already high. Josef had left for the greenhouse at the crack of dawn, and the Bauer children as well had long since left for school. Anni was bustling around the kitchen, preparing breakfast for her young guests. Anni felt so good, being able to help her niece through a difficult time. She and Josef were determined to lift Lisbeth's spirits. Rested and relaxed after a long journey and the stressful time preceding it, Lisbeth and the girls enjoyed a hearty breakfast and the bright beginning of a sunny day.

Before long, Anni loaded her visitors into the car for the short ride into the country. In the brilliant sunshine the countryside looked fresh and green. The Bauer enterprise consisted of two large greenhouses in which a variety of flowering plants and vegetables were growing. Soon customers would come from far and wide to buy all that was needed for spring planting. There was everything from anemones to zinnias, gardening supplies, fertilizer and tools of all kinds. Adjoining the greenhouses was an acre of shrub and tree plantings. Anni explained that the adjoining acres had once been an apple orchard belonging to the family of Jim Harding, who was now their young business partner. He still lived in the farmhouse on the other side of the orchard. Jim had worked for the Bauers since he was in high school and had returned after college. His father had died years ago, and his mother had leased out the property. In time she gave Jim the apple orchard as his payment for a partnership with Josef. This partnership had worked well for both of them as the Bauer Garden Center became a well-known success story in the area. Since his mother's death two years ago, Jim lived alone but felt very much part of the Bauer family.

When Lisbeth entered the greenhouse, she breathed the sweet humid air and could almost feel the plants growing. Jim was working on a multitude of tiny tomato plants. His tall lanky frame was bent over the plants, and with deft fingers he was trimming the unwanted shoots. When he heard Anni call to him, he straightened and a big smile spread across his face. He had friendly, regular features, and his skin sported a healthy outdoor look. His light hair fell in soft waves onto his forehead. When Lisbeth was introduced to him, his open and friendly smile made her feel as if they had known each other for a long time.

"Welcome to America! Happy to meet you," Jim said in his friendly, easy way, extending a dusty hand.

"Sorry," he smiled self-consciously, wiping his palm along his jeans. He bent down and spoke to Rosalinde who, suddenly shy, hid behind her mother. But Angelina responded to his friendly gestures by blowing a little bubble at him. That was the beginning of a gentle and warm relationship between the two of them.

After touring the greenhouse and the shrub nursery, Anni took them around the corner to an old farmhouse. The Bauer family had lived in this small house until their move closer to town the previous year. At the moment the house was empty, but part of the main floor was used by Anni as her office. Every day while her children were at school, Anni spent several hours placing orders, keeping the books, and taking care of the paperwork. At this time of year, things were still relatively quiet, but the busy season would begin in a few weeks and end in October with the fall sales of pumpkins, apples and cider.

Lisbeth fell in love with the old farmhouse at once. "How could you leave this beautiful little place?" she exclaimed. There were two small bedrooms and bath upstairs, a living room and a large dining room, a small kitchen and a screened-in back porch. A covered veranda ran along the front of the house where an old swing was attached to the ceiling rafters. Rosalinde made herself comfortable on the swing and smiled for the first time.

"Are you leaving the house empty from now on?" Lisbeth wanted to know. Anni explained that they had plans for the future, but for now it would remain the office and a place where the employees could rest and eat in the little kitchen.

"What are your plans for the future?" Lisbeth could not contain her curiosity. But Anni dismissed it with a wave of her hand. "It will be a long time before we can think about that. For now we are making good use of it."

Lisbeth turned and looked back at the house. It was painted bright yellow with dark green shutters. She could imagine Anni and Josef being very happy living there with their children. But now the family had outgrown this first home and seemed very content in their new place.

"Look, Lisbeth," said Anni. "Here in the back yard is still the old sandbox and play set. I'll have Josef or Jim get some clean sand for Rosalinde and Angelina to play in."

"Oh, what fun my little girls will have here!" Lisbeth replied. After their tour, they returned to Anni's house where they made lunch and put the girls down for a nap. Later in the afternoon they drove to the post office so Lisbeth could mail all the letters she had written on board ship. It was amazing to her that Anni drove her car everywhere and how much they had accomplished in one day. Back at *Bien Cielo* it would have taken half the day just to ride back and forth to the post office in Baradera. Of course, she could have had Juan or Manuel drive her, but all that seemed too complicated.

How different life was here in the United States. She liked what she saw and knew it would not take long to adjust to life here. It would be so much easier than adjusting to *Bien Cielo*, although there she had had Lorenzo's loving presence.

Lisbeth was very impressed by the Bauer enterprise. Everything was so neat and orderly, and one could feel the pride of accomplishment, hard work and perseverance. Aside from that, she could sense that the Bauers were a happy lot who were accepted and respected by their neighbors and townspeople. Anni and Josef had come to Springbrook in 1923 after working as cook and gardener at a large estate in upstate New York. With Anni's inheritance safe in the bank and their meager savings, they had set out to find a business of their own as soon as they could command the English language. They had been fortunate to find Springbrook and buy the property from Mr. Max, a retiring gardener without heirs. They were even more fortunate to complete the purchase before the collapse of the banking system a few years later.

Their present partner, Jim Harding, had been a friend of Mr. Max and had learned many things from him over the years. Finding the greenhouse and knowing Jim had been like a miracle for the Bauers. They had become friends first and partners second. Their teamwork and congeniality had made them successful.

Anni and Josef had never regretted immigrating to America. Her parents had not been too eager about her plans to marry a gardener and sail off to a foreign land. But finally they had relented, knowing Josef to be a good and hard-working man. So they had given their blessing and let them go. As Anni told Lisbeth her story, she realized that Lisbeth had done the same thing.

"Yes, Liesl, you and I, we both got our way in love, didn't we? I hope you are as happy as I have been with my Josef. Your Papa has written me how much he misses you, yet understands that you had to follow your heart and be with Lorenzo. It is just so sad that this war had to break out when we are all so far from each other."

Lisbeth nodded.

"But while you are here with us, we will enjoy each other. Try not to worry so much, Lisbeth. Promise me, try to enjoy your time here. God will look after our family," Anni added.

Lisbeth knew that Anni was right. No amount of worry would stop the war and make things right again. "I know,

Anni. I'm so happy to be here. I feel better already. What will be, will be, and Papa would want me to be strong and not despair as I have been doing. This time here will help me in so many ways, and when I see Lorenzo again I will be happy to go on with our life and not give up. Let's hope and pray for that."

THRITY-FOUR

It didn't take long for Lisbeth's life to fall into a routine. In the morning after everyone had left for work or school, she cleaned up the breakfast dishes and took her little girls for a walk. She was glad she had brought her baby carriage all the way from *Bien Cielo,* but sometimes she put both girls into the little pull wagon Josef had brought down from the attic. She remembered her walks to Oma-Maria's house, struggling with the carriage on the rough country road. Here, walking was a great pleasure, the wheels rolling smoothly along the pavement. She loved strolling around the neighborhood, marveling at the green lawns, the beautiful shrubs and the leafy trees, reminding her of Hamburg.

She had forgotten how relaxing it was to wander along under a canopy of green. How she enjoyed the abundance of trees and flowers compared to the treeless plains of the Pampas! Sometimes she walked along the road to the greenhouse where the children played in the back yard of the old farmhouse. Often Rosalinde curled up on the veranda swing and promptly fell asleep. Usually Josef or Jim drove them back to the Bauer house. Lisbeth felt very comfortable in her aunt's home, and for the first time in her young life she could attempt cooking under Anni's tutelage. She was happy to help in the household and be part of the family. Never, ever, did she miss the cooks and maids doing everything for her back at *Bien Cielo*.

Every week she continued to write to Lorenzo, to Oma-Maria, to her parents and sister. And every day, as she had done at *Bien Cielo*, she waited for the mail. Two weeks after her arrival at Springbrook she finally received a letter from her husband, very short and formal. Lisbeth knew he was not the letter writer that she was, and therefore was content with the short notes that continued to arrive periodically. Oma-Maria, on the other hand, wrote long and newsy letters, although most of the time there was nothing new to report.

The days flew by, and suddenly it was May, the country exploding with blooms and sunshine. Rosalinde and Angelina were happy little girls and were growing and thriving in the attention and companionship of their three cousins. Soon school would let out for the long summer vacation. Monika in particular was looking forward to the break. She offered Lisbeth her baby-sitting services and hoped to find time for her favorite pastime, reading. Willy couldn't wait for the promised trip to New York later in the summer, and Little Joe was happy simply to be out of school.

"What a fantastic summer this will be!" Lisbeth thought

to herself. She too was anxious to see something of the country. Anni and Josef had planned a number of excursions in the area as Josef loved to drive, and Anni loved going to antique and estate sales. She loved collecting old and unusual things, and her home was filled with many pieces that had histories of their own. Lisbeth was interested in her aunt's hobby and hoped to learn many new things from her. The next few months promised to be a storehouse of small adventures, and Lisbeth welcomed them. Her thoughts and prayers traveled across the ocean daily, remembering her far-flung family. But the intensity of her former fear, her near panic, slowly receded, making way for growing acceptance and optimism. Her children were amazingly content and happy in their new environment. But it surprised and slightly disturbed her that even Rosalinde rarely asked about her father.

"How quickly little children forget," she thought in wonderment, hugging her little girls close and telling them how much their father loved them. She herself thought lovingly of Lorenzo, thanking him daily in thoughts and letters for his love, his kindness, his willingness to give her this precious time with her family. She had not imagined it possible, but now with thousands of miles separating them, she loved him more than ever.

But Lisbeth could not shake her old habit of anxiously waiting for the mail. After several weeks she received a long letter from Emilio Alvarez. He and Paulina had enjoyed their week in New York, and Emilio had satisfactorily concluded his business there. Of course the return journey had not been nearly as pleasurable without Lisbeth and her darling girls. Emilio, kind and concerned as always, had contacted Lorenzo and told him about the voyage and the happy family reunion in the States. He reported that all was well at *Bien Cielo*, and that Lisbeth and her children were greatly missed by everyone. Lisbeth smiled, rereading the letter. Señor Alvarez reminded her of her Papa, always concerned for her welfare, and always taking care of everything.

"If you need anything, please let me know. If you need more money, you know that I can cable it from your account," Emilio wrote, adding best wishes and greetings from him and Paulina.

"How very lucky I am! So many wonderful people caring for us," Lisbeth reflected, looking forward to the pleasant weeks ahead. She began to relax; from day to day she felt better. She no longer awoke daily imagining the worst happening in Germany.

The American newspapers reported many more details and photographs of the war in Europe than the Argentinean press. Worrisome as these reports were, there was never news of Hamburg. Josef scanned the papers daily for news of that specific area. So far nothing had been reported.

"No news is good news," Josef was fond of saying. "There is nothing about Hamburg. Your parents are safe. I just know it, or we would hear something."

Lisbeth hoped and prayed that he was right. His calm and reassuring manner was infectious, and there were days when she actually forgot to worry about the war. She was busy with her children, involved in her aunt's activities, excited to be a part of a happy and close-knit family.

Quickly the wonderful days of summer flew by. The Bauer children were enjoying their long vacation. Now Monika took her little cousins for their daily walks. Almost every day Lisbeth and all the children went to the local swimming pool where they cooled off with shrieks of joy. There was time to read, play games, or just be lazy. Once a week Lisbeth joined Anni and Josef going to the movies. It was not only to see the latest Western; watching the weekly newsreels of war-torn Europe was of greater importance. So far Hamburg seemed to have been spared as it never made the news. But what made everyone ecstatic was a letter from Margarete which had miraculously appeared in their mailbox. Just when Lisbeth had given up hope of ever receiving news from home, there it was, a tattered envelope filled with joy.

Margarete wrote that everyone was well—worried and scared, but well. They were anxious and uncertain but so far their lives had not changed and they were safe. They had received Anni's letter, informing them of Lisbeth's upcoming visit. They were puzzled as to the reason, but nevertheless happy that they would be together. A great weight was lifted off everyone's chest. Lisbeth especially was giddy with relief. She felt that life just could not get any better. All was finally well in her world.

THIRTY-FIVE

Soon after this happy event, it was time for the Bauer excursion to New York City. According to Willy, the main reason was to visit the Statue of Liberty. His class had studied American history of that era, and he begged and badgered his parents to actually see and experience it. Lisbeth had seen the large statue as *La Paloma* was sailing into New York Harbor, but she had no idea of its history or significance. Willy planned to write a special report to his class in the fall.

It had been decided to take a bus into the city as there were too many of them now to go in the family car. This in itself was a great adventure for young and old alike. Jim Harding had repaired an old collapsible stroller which had stood on three wheels, dusty and broken in the garage. Lisbeth had cleaned it and made soft new cushions for baby Angelina. Everyone was packed and ready to go. Jim Harding would handle the greenhouse operation alone for the day. He drove the family to the bus depot, making two trips. Then he waited until the Greyhound rolled out of the station, and waved a friendly goodbye.

Anni's children had never been out of Springbrook and just riding along in comfort, watching the scenery roll by, was exhilarating for them.

Lisbeth remembered very little of her ride from the New York harbor to Anni's house as she had been dead tired. Now she saw everything for the first time. She was struck by the beauty of the countryside, the gentle hills, the well-tended farms and small towns. She wished Lorenzo could be with her to experience this green world, remembering the cooler, rainy season in the Pampas right now.

"I hope all is well at *Bien Cielo*," she thought, not having received any mail recently. But she knew that the postal service in Argentina was unpredictable and slow. "I really do miss him. I wish he could see this beautiful place. Soon, much too soon, this time with Anni will come to an end. But then I will look forward to being with my Lorenzo again, and everything will be good between us."

After the thrilling drive through the Lincoln Tunnel, the bus soon arrived at Battery Park in the city, and the Bauer children could hardly wait to board the ferry that would take them to Liberty Island. Rosalinde and Angelina had been sleeping peacefully, but they were quickly ready for the upcoming adventure. As the ferry approached the island, the family was overwhelmed by the size of the statue. Amid oh's and ah's, they stood mesmerized at its impressive beauty. They continued to marvel at its size and elegance as they strolled around its gigantic base. Willy explained that this huge statue was a symbol of freedom and opportunity to arriving voyagers and immigrants.

"Just like us," Josef declared solemnly. "Just like us, giving us the opportunity for a good life." And Anni nodded in agreement. Even Lisbeth, only a visitor to these shores, felt welcomed as she recalled seeing this beautiful lady greeting her in New York Harbor.

The next highlight was the elevator ride up to the statue's pedestal. From there two spiral staircases climbed through the hollow statue into the figure's crown. Josef and Willy were the only two of the group to undertake the climb to enjoy the panoramic view of the harbor and beyond. For the others, the view from the pedestal was spectacular enough. As Lisbeth looked out over the Atlantic, her thoughts turned to her family on the other side. But cherishing the recent news from Margarete, she could take a deep breath of comfort and enjoy this magical day. Returning to the base of Lady Liberty, the Bauer clan gathered once more to read the inscription on the bronze plaque. Willy stood boldly in front of the tablet and surprised everyone by reciting the entire verse which he had proudly memorized. Especially the last part of the verse touched all who heard young Willy. He was warmly applauded by the onlookers. Lisbeth's eyes misted as she heard Willy recite:

> "Give me your tired, your poor,
> Your huddled masses yearning to breathe free,
> The wretched refuse of your teeming shore.
> Send these, the homeless, tempest-tost, to me.
> I lift my lamp beside the golden door."

"What a country," Lisbeth thought, "welcoming all, even me, to this great land. Look what it has offered my aunt and Josef. How proud and happy they are, and look at Willy, the patriot! I could be happy here if only I had my Lorenzo with me." She smiled at Willy who had made this a day to remember.

After lunch of hotdogs and ice cream cones, they strolled through the park and then boarded the ferry back to the city. They marveled at the beautiful tall buildings, the size of Macy's Department Store, and all the activity on the streets. Visiting the Empire State Building was left to a future trip. A tired but happy group boarded the bus home late that evening with promises to return soon.

As the bus rolled toward Springbrook, most passengers had fallen asleep. But Lisbeth was too excited to sleep. Holding her children close, she replayed the events of the day in her mind. Seeing Willy recite the poem at the Statue of Liberty made her smile. She was learning a lot from Willy. He had already told her about another American holiday, coming up in July. He and Little Joe were going to participate in a parade on the Fourth. Although Lisbeth did not yet understand the historical significance of that holiday, she and her girls looked forward to a parade and big picnic in the Springbrook Park. Little Joe told her about the fireworks to be held in the evening, and how everyone in the whole country celebrated. That was enough to look forward to with great anticipation. Lisbeth closed her eyes, knowing the happy memories of New York and Liberty Island would remain in her heart forever.

THIRTY-SIX

The days passed quickly as June slid into July. Soon Lisbeth would have to face her return journey to Argentina. It would be more difficult this time for several reasons. Emilio and Paulina would not be with her, helping her with the children and keeping her in their watchful care. This time, she would be alone, with her babies depending only on her. But at the end of the voyage, there would be Lorenzo waiting for her with open arms. Leaving Anni and Josef would be very difficult. They had all melded into one large happy family, and Lisbeth dreaded having to leave them. But she knew what she had to do. At the end of August she would return to her real life at *Bien Cielo* with Lorenzo. She had done a lot of thinking during this time away, and she knew she was ready to return where she belonged. She realized that her immature behavior had caused the rift with her husband. She could see that now. She wanted more than anything to rebuild her marriage, regain the love she and Lorenzo had pledged each other on their wedding day.

"I'll write Lorenzo today, telling him how I can't wait to see him. I'll tell him that I will be home in August. I know that will make him as happy as it makes me."

On a hot afternoon, Lisbeth was home alone with her children. She had just put them down for a nap, and was enjoying the stillness. Monika and the boys had left for the swimming pool, their packed lunches in their bike baskets.

Looking out the kitchen window, Lisbeth saw Jim Harding's truck pull into the driveway. Wondering what he was up to at this time of day, she ran to open the front door.

"Hi, Jim. How are you? Please come in." Lisbeth greeted him. Smiling, Jim entered the living room, handing Lisbeth a packet of mail.

"I had to go into town, and I stopped at the post office. Melba gave me the mail as she knew how anxiously you always look for letters from Argentina." He winked mischievously at her. "I spied one airmail letter and told Melba I would bring it out right away."

"Oh, thank you! Please let me get you some iced tea."

Jim sat down in Anni's rocking chair, stretching out his long legs. He looked around the cozy room. He felt at home here with the Bauers and had spent every holiday with them since his mother's death. During the winter months, he had dinner with them once a week, usually staying for a game of checkers or monopoly with the kids. He was too busy right now for these family nights but stopped quite often on his way home. Since Lisbeth's arrival he had only been here a few times, but he loved playing with the little girls when they came by the greenhouse. Usually he had a treat for them in his pocket, and today was no exception.

"Are the girls asleep?" he asked Lisbeth as she set down his glass of iced tea.

"Oh yes, they were tired. We were at the playground this morning. Now let me see about this mail you brought." Lisbeth quickly found the letter she was looking for. "A letter from Oma-Maria," she exclaimed, ripping the envelope open. Jim stood up suddenly.

"I'll be on my way then," he smiled awkwardly. Handing her two lollipops for Rosalinde and Angelina, he headed for the door.

"No, no, please stay. You don't mind if I quickly read my letter, do you? Stay, please, and drink your tea."

Jim sat down again, watching Lisbeth's happy face as she quickly scanned the letter. As usual, Oma-Maria's letter was cheerful and full of love. She missed Lisbeth and the girls very much and hoped they were all well and happy. Much as she missed them, however, Oma-Maria suggested in the next paragraph that Lisbeth stay at Anni's longer than planned. Lisbeth frowned. Stay longer? But knowing Oma to be a practical woman, Lisbeth understood that a longer stay seemed more worthwhile to her. This was a once-in-a-lifetime experience, and Oma-Maria wanted her to get the most out of it. What a wonderful woman, her Oma-Maria!

She folded the letter and smiled at Jim. She had almost forgotten that he was still sitting there.

"What a nice letter! Thank you, Jim, for bringing it. Oma-Maria is like my own grandmother. I just love her. Can you imagine? She thinks we should stay even longer, as I may not get this opportunity again. But I'm ready to leave in August. I need to get back to my Lorenzo. He has been missing us long enough."

Jim nodded agreeably. "There is no way in the world I would let my wife and two little ones leave without me!" he thought. "If it were my family, I would want to be with them every day. I would not let them go so far away! Never!" But it was not his family. He was alone with only his dreams.

After Jim left, Lisbeth sat down to read the letter again. Much as she loved living the American way of life with the Bauers, her longing for Lorenzo grew with every passing day. She was ready to go back and begin a new chapter with him. Strangely enough, since living with her aunt, her tormenting worries about her parents and Margarete had subsided. She thought and prayed daily for their safety. She wished that she could see them, but it no longer consumed her. She had learned to accept, to trust, and to cope.

Resolutely, Lisbeth rose and went into the kitchen. She could cook dinner for the family tonight. Anni had been teaching her so much--especially cooking. She smiled to herself, planning to teach Marta back at *Bien Cielo* a few of Anni's recipes. She actually began looking forward to going home.

When the Bauers came home that evening, they found Lisbeth singing to herself as she banged her pots and pans around, cooking what she hoped would be a good dinner for them. Seeing her so happy brightened everyone's day.

THIRTY-SEVEN

Oma-Maria was restless. Lisbeth and the children had been gone a long time, and she missed them terribly. Her head told her that this trip was good for Lisbeth, but her heart could not understand the reasons for Lorenzo's approval. She simply could not get Lisbeth out of her head. They had bonded so tightly in the last four years, and Lisbeth had become the daughter she never had. Maria missed her beautiful face, her sweet accent, her happy smile. But she had to admit in the last half year, Lisbeth had hardly ever smiled anymore.

Oma-Maria missed their visits to town, she missed their horseback rides, she missed the opportunity to speak a little German again. She missed everything about Lisbeth and the children. The beautiful little girls were a special bonus for her, and she could never get enough of holding and loving them. Now they had gone thousands of miles away, and the weeks seemed endless and lonely. She could not understand why or how Lorenzo had agreed to such a long absence. But when she brought up the subject, Lorenzo tossed his head and said coldly, "It's what she wanted. It's for the best."

Still, Oma-Maria could not understand it. Didn't he miss them as much as she did? Why did he let her go for so many months? There were too many unanswered questions. "I'm an old woman now. These young people have different ideas today. In my day my husband would never have let me go away for so long, or he would have gone with me," she said to herself, shaking her head. She could, however, understand Lisbeth's restlessness, having to adjust to a new country and a new life, the outbreak of war in her homeland, the worries about her family, and having two babies in two years. That was a heavy load for anyone's shoulders. Oma-Maria became as anxious as Lisbeth had been, waiting for the mail, and often driving into Baradera for no reason except a stop at the post office. Of course, she also needed and enjoyed her visits with Juliana, talking about Lisbeth and sharing any news.

Today Maria was getting ready to drive into town, mostly to visit her old friend Emma whose birthday was today. Several other ladies were going to meet and have tea together. Maria was looking forward to a little diversion and relaxation. Her friends in town always had something new to talk about, and these gatherings were greatly anticipated. But first the stop at the post office. As usual, Juliana was happy to see her, but unfortunately there were no letters today. When Maria shared Lisbeth's last letter with her, Juliana was as happy as if she had received one herself.

"I'm glad Lisbeth had a safe trip and is having a good visit with her relatives. I'm happy for her that she went, no matter what people say about it. It was the best for her."

Maria wrinkled her brow. "What do people say?" she asked.

"Oh, nothing," Juliana stammered, a bright red flushing her pretty face. She clamped her mouth shut, and there was no way to get anything out of Juliana if she did not want to talk. Perplexed, Maria walked to Emma's tea party, but somehow the wonderful day she had expected had been spoiled for her.

Maria's friends had already assembled when she arrived. After the customary greetings, the five ladies settled down to the serious business of enjoying tea, cake and conversation. First the general news around town was covered, health and family came next, and of course, Lisbeth's departure had to be discussed all over again.

"I'm pleased she had the opportunity to go, but I miss her just terribly!" Maria commented.

Alma agreed, saying that without Lisbeth's weekly lessons, her job at the library seemed to be just an ordinary routine job. Francesca, who had been quietly listening, asked in a sweet voice, "And how is poor Lorenzo doing?" with fake concern in her voice.

Knowing Francesca and her occasional back-stabbing ways, Maria replied openly, "Poor Lorenzo? Of course he misses her, but being the good and loving husband that he is, he let her go to help her."

Pilar interrupted, "Let her go? I understood she left him, took the little *bambinas* and just left him."

Maria was stunned. "What is going on here? What is the talk around town? Please tell me, please..."

Maria's friends looked at each other, all speaking at once. What was totally new to Maria seemed to be old gossip to everyone else. Apparently word had spread through Baradera that Lorenzo's foreign wife had simply taken their children and left him. The talk was that her "city friends" had helped her and that she had gone to America for God knows how long, perhaps forever. The fact that Lorenzo himself had taken his family on the train to Buenos Aires seemed immaterial.

Lorenzo was being pitied by everyone, and it was only natural that he was consoling himself by seeing Elena and spending many evenings at the cantina with his friends. Francesca scornfully mentioned that her son had spotted Lorenzo and Elena at the races in Pergamino last weekend.

Maria was speechless. Had she been living on the moon not to have heard any of this? The tea party broke up earlier than usual, and Maria began her ride home with confusion and sadness. "Who has spread this vicious rumor?" she had demanded of her friends, but no one seemed to know. However, each one quietly suspected Elena herself.

When Maria finally confronted her grandson a week later, Lorenzo just laughed. "Why do you bother with old ladies' gossip? Yes, I go to the cantina, and yes, I do meet my friends there, and I even see Elena there sometimes. But why does it concern anybody? It is not anyone's business but my own. My wife is gone and I am bored. Can't I have some entertainment too? Whom does it hurt?" Lorenzo answered with a raised voice.

But his Nonna looked at him with mournful eyes and said, "You know who gets hurt. Your wife and your children get hurt, your reputation—we all get hurt. What are you thinking? Have you forgotten what you have been taught, what is right and what is wrong?"

His grandmother's reproachful look suddenly touched his heart and, dropping his head into his hands, Lorenzo began to sob. Gently the old woman placed her hand on his head. She had never seen an adult man cry before.

"What is it, Lorenzo? What is wrong? Please, what is it?"

Finally Lorenzo raised his head and spit out with a despairing voice, "What am I expected to do? Ever since last fall my wife, my Lisbeth, is not my wife any more. All she does is cry, complain, worry and talk about her family. All she worries about is them, the stupid war, the stupid war! Doesn't she have a family here too? Who am I to her? Nobody! She gets so involved with the girls she hardly has time for me."

Lorenzo lifted his tear-streaked face to Nonna as if she could help him as she had so often done when he was a child.

"But, Lorenzo, you must understand..." Maria began.

"No, no! I do not understand." Lorenzo interrupted impatiently. "She is not the same, I tell you. She doesn't want to go anywhere with me, do anything with me. She didn't even go to the Christmas Fiesta with me. She used to enjoy it so much, but now everything is different. She has Nina to help her. Why can't she be there for me?"

Maria had never seen Lorenzo rave and scream like this since he was a boy. Oh, what tantrums he used to throw when he did not get his way! Nonna remembered well. She was pulled out of her reverie as he continued more quietly now.

"I tell you, I don't count with her anymore. I am nothing to her. But I am ME, ME, and I want a life. I was so happy when I met her. We were so in love. I don't know what has happened to us, but things are not the same. All she thinks about is them back in Hamburg, never me." He screamed again. He barely caught his breath, then continued defiantly, "So I went to the Fiesta by myself, and I had a good time without her. That's what she wants anyway. Yes, I met Elena there, and I have been seeing Elena ever since. I have known her all my life, and she understands me. I don't have to explain anything to her. She knows what makes me happy."

Maria held up her hands. "Stop, Lorenzo, stop. I can't listen to this any longer. I don't care what is going on between you, but you are a married man. You have two children. You must try to make your marriage work. You cannot throw everything away. Try to understand Lisbeth, how difficult things have been for her too. Have you tried to help her? Can't you understand what she has been going through? Did you forget that for loving you she left her family, her country, to be with you? Don't you call that love? She needs your help and your love, not your childish, selfish behavior!"

But Lorenzo was not listening. All he wanted to do was to justify himself, blaming only Lisbeth. "Didn't I let Lisbeth and the girls go up north for a few months? Didn't I give her a chance to see her family there? Maybe she will think about me and change her ways, and maybe I will feel differently about her too. But I'm not suffering for all her mistakes!" he stormed.

Maria shook her head sadly as tears ran down her cheeks. "Have you talked to your parents about this? Do they know what you are doing? Do you know that the whole town is talking about you and Elena? Do they know how you feel?"

"No, not really," Lorenzo replied slowly. "But I know when Father saw me at the Fiesta without Lisbeth, he did not approve. But he doesn't know everything..."

"What is everything?" Maria asked, alarmed.

"Every thing is that... that..." Lorenzo began to stammer, breaking into more dry sobbing moans. "Elena is pregnant. She told me several months ago. She is going to have my baby in September."

"Oh, my God!" Maria gasped. "What have you done to your family? Now I see, you think if you send your wife and your *niñas* (little girls) away, far away from here, she will just be conveniently out of the way while you and Elena continue your affair and have a baby! Lorenzo, Lorenzo, what have you done? What are you going to do?" Now Maria was sobbing too.

"I don't really know what I can do, but I know I have to stand by Elena for now. I know only that I need to be with her," he added, finally becoming calmer.

"Lorenzo, you can't have it both ways, you know. You must talk with your father. You must talk to Padre Dominicus. And you have to be honest with Lisbeth. Oh, Lorenzo, I don't know what to do. God help us!" Nonna sat down heavily, totally drained. Now she understood why Lorenzo had been so generous, so cooperative about Lisbeth's trip. She finally knew why Lorenzo was so eager to see Lisbeth and the children go to the States. What she had perceived as love and generosity was really only an act of great cowardice. "Lorenzo, how could you..."

But Lorenzo did not allow her to finish the sentence. "Nonna, I don't know why I told you all that. There is nothing you can do. There is nothing anybody can do. I will have to figure it out all by myself. I know you think badly of me for sending Lisbeth away, but what else could I do? It seemed like the best solution at the time. Now I don't know. I miss the children, and I miss Lisbeth. I am confused. I don't know what to do. But it is not for you to worry about, Nonna. Please forgive me and let me work it out somehow."

With that Lorenzo rose and without a goodbye turned to go.

Maria sat in her old rocking chair, letting the shattering news sink in. Her initial shock gave way to worry and helplessness. How could things change so quickly? One day Lorenzo has a beautiful wife and family, the next they are shipped off, and Lorenzo is involved with another woman. Elena of all people! And in all this, another innocent child caught up in this web of deceit!

"Now I understand why Lorenzo was so agreeable, even eager, to send Lisbeth on this distant and arduous journey. And poor Lisbeth thinks her wonderful husband only has her welfare in mind. Oh, I am too old to deal with this, and there is nothing I can do. I love Lorenzo, but I also love Lisbeth like my own. Even if she was at fault, she did not deserve this, nor her daughters. What will happen to them? Will they ever return when the truth comes out? How will Elena fit into all this? It will break Lisbeth's heart, I know, as it will break mine if I never see her again. Oh my Angelina, oh my Rosalinde, oh my Lisbeth!" she cried.

Too many problems were crowding Maria's thoughts as she sat helplessly. She knew Elena was a headstrong and temperamental person, in many ways similar to Lorenzo. Surely there will be fireworks in that relationship too, Maria knew. "Why did he tell me? Why bother me with these problems? It is not my affair, and there is nothing I can do."

Her loyalty toward Lisbeth was very strong, wanting to protect her and keep her in the family. Maria began to pray—pray that what she had been told today was just a horrible nightmare.

Slowly a plan crystallized in her brain, and resolutely she walked to her desk to write a letter to Emilio Alvarez. Two weeks later, Maria boarded the train at Baradera. She met Emilio at the bank and with his help and advice concluded her business swiftly and without regret. She spent the evening with Paulina and Emilio, sharing whatever news they had about Lisbeth's stay with her family. Maria was careful not to mention the upheaval and troubling events back at *Bien Cielo*. They would find out soon enough. Maria was ashamed of her grandson's actions. She was saddened by the loss of three innocent people who had come into her life for such a short time and now were gone from her forever. She could not shake the thought that Lisbeth would never return to *Bien Cielo*. She was frightened that now Lisbeth had no home, not in war-torn Germany, and not in Argentina where she had been so heinously betrayed.

Riding back home on the train, Maria could not think straight. The only thing she was totally certain of was that what she had done in Buenos Aires was right. She had no control of the future, but she had done the one thing that she had control over. "What will be, will be. *Que sera, sera.*"

"I will go home and take care of Lisbeth's roses. Yes, that is what I'll do. As long as I live I will tend her roses. That is all I have left of her."

THIRTY-EIGHT

Every day Josef followed the war news in the papers. So far there had been no mention of Hamburg. What shocked him the most was the report that Nazis had taken Paris in mid-June and were pushing toward the English Channel. The war was escalating rapidly, but as concerned as he was, he knew how easily Lisbeth could panic, and carefully kept the news from her.

Both he and Anni continued to be optimistic, involving Lisbeth and the children in their busy daily routine. Lisbeth finally was calmer and stronger, and they intended to make her visit with them as rewarding and as memorable as they could. She had blended into their family so effortlessly and seemed to be resolving her problems of homesickness and loneliness. In fact, she appeared to look forward to her return to *Bien Cielo*, intent on rebuilding her marriage.

But a conflict of major proportions was also brewing at *Bieno Cielo*. Lorenzo's father José was devastated by the rumors which were now known to be fact. Cecilia remained steadfastly silent, as was Lorenzo, unable to take action.

José tried repeatedly to discuss the situation with his son, but to no avail. Lorenzo simply did not seem to care. He continued seeing Elena as if he were a free man. But José was a man of action. He insisted something had to be done, and soon.

"Be a man, Lorenzo! You must be honest with your wife before she returns. You have to decide how to resolve this situation. Do you love Lisbeth? Do you want to save your marriage, hoping your wife will forgive you? What about Elena? Do you want to continue to give her false hope? Whatever it is, you must first of all be honest with Lisbeth. She needs to know what is happening here. She deserves to know the truth—now!" José insisted.

But Lorenzo was confused. On one hand, he was torn between his commitment to Lisbeth and his duty to Elena. His wife and daughters were so far away that at times they seemed unreal to him. Elena, however, was here. She was real, flesh and blood, and she was carrying his child. He was pulled by a strange fascination toward this new being, perhaps, even a son.

Selfishly he blamed Lisbeth for all their problems and misunderstandings, never once admitting to a shared portion of the blame. He continued to justify his infidelity by placing the guilt on Lisbeth alone. It was she who did not understand him and his ways—she who was not happy with him—she who always put her family before him. What did the war in Europe matter to him? Why were her thoughts over there instead of here with him? For now Lorenzo continued to procrastinate, doing nothing, wishing to prolong Lisbeth's absence and delaying the final confrontation with her.

As Elena's pregnancy became public knowledge, the townspeople divided into two camps. There were those who felt sorry for Lisbeth and yet could not understand her hasty departure. There were others who thrived on scandal and were eagerly awaiting the outcome of this volatile situation. Elena, enjoying being the center of attention and the talk of the town, proudly showed off her expanding figure, a smug smile on her face. In her heart she knew that if she had a son, her place as mistress of *Bien Cielo* would be assured.

THIRTY-NINE

Lisbeth, however, unaware of the disasters mounting all around her, continued to live in blissful ignorance. Day by day as she became stronger and more self-confident, life as she had known it at *Bien Cielo* was falling apart. She savored each day in Springbrook, keeping her memories as precious treasures in her heart. Her children were thriving, blossoming in the attention they received from everyone in the Bauer family, and their friend, Jim Harding. He often stopped at the house on some pretext or another, always bringing special treats for the girls. Rosalinde smiled her sweet, shy smile, opening up to him as she sat on his lap while he read stories to her. Angelina would clap her fat little hands and squeal with pleasure whenever he came into view. Jim always had time for a piggy-back ride or a special hug. Lisbeth thought sadly of Lorenzo and wondered why he had seldom found the time or interest to play with his children.

"Perhaps that's part of his upbringing," she thought,

remembering what he had once said to her: "When they are small, they belong to you. When they grow older I will do things with them, you know. I'll take them riding and things like that."

Still it warmed her heart to watch Jim, a stranger, so relaxed and playful with them. One day, when Lisbeth and the girls had walked to their private little playground behind the old farmhouse, Jim stopped by, and as he often did, offered them a ride back home. Lisbeth was very happy today to take him up on his offer as the pleasant morning hours had now turned into a blazing hot day.

"I can't wait to get home and get a cool drink for all of us.!" Lisbeth commented as she settled the girls in the truck, wiping her brow. Jim stowed the baby carriage in the back of the pickup and with a happy grin began the short drive to town.

"I have a much better idea," Jim said, winking at the girls. "Let's drive to the ice cream parlor first. We can get a cold drink there, or better yet, a super deluxe chocolate sundae!"

"Ice cream, ice cream!" Rosalinde cried out with pleasure while Angelina clapped her hands and laughed in agreement.

"Well, Jim, if you have time, it does sound good."

"Sure, I have time," Jim replied. "You know my work at the greenhouse is never done, but it will wait for me. I can finish it anytime. Right now I'm ready for some ice cream."

"Isn't it great when you have a car, being able to drive wherever you need to go? To get ice cream on the spur of the moment! Imagine that! I could never do that at *Bien Cielo*.

Everything seems so much simpler here," Lisbeth said, speaking more to herself than to Jim.

Jim gave her a puzzled look. "Are there no ice cream parlors in your town—what is the name—Bara...?" he asked her. "And I know there must surely be a car at *Bien Cielo*. I don't see why..."

"Oh, Jim, you don't understand. There is no such thing as an ice cream parlor in Baradera. Maybe in Buenos Aires. And yes, of course there is a car at *Bien Cielo*. A beautiful black car. But you don't understand how life is there. Even if there were such an ice cream place, and even though there is a car, I cannot drive. I cannot just go as I please unless I ride my horse or ride with Oma-Maria in her carriage. Otherwise I need Lorenzo, or Manuel or Juan to drive me to Baradera. That is all too complicated. That's why I say everything is so much simpler here."

"Then, why don't you learn to drive while you're here? Then you wouldn't have to ask anyone for favors. You could drive yourself. Wouldn't that make it simpler for you? I would be glad to teach you. It isn't that difficult. You'll see."

Jim was getting more excited and enthused as he spoke. Lisbeth could not believe what she was hearing. Learning to drive! Her secret wish for a very long time! "Are you a mind reader, Jim? How I wish I could learn!" Remembering her life in Germany, Lisbeth had once jokingly asked her father if Johann might teach her. Her Papa had laughed and said, "What a silly girl you are. As long as we have Johann, why would you want to drive?" And that had been that.

She remembered asking Lorenzo the same question and also being refused.

"Lisbeth, what do you say?" Jim prodded, pulling her back to the present.

Learning to drive! What a dream come true! But Lorenzo had firmly and finally denied her that wish. And suddenly, here was Jim, a stranger, offering to teach her, simply, so sincerely! "Would you really do that for me?" Lisbeth was overcome. "But there probably is not enough time anyway," she added sadly. "You know I'll be leaving at the end of August."

"Sure, there's enough time. You still have six weeks. You can do it. I'll bring you the book tonight, and you can study the rules and get a learning permit. I'm sure Josef and Annie will help you if there is anything you don't understand. I'll take you out on the country roads to practice. It will be fun, I know. Just think what a nice surprise that will be for your husband and his family! You can show them what you have learned in America. You will be independent. Your husband will be very proud of you."

Lisbeth was not so sure that Lorenzo would be proud of her, nor would he want her to be more independent. But the temptation was too great. Learning to drive was something she had wished for ever since she had begun her life in the Pampas of Argentina. "Yes, yes, Jim! Let's do it! Let's get our ice cream first, and then you can teach me to drive."

Jim nodded and smiled. He was thrilled to have acquired his first student driver. Looking at Lisbeth's happy face, Jim knew that he was giving her a big gift.

And so began the routine of the evening driving lessons. Several times a week Jim showed up after supper to take Lisbeth out in his old Ford. There were miles of country roads without traffic where he taught her the intricate maneuverings of starting the engine, shifting gears, and coming to a smooth stop. Lisbeth had studied the rule book carefully and was slowly becoming a prudent and observant driver.

Jim was extremely patient and kind, even when a sudden stop caused both of them a bump on the head. After each lesson Lisbeth returned home beaming, radiating a sense of accomplishment. She was a quick learner and before long was adept and confident enough to drive the streets of Springbrook. Soon Lisbeth did all the driving whenever she and Anni went shopping, to the post office, the movies or the swimming pool. She looked forward to these outings, enjoying driving and feeling in charge.

One Sunday afternoon, Jim wanted to show her more of the countryside. Angelina was sleeping, but Rosalinde was eager to come along. Jim directed Lisbeth down a narrow country lane, showing her his family's acres which were still leased to a neighboring farmer. There was also a small lake where he liked to go fishing in the evenings. He explained that his father had taught him to fish when he was a very young boy, and he in turn had taught Willy and Little Joe.

"Ah, so this is the spot where the boys come with their bicycles and fishing poles. Just last week they caught two fish."

"Yes, I think they enjoy it as much as I do. Even if I catch nothing, I enjoy being out here. It's quiet and peaceful and gives me time to think and relax."

Yes, Lisbeth could understand that Jim was a man who could enjoy simple pleasures. Being there for others was one of them. Returning home, they passed Jim's home, the family farmhouse where he had grown up. Lisbeth had never been inside, and Jim did not invite her in. But it looked well loved and cared for with beautiful flowers all around it.

"When do you find time to tend your own flowers when you work at the greenhouse all the time?"

"Oh, it's easy, and I need to show my neighbors what beautiful flowers they can buy at our greenhouse!" he joked.

"Do you have roses in your garden too?" Lisbeth wanted to know, remembering her mother and her spectacular rose garden.

"Yes, there are roses in the back of the house. I'll show them to you some other time. We should head home now. Anni wanted me to stay for dinner tonight."

Lisbeth smiled. Angelina would be awake by now and ready for a piggy-back ride on Uncle "Immy" as she called him.

Speaking of roses brought Lisbeth's thoughts back to her family. Were they well? How was their life going now that there was war? In Margarete's lone letter she hadn't really said much specifically. What was really happening?

Lisbeth shook her head and concentrated on her driving. But her thoughts wandered to Lorenzo and Oma-Maria. She was unsure about Lorenzo, but she was certain that Oma-Maria would indeed be very, very proud of her. Imagine, driving a car!

"Well, Jim, is Lisbeth ready to take her driver's test?" Josef called out as Jim walked up the steps, holding Rosalinde's hand.

"Yes, I think so. What do you say, Lisbeth? Shall we go tomorrow and get your driver's license?" Jim asked, turning to Lisbeth who was coming up behind him.

"Tomorrow already? Do you think I can do it?"

"Certainly. I have time tomorrow. Let's do it." Encouraged by everyone, Lisbeth agreed: "Tomorrow is the day." Willy and Little Joe patted Lisbeth's shoulder, wishing her good luck as everyone happily walked into the house, ready for dinner.

Passing her driver's test was another highlight in Lisbeth's summer. "I did it, I did it!" she squealed happily, waving her license. Wishing Lorenzo were with her, sharing her amazing feat, she still felt a pang of uncertainty and doubt. Would he be as happy about it as she felt right now? A sudden frown crossed her face. But looking up, she saw a very proud, smiling Jim.

"I knew you could do it. I'm so very proud of you," he said, and the look on his face said it all.

"I couldn't have done it without you," she exclaimed, impulsively hugging him and kissing his cheek.

Jim blushed to the roots of his fair hair, feeling a gamut of emotions. Proud and happy for Lisbeth, he felt sad that the driving lessons had come to an end. At first it had been a welcome diversion after a long day's work, but he was soon looking forward to his outings with Lisbeth as a rewarding pleasure. From now on she wouldn't need his help. Soon, too soon, she and her sweet little daughters would be leaving, sailing back to Buenos Aires. He knew that was where she belonged, yet he had conflicting emotions about it. Over the course of the summer he had grown to love them all. It was as simple as that. He was all too aware that he had no right. Still, they had unexpectedly entered his life and had gently and tenderly found a special place in his heart. Every moment he had spent with them was a treasure.

Lisbeth could not sleep that night. She was too excited, too happy, and very proud of herself. She thought of the many problems she had overcome this summer. She realized how much she had grown in confidence and maturity.

She had learned from Anni that her husband and children had to come first. Without loving her family in far-away Germany any less, her life was with Lorenzo, and he had to be her first consideration. She had watched how Anni and Josef had become one unit, how close they were to each other and their children. Their optimism transferred to her, and being surrounded by positive people she could trust, helped her mature and face whatever lay in store. Even Jim's calm and helpful demeanor had a decided influence on her and the girls.

Rosalinde was now almost three years old and Uncle "Immy" had become a special friend. Lisbeth was grateful to all around her, thanking God every day for their loving presence in her life.

FORTY

One hot July afternoon in Hamburg, Marianne was slowly walking home after meeting three of her friends at Café Mozart. The ladies had a standing date once a month to catch up on family news and enjoy coffee and cake. They had been friends for ages and were extremely close. They shared each other's joys as well as sorrows and were always there for each other.

"I wish Johann could have picked me up like in the old days," she thought, fanning herself with a handkerchief. But today she had actually wanted to walk, to be alone with her thoughts. Still it was too hot, and Marianne felt unsettled. Today's conversation had not covered the usual light subjects. Marianne was disturbed by the constant discussion of the war. She wanted to forget it. She wanted her old life back, peaceful and calm.

It seemed that ever since Lisbeth had met Lorenzo there had been one thing after another upsetting their family's life—Wilhelm's heart attack, then Lisbeth's impulsive and, in Marianne's mind, hasty marriage and departure to a strange and foreign land. Losing her daughter had been very difficult for Marianne, but the hope of seeing her soon had eased the pain. Now that hope was gone. There would be no trip to see Lisbeth and the two young granddaughters. There was even no hope of a letter.

The war had done that to her. She was very disturbed by the constant discussion of it. Today's meeting with her friends had been no different. Although the women didn't scan each newspaper as their husbands did, they were still anxious and concerned about their lives. It was difficult to ignore the daily broadcasts, reporting new developments on the front lines, and the continuous invasion of neighboring countries. The women were fearful for their safety at home, the quality of life in store for them. None of the women had sons in the military, but each knew of other families whose sons were battling in far-away places.

Already they were noticing certain shortages not only of imported items but of everyday necessities. Everyone realized that things were bound to get worse. Even Frau Müller, the owner of the café, had jokingly reminded them to enjoy their coffee as such luxury items might become scarce or unavailable if this war continued.

Instead of being an uplifting afternoon, it had put Marianne in a somber mood. She knew that her Wilhelm would shield and protect her, even if it meant keeping the truth from her. Even so, Marianne knew that after the fall of France, Hitler's plans would include the invasion of Britain. What would this bold undertaking mean to all the innocent people on either side of the Channel? Marianne could not imagine the horrors to come, but she knew they would come. Much as she missed Lisbeth and the little girls, she was thankful they were safe and far away from the present terror.

She no longer thought Johann had been overly pessimistic planning his vegetable garden and putting in rows and rows of potatoes. The two apple trees in the back yard were full of ripening fruit, and Johann was already talking about putting up jars of applesauce. Marianne smiled. What a treasure old Johann was! He and Wilhelm were planning to clean out part of the cellar and prepare an air raid shelter. Marianne and Margarete were strongly resisting the idea, but this time Wilhelm was firm. He and his Skat-playing friends had already discussed various ways to protect their families without alarming them. He knew that Lars had a walk-in safe in his house, and that Hans Birkner had constructed a shelter at his factory and was preparing one at home now. The only one who had not prepared was Judge Hoffmann; he refused to let himself get caught up in the pessimistic preparations. He truly did not believe it would come to such serious consequences and the immense deprivations everyone else feared. Christian Wagner, on the other hand, had already evacuated his family to an isolated farm community. He remained in the city for the time being but prepared to do what was necessary to survive.

Marianne shook her head sadly. At least Margarete's life still had a semblance of order. She spent four days a week at rehearsals and was involved in two performances. So far the opening of the opera season was scheduled as in peacetime, but nothing was certain. Many of the young male singers had been drafted, but so far the lead actors were exempt from the service. Even so, how long would the public feel free to venture out and enjoy an evening at the opera?

Marianne was glad that Margarete was busy, doing what she loved, pretending to have a normal life. She lived for mail from Peter, much as Marianne had lived for mail from Lisbeth. At least, so far Peter's letters had been arriving regularly. However, he hardly ever wrote of his duties or what he was experiencing, and was vague about his location. All Margarete knew was that he was on the Eastern Front. But he was well and still hoping for a speedy resolution to the conflict, as he called it. "I pray he is right," Marianne thought now as she reached her front door.

Wilhelm was at home reading the papers and listening to the radio. Hearing his wife enter the house, he rose to greet her. "Well, Marianne, did you have a nice afternoon with your ladies?"

"Oh, it was good to see them, but it was more depressing than relaxing," Marianne muttered, dropping tiredly into a chair.

"There is a letter from Kurt," Wilhelm said, pointing to an envelope on the table. But Marianne was not interested in reading more news about the war. She was glad Wilhelm and Kurt kept up a correspondence; it gave her husband something to do. Since the glass works had been closed at the end of last year, Wilhelm had become more quiet and somewhat dispirited. He had not been ready for this forced retirement although he knew that closing the factory was the only solution at the moment. Still he missed the daily routine and the satisfaction of running his business. He also missed Kurt. More than his business associate, more than his general manager, Kurt was his friend. He thought of him daily, wishing him well. Writing to Kurt gave him a link to the many productive and memorable years they had worked together. All he knew of Kurt at the moment was that he was in France and had been assigned to the supply division. "Keep those letters coming. Keep them coming until you come home yourself," Wilhelm had written in his most recent letter.

Marianne rose and sighed. Wilhelm looked up from his paper, noticing the worried look his wife wore every day now. "What is it, Marianne? Try not to worry so much. There is nothing we can do. Just be grateful Lisbeth is safe, her babies are safe, Margarete is here with us, Peter and Kurt are both well, and we have each other. Please, Love, cheer up a little. I hate to see you so sad all the time."

"Oh, Wilhelm, how can you be so calm? Everyone we love is either far away or in danger. Everything is so uncertain. And you say I should be grateful? This war, it's terrible. It's stupid. It is ruining everybody's life."

"I know, Marianne. Everything you say is true, but we must not despair. Even if we have no news of Lisbeth or from Anni, we know they live in safe places. Nothing can happen to them. We will see each other again, I know it. Be brave. Everything will work out." Wilhelm put his arm around Marianne and kissed her gently.

"I know you're right. What would I do without you? We are lucky, and we have each other. When the war is over..."

Wilhelm kissed her again. Yes, more and more the phrase, "When the war is over" was creeping into everyone's conversations, as they hoped to resume their previously secure lives once again.

FORTY-ONE

The months of June and July were dragging for Oma-Maria. She lived for Lisbeth's letters but with each one she felt her moving further and further away from her. Each writing spoke of a certain contentment, a happiness, without a trace of the old melancholy. "She is really happy up there in the U.S. She must have found something there she could not find here," she thought sadly.

Ever since Lorenzo had disclosed his relationship with Elena, Maria had been in a constant state of agitation. She could not sleep, nor could she keep Lisbeth and the children out of her mind. What would it do to her, finding out what was going on between her husband and that woman Elena? How often had she asked Lorenzo if he had at least written to his wife, explaining the chaos he was creating here at home! But Lorenzo was quiet and sullen, refusing to discuss anything with her. She knew that her son José was equally disturbed and disappointed by Lorenzo's behavior. But even he had no influence on him. Cecilia kept quiet and refused to discuss anything with Maria. It was clear that in Cecilia's eyes her son was still perfect and that, by her silence, she supported him. Maria was tempted to write to Lisbeth herself, but she knew it was not her place to do so. Nevertheless, she thought about it constantly, feeling almost like a traitor, not telling Lisbeth the awful truth.

As the time of Elena's confinement came closer, as well as the possibility of Lisbeth's return, Maria became even more nervous. She almost had to force herself to ride into Baradera, knowing that everybody was talking about her family. Elena and Lorenzo were the hottest topic in town as speculation and rumors grew around them. Lorenzo's nonchalant attitude, his seeming disregard of his marriage and Elena's shameless behavior continued to fuel the fires of gossip.

Maria was restless. Finally she saddled her horse and rode into town. Perhaps there was a letter from Lisbeth waiting for her. When Juliana saw Maria approach the post office window, she shook her head sadly.

"Nothing today, Señora Moncrief," she said, knowing how disappointed the old woman would be. They looked at each other sadly, both remembering Lisbeth and her frequent stops here.

"Does she know yet?" Juliana whispered, knowing they were alone. Maria shook her head sadly, ashamed of her grandson's cowardly behavior and total disregard for his wife and children.

"But what will my friend Lisbeth say when she returns and finds out the truth? She needs to know. Do you think she will come back? How can she live here with Elena making her life miserable? Poor Lisbeth! What can we do for her?" Juliana lamented.

"There is nothing you or I can do, only pray for her. Lorenzo is the one who needs to tell her. He must beg for her forgiveness if he wants her to return to him. But he is doing nothing. He is not telling me anything. How can he be so cruel to his wife? I do not understand it." Maria began to cry as Juliana's eyes brimmed with tears. Helplessly the two women hugged briefly as Maria turned and left the post office, hoping not to meet anyone she knew. She mounted her horse and slowly rode back to *Bien Cielo*.

Passing the stables, she decided to dismount and look for Lorenzo. But neither he nor José was anywhere to be seen. Reluctantly she walked up to the house, finding that Cecilia was upstairs taking a siesta. Lost in thought, Maria walked out onto the terrace. She was suddenly very tired. She sat down on the nearest chair and closed her eyes. She was frustrated that nothing was being done for Lisbeth.

It seemed to her that nobody cared, that Lisbeth and the children were suddenly forgotten. Didn't anyone miss Lisbeth, what she had brought to *Bien Cielo* years ago—her happy smile, her adoration and love for Lorenzo? Had they forgotten Rosalinde and the happy squeals of Angelina? Had everyone forgotten the happy little family that had once lived here? Maria began to cry again. Her love and loyalty to Lisbeth were very strong, and she could not bear to see them hurt. All she could do for them, she had done already. Now there was nothing left but to wait and hope. "I'm not a meddlesome old woman, but I have to keep trying. Somehow I must get Lisbeth and the girls back!" she vowed.

Maria looked across the garden, suddenly remembering Lisbeth's roses at the side of the house. Quickly she got up and walked around the corner. Lisbeth's rose bushes were a sorry sight. Obviously they had not been watered or pruned for some time. Feeling somewhat guilty herself, she marched over to the garden shed, looking for shears and a trowel. She found both as well as the rusty sprinkling can and resolutely began working on the neglected rose bushes as tears ran down her wrinkled cheeks. Lisbeth had been so attached to these scraggly bushes, her link to home. Now that she was gone, no one had bothered to tend her roses, and unless she returned soon, they would surely fade and die.

Maria had a strange premonition; she would never see Lisbeth again and Lisbeth would never see her roses again. Suddenly determined, and with renewed strength, Maria began to dig deeper, carefully pulling the roots out of the ground. Nobody seemed to care about Lisbeth or her roses, and it was up to her to preserve this last and very special link to the young woman she loved like her own granddaughter. Carefully she wrapped the rose bushes into her full skirt, determined to care for them in her own garden. Fervently hoping that Lisbeth would once again be with her, she would love and tend two lonely rose bushes. They became a symbol for her; if they survived and bloomed again, her Lisbeth too would survive, come home again and all would be well.

August was approaching, and Maria still knew nothing of Lorenzo's plans. He and his parents simply did not speak of the looming disaster that was about to befall their family. Maria wondered when Lisbeth was returning or if at all.

Rumor and gossip continued to spread around town until there was suddenly no more room for speculation.

Late one evening, one of the townspeople came riding up to *Bien Cielo* with the news that Elena had gone into premature labor. In shock, Lorenzo jumped into his clothes and rode into town in a flash. He was not ready for this sudden turn of events. In his mind there were at least six more weeks until Elena's due date. He still had not written to his wife. He still did not know what to do. There was no time even to think about a decision. All he knew was that he had to be with Elena now.

He arrived at the cantina, breathlessly running up the stairs to Elena's room. But Frida, the midwife in charge now, would not allow Lorenzo to enter. Elena's screams and moans could be heard through the closed door and all through the house. Lorenzo pushed Frida aside forcefully and entered the hot, stuffy room. Elena was crouched on her bed, her black matted hair spread across the pillow, her eyes wide open in fear and pain. Lorenzo knelt on the floor next to the bed, gently reaching for her hand. Just then another painful contraction washed over her, and with a piercing scream, Elena pushed Lorenzo aside. At that moment Frida entered the room with Gilberto, Elena's father, and together they pulled Lorenzo out of the room.

"Come, Lorenzo, let's wait downstairs. This is women's business," Gilberto muttered as the men stumbled down into the cantina. Wordlessly someone handed Lorenzo a tall drink which he gulped down thirstily. For hours the men sat and drank as Elena's screams and cries wafted down from above. Occasionally Frida came downstairs, getting something from the kitchen, to shrug her shoulders helplessly, to shake her head and disappear upstairs again.

By morning Lorenzo was asleep from exhaustion as well as from alcohol consumption. By mid-morning the news leaked out that Elena was close to giving birth. The cantina filled with curious onlookers waiting for news, anxious to observe Lorenzo. It was as if everyone in Baradera was holding his breath awaiting the outcome of some spectacular event. Nothing had caused such interest and fascination in town in a very long time—not since news came of Lorenzo's marriage to a foreign bride. But this event today concerned one of their own, Elena, whom everyone had known since childhood.

Shortly after noon, after another piercing scream, there was finally a baby's cry. Everyone fell silent, Lorenzo suddenly alert as he started to race up the stairs, the baby's wail becoming even louder and stronger. Lorenzo burst into the bedroom, ignoring Frida's and her nurse's protests. He stumbled toward Elena, grabbing her hands and looking into her exhausted, pale face. Barely audible, Elena whispered, "Lorenzo, the baby, you have a son, you have two sons."

Lorenzo stared at her unbelievingly. What had she said? "I have a son, I have two sons?" Too overcome to speak, he buried his face in Elena's arms.

Frida's shrill voice brought him back to reality. She yelled angrily, "Go away, Lorenzo. I am busy here. Go away. Go away and come back later. Elena needs me now, not you. This is no place for a man." She tried to pull Lorenzo to his feet.

By this time, Gilberto had also run up the stairs to see about his daughter. Above the commotion taking place in the crowded room, there was again the insistent cry of the babies. Gilberto and Lorenzo both looked up, seeing the midwife's nurse, busy swaddling not one, but two tiny babies on a large dresser in the corner. The young woman lifted each baby into her arms and smiled broadly as she walked toward Lorenzo and Elena.

"Here are your babies," she told them proudly, "*Gemelos* (twins)! Here are your sons. Look how beautiful they are. *Gemelos!*" she repeated proudly.

Lorenzo stared at the two bundles in the nurse's arms. Two dark-haired infants were sleepily yawning. A feeling of unbelievable pride welled up in Lorenzo as he had never experienced before. He gently touched each baby's cheek, then turned to Elena, kissing her eyes, her wan face, her dry lips.

"Elena, *Gemelos!* You are so wonderful. Thank you, thank you, for our sons."

Elena smiled tiredly but triumphantly. She had done it! She had given Lorenzo not only one but two sons, something Lisbeth had not been able to do. The long labor, all the pain, all the gossip and speculation, all she had had to do to get to this very moment, were worth it. She, Elena, had delivered the grand prize and was now sure that Lorenzo would be hers forever. Tiredly she closed her eyes as she let Lorenzo's kisses and words of love wash over her.

Interrupting this tender exchange, Frida was now yelling again, shooing everyone out of the room. "*Si, si*, I know you are all happy and excited. But you must all leave now. Elena needs her rest. The babies need some quiet, and we have much work to do here. Go away, everybody. Come back later tonight when we are finished here and Elena feels like having company."

With that she pushed everyone out of the room and closed the door firmly. A beaming Gilberto silently embraced Lorenzo in the hallway, kissing him on both cheeks.

"I am a grandfather now! And you have two sons. Bravo! What a wonderful day for us!" he beamed as the two men stumbled down the stairs, arm in arm, eager to share their news with the waiting patrons in the cantina.

"Drinks for everyone! I have two sons. *Gemelos!*" Lorenzo yelled across the crowd which erupted in cheers and whistles. He openly admitted paternity of the sleeping infants upstairs, drinking to Elena's health and achievement. Sadly nobody remembered excitement such as this when Rosalinde and Angelina were born at *Bien Cielo*. At this moment of jubilation, everyone including Lorenzo seemed to have forgotten that he had a wife and children. In this heady rush of pleasure, they were totally dismissed, ignored, as if they were non-existent.

Later in the day, as Lorenzo rode toward *Bien Cielo*, he made the decision that had eluded him for months. Eager to tell his parents about the birth of his sons, Lorenzo galloped faster. Having made up his mind, he was eager to discuss his decision with his father.

One of the *gauchos* who had been to Baradera had already brought the news about the birth to his parents. He found them sitting the parlor, stunned. Reluctantly his father rose and congratulated Lorenzo quietly. Cecilia was crying softly; Lorenzo was not sure if they were tears of joy or sadness. He had expected his parents to be jubilant. It was as if the enormity of today's events had finally become a reality to them. There were two new grandsons sleeping in Baradera tonight, and there were two granddaughters far away in a foreign land. They knew a major decision had to be made soon that would affect all their lives. It was a bittersweet joy they felt.

Late that night, Lorenzo sat in his room, drinking and brooding. The first heady rush of excitement had worn off, and now he had to face the future. Right or wrong, he had to do what he had to do. He finally found the courage to sit down and write some letters, to Lisbeth and to Emilio Alvarez.

He wrote to Lisbeth, page after page, then tore up the letter, loathing himself. He could not find the right words to explain his actions, to extricate himself from the distasteful situation he had created. He was not as sure about his decision now as he had been earlier in the day. Torn by guilt and selfishness, torn by indecision and needing a resolution, Lorenzo's need for his own gratification won out in the end.

An odd feeling of pride and vanity made him incapable of giving up his two new sons. Yet happy memories of Lisbeth and his two adorable daughters continued to flash through his mind. Forcefully pushing aside these haunting reminders of love and loss, Lorenzo settled on a businesslike approach. Coldly and matter-of-factly, he wrote about the recent events that had taken place in his life, stating just the facts, announcing his decision. There were no words of remorse, regret or sadness; no plea for forgiveness, no reference to the good years they had spent together or the children they had created. Lorenzo's last letter to Lisbeth was as emotionless as a legal document. His heart was pounding as he sealed the envelope, knowing in his heart that he was a traitor. Thinking only of himself and the two sons born to him today, he ignored his conscience and stuck to his decision.

The second letter, to Emilio, flowed much more easily. All his life Lorenzo had been surrounded by people who were there to serve him, solve his problems, easing his way. Now he looked to Emilio to handle legal and financial matters without great inconvenience to himself. In his mind it was a simple fact that with enough money and the right people, any difficulties could be overcome. Having come to this cold decision on his own, he was now prepared to let others handle the practical matters for him.

Lorenzo sighed as he finished his correspondence. He poured himself another drink, wanting to relax and bask in the contentment of being the father of two sons. But hard as he tried, he could not put his former life aside so easily. Memories and old promises continued to haunt him, uncertainties about the future continued to plague him, and the love of two little girls that would be denied him forever continued to tug at his heart. And lastly, the image of his beautiful Lisbeth could not so casually be banned from his mind. He remembered their first meeting, her cold and shivering body next to his on Hans Peter's sailboat, her adoring smile on their wedding day, and the love they had shared with total abandon. He recalled the sadness at their parting at Hamburg Harbor, and the deep and unbearable longing he had felt until she arrived in Buenos Aires. When he saw the *Neue Welt* gliding into the harbor that morning, Lorenzo had thought his heart would burst with happiness.

Tears welled up in Lorenzo's eyes. He remembered the births of Rosalinde and Angelina, how proud and happy he had been then. But something had happened, something had changed. Somehow Lisbeth was no longer the same. Lorenzo, as always, found a way to put the blame on others: life had only changed because of Lisbeth. Restlessly he tossed, trying to find ways to exonerate himself. He realized that he was tossing Lisbeth's love aside, all that she had given up for him, thrown aside for an unknown future with Elena and two innocent boys caught up in a web of lust and lies.

In the end, he could not go back, could not undo the sins he had committed. As dawn broke he finally fell into a fitful sleep.

FORTY-TWO

When Anni arrived home that hot August afternoon, she found Rosalinde playing quietly on the living room floor. Angelina was crying in her crib. After a quick search she found Lisbeth, sobbing her heart out on the chaise on the back porch.

"What is it?" Anni asked gently. "What is wrong, dear?"

Lisbeth could not utter one word, but instead began crying even harder. Then Anni saw that she was clutching a letter with an Argentine stamp.

"What is wrong? Did something happen to Lorenzo or to Oma-Maria?"

But Lisbeth was not able to answer. Anni patted her shoulder as she turned to go inside and look after the children. "What could it be? In a few weeks Lisbeth will be returning to Lorenzo. What could be wrong?" Anni wondered.

Drying little Angelina's tears and muttering soothing words to her, Anni took her out of the crib and carried her into the kitchen. She placed her in the high chair and gave her a snack. It did not take much to make Angelina smile again.

"Why is Mommy crying?" Rosalinde wanted to know, but Anni had no answers for her. Rosalinde stepped out and hugged her distraught mother. "Mommy, stop crying. Are you hurt? Why are you crying?" Rosalinde was about to burst into tears herself. Lisbeth sat up, hugging her little girl.

"It's all right, Rosalinde. Everything is fine. Mommy just doesn't feel well, that's all." With that, Lisbeth wiped her tear-stained face, kissing Rosalinde. "Go play with Monika or the boys. They are at the neighbors', I think."

Anni gently took Rosalinde's hand and walked out into the yard. She could hear her children playing in the neighbors' yard, shrieking with joy as they sprayed each other with the garden hose. She opened the gate and called to Monika: "Hi, look who is here just up from her nap. Keep an eye on Rosalinde for me, will you please? I have some things to take care of with Tante Lisbeth."

"Sure, Mother; come Rosalinde, have fun with us!" Monika replied, wondering about her mother's troubled expression.

By the time Anni returned, Lisbeth was somewhat composed. She looked at her aunt with swollen tear-filled eyes, shaking her head and balling up her fists. "That jerk! What a stupid fool! What a terrible, horrible liar he is! How can he do this to me? Oh, Lorenzo!" Again she began to cry uncontrollably, throwing the letter on the floor.

"What is it, Lisbeth? Tell me, please tell me, what is it?"

"Yes, I'll tell you, Anni! You will never believe what has

happened. I cannot believe Lorenzo could do this to me. Now I know why he wanted me to come and visit you! Now I know why he was so agreeable. He just wanted me out of the way!" Lisbeth began sobbing again, and all Anni could do was to hold and console her, not understanding anything Lisbeth had said. What could be so dreadful, so heartbreaking, so upsetting? What Lisbeth had just uttered made absolutely no sense to Anni.

"Lisbeth, calm down, please. What is it? I don't understand. What has happened to Lorenzo. What is going on?"

Lisbeth caught her breath, wiped her nose and said sadly, "Tante Anni, to make it short, Lorenzo does not want us anymore. He does not want us to come back. He does not want us back at *Bien Cielo* with him. He does not want us!"

Anni looked at her niece in shock. "What do you mean? You are his wife. He has two children. He doesn't want you?" Anni gasped, not believing what she had just heard.

"Yes, Anni, it's as simple as that. He doesn't want us. He has been thinking about it for some time. He says I was never really happy there. I was always thinking of home. I did not try to fit in. We probably married too quickly. Whatever it is, it's all my fault!" A new bout of tears overcame Lisbeth as Anni tried to absorb and understand what she had just been told. Nothing made sense to her except that her niece had been dealt a terrible blow.

"But Lisbeth," Anni tried to console her, "you can still work things out with Lorenzo. You must go back and work things out. You have two children. You can't let everything just fall apart, no matter whose fault it is." Anni couldn't think of anything else to say to her devastated niece.

"There is nothing to work out, Anni. Lorenzo does not want us. I know we had some problems. I was so worried and homesick, but I loved him and he loved me. When he said I should join Emilio and Paulina and come to visit you, I thought he was the best, the most considerate husband to let me come to see you. He said it would help me. He wanted me to take the girls and go on this trip. He insisted that we go. And now he says I left him, and it's all my fault!"

Anni was speechless. How often had she and Josef commented on Lorenzo's generosity, his concern for her, his love for her. They credited him with trying to find a way to overcome Lisbeth's homesickness when, instead, it now looked as if he wanted his wife and children to leave for other reasons. Anni shook her head.

After a long silence, Lisbeth, all cried out, looked at Anni's face and said, "I'm sorry, Anni, I could not understand or believe myself. I've read this letter over and over, and it is still like a bad dream. I know you don't understand either. But it's very simple: Lorenzo does not want me back. He has someone else. He has been seeing her since before Christmas. It doesn't matter what I say or do. He has someone else. He wants to be with her, not with me. I think he has even forgotten our two children. He does not even mention them in his letter. Now I know why he wanted us to leave—so he could have time with her."

Anni was shocked by this cruel and devastating turn. "What do you mean? He is married to you. He can't push you aside just because he was lonely and made a mistake. He will come to his senses. He must."

Composing herself, Lisbeth gave Anni the last piece of her devastating news, as Lisbeth spit forth the final blow that had been dealt her. "Anni, there is even more. Lorenzo's new woman, Elena, has just given birth to twin sons! Can you imagine? Sons—just what Lorenzo always wanted—a son. Now he has two sons. That is why he doesn't want us anymore. He wants to be free so that he can marry her and legitimize his sons."

Anni was stunned. She could not find words to console her niece. Instead she held her close as they rocked back and forth, smoothing her hair as both women cried for the loss of what could have been.

Lisbeth, finally calm again, suddenly had an overwhelming desire to hold her children. She walked into the kitchen where Angelina was still sitting in the high chair, blowing bubbles and crumbling crackers on the tray. Anni went next door to fetch Rosalinde.

As she hugged and kissed her girls, thanking God for having them in her life, Lisbeth was determined to make some sort of a new life for them. She would fight for them if need be, and she would never let Lorenzo take them away from her.

She sat holding her children for a long time. The shock of Lorenzo's letter caused a physical pain almost taking her breath away. She felt lost and abandoned. Why had nobody warned her? Why had nobody told her? "Why did Lorenzo wait so long to tell me the truth? Why did Oma-Maria, whom I love and trust, keep silent for so long?" Lisbeth felt totally lost and betrayed. "Where can I go now? I have no home anywhere. Where do I belong? I can't go back to my parents. There is a war over there. I will not return to Argentina. I am not wanted there.

I'm not even sure that I can stay here. I am only a visitor."

Evening came. After Lisbeth and her daughters had gone to bed, Anni and Josef sat up for hours, trying to find answers, trying to find a way to help their niece. At the moment, there was nothing any of them could do. "Let's go to bed. Tomorrow is another day," Josef finally said. "We will find a way tomorrow."

In the morning, Josef in his calm and practical way said, "Anni, there is really no choice for her. Lisbeth and the girls cannot go back to Hamburg. That is clear. She cannot and will not return to *Bien Cielo*. That is clear too. She can stay here with us as long as she needs to, and when the war in Europe is over, perhaps, if she wants to return there, she can. But in the meantime she is part of our family, and we will take care of her."

Anni smiled in agreement. Her Josef always found the best way. Together they would somehow overcome this great heartbreak by keeping Lisbeth and her girls safely in their midst.

All night Lisbeth tossed and turned, at times crying, at times giving in to her great anger. She wavered between her own guilt in the failure of the marriage, and anger, not only at Lorenzo, but at Elena as well. She was disappointed and bitter at everyone who had kept the truth from her. Why had Oma-Maria not told her? Why not her friend Juliana? Perhaps in time she would understand or even forgive them. But right now the pain was too great. Exhausted, with a deep ache in her chest, she thought again of her beautiful children sleeping peacefully beside her. For them alone she had to overcome this blow and make a new future for them, although at the moment she could not think of a way.

FOURTY-THREE

The next weeks were a blur for Lisbeth. After the first few days of tears and lament, of hateful outbursts and helpless frustration, she realized that she had to put the past aside and think of the future. Crying for what might have been was useless. Somehow her anger and rejection infused in her a strange kind of energy. Knowing that she and the girls were welcome to stay with the Bauers calmed her initial fear and panic immensely.

A letter soon arrived from Oma-Maria. She wrote of her love for Lisbeth and her disappointment in her grandson's actions, her own helplessness in the situation. This letter brought forth another flood of tears as Lisbeth truly loved and missed her too. She remembered early conversations when Maria had expressed her own concern about the way Lorenzo had been raised. As an only child of well-to-do *estancieros*, he never knew what it was to do without or not to get his way. Maria remembered how hard she and her young son, José, had worked to keep the *estancia* going after the untimely death of Anselmo. José had never had time for personal pleasures. His mind was totally focused on work, work, work. By the time Lorenzo was born, everything had improved immensely, and the addition of the race-horse operation had brought unusually high profits for the Moncriefs. Lorenzo grew up having fun, playing sports, and enjoying his youth. His university years in Buenos Aires were carefree years; he barely passed his final exams. With his charm and good looks he had been able to bewitch everyone.

'So, he was a spoiled little rich kid. Is that what you are telling me?" Lisbeth had asked Oma-Maria, and with a shrug and a smile, Oma had agreed.

"Yes, he always gets what he wants, and this time I am so happy that he got you!" she had replied, enfolding Lisbeth in her loving embrace.

"Those were happy days," Lisbeth thought. "How quickly they have disappeared from my life!"

The next letter was from Emilio Alvarez. He had been contacted by Lorenzo who had informed him of the events that had taken place since Lisbeth had begun her journey north. He expressed his deep sorrow and disappointment and offered his help. He would contact an attorney who would represent Lisbeth's interests. Apparently Lorenzo wanted a dissolution of the marriage as soon as possible, assuming Lisbeth was agreeable and not contesting his wishes. He was willing to settle an amount into a fund for the care and education of his daughters but had not voiced a desire to have them return to Argentina. At this time, Emilio suggested that Lisbeth send him copies of all her documents, her marriage certificate, passport, children's birth certificates, and especially, a copy of Lorenzo's signed statement allowing Lisbeth to take the children out of the country. Emilio promised to do everything possible to assist her and to simplify the procedure from his end.

Almost as an afterthought, Emilio told Lisbeth about a special provision her father had made for her in case of a future emergency. Emilio considered this time in Lisbeth's life to be a great emergency.

> "Do you remember the package your father sent with you when you first arrived in Buenos Aires? The business matter he wanted me to handle for him?"

Lisbeth recalled her first meeting with Señor Alvarez very well. How young, how trusting, how confident she had been then! She had never wondered about the contents of the envelope she had delivered to Emilio. Now she was about to find out what these contents meant to her.

> "Your father sent funds for me to invest in your name, for emergencies, and for your own financial security and independence. I believe the time has come for these funds to be made available to you. I can suggest a bank in New York, or you can open an account in Springbrook. Please let me know where to transfer your funds. I am sure your father would agree that this is the right time."

Lisbeth reread the letter many times. This news was completely unexpected. She could not believe how Emilio, as well as her father, were looking out for her welfare. Even from a great distance, living in the uncertainties of war, her parents were taking care of her. Her father had planned ahead for any eventuality. But surely her father would not believe what was happening to her now. Or had he had his doubts after all? Or was it her mother's constant worry that had caused her father to provide for her future? Whatever the reasons, her father's forethought and love enveloped her like a warm blanket, making her feel calm and secure. "What a carefree girl I was only a few short years ago, falling in love, married a few weeks later, and setting out on my life's adventure in far-away Argentina. The possibility of misfortune or unhappiness had never entered my mind. That Lorenzo would abandon me in this cruel manner was unthinkable. What would I do without my family's help?" she reflected sadly. Again she thanked God for her good fortune in the midst of betrayal.

With September's arrival, a sense of normalcy was returning to the Bauer household. Monika, Willy and Little Joe went back to school, and the house was quiet most of the day. Robot-like, Lisbeth performed her daily chores, took her children on long walks and wrote letters. She had sent the required papers to Emilio but refused to discuss Lorenzo. She left everything in Emilio's hands, knowing that he was the only person she could trust. She continued to write to her parents and sister, hoping that some mail would get through. She also wrote to Oma-Maria, but never mentioned Lorenzo and his abandonment. Despite his unfaithfulness and cruel conduct, Lisbeth loved his grandmother and wanted to remain in touch. Lisbeth slowly began to realize the severity and finality of Lorenzo's actions. She became more quiet and introspective, unable to join in family activities as before. She was no longer interested in going anywhere with the Bauers, be it to the movies or the county fair. She dealt with the pain of rejection, of loss, by going inside herself.

Jim Harding continued to stop by the house several times a week, bringing Lisbeth's little girls a treat of some kind and then quietly disappearing again. He had not seen Lisbeth since that fateful letter had arrived and did not want to intrude, but he faithfully came by to see Rosalinde and Angelina. Of course, Jim had heard that Lisbeth would not be returning to Argentina. He knew no details of the situation, but in his mind he pictured Lorenzo as a cold and heartless man. How else could he forsake his wife and two beautiful children? He wished he could do something for Lisbeth, but Anni told him that only time would heal her wounds. Still, Jim wondered whether Lisbeth could remain in the United States. Working with Josef in the greenhouse one day, he dared to voice what was on his mind. "Tell me, Josef... I have been thinking...about Lisbeth. I mean, will she stay here in the U.S.A. now or go back?"

"No, no. She is not ever going back to Argentina. We have told her she can stay with us as long as she likes."

"But that's not what I mean. I know she can stay with you. I was just wondering about her passport or her visa. Can she just stay here, or does she need some special permit? She told me a long time ago that she was here as a visitor and that she could stay up to six months. Isn't that time up fairly soon?" Jim was actually happy that the little family was staying in Springbrook, no matter what the reason.

Josef looked at him aghast. In all the upheaval during the last weeks, no one had bothered to check on Lisbeth's status; as far as Josef knew, she was only a visitor with a short-term visa. Josef dropped the pruning shears in his hands and stared at Jim. "Oh, Jim, you're right. We must see a lawyer and check Lisbeth's passport. We want her to stay here with us; I hope it isn't too late. Thanks, Jim, for reminding us. I must go home right away and discuss this with Anni and figure out what we have to do."

The very next morning Josef and a very nervous Lisbeth set out to see an attorney. Lisbeth's visitor's visa was expiring in a few weeks, and only through Jim's reminder were they aware of the problem. Now she was seized by a new panic. "Josef, what will happen to us? I can't go back to Hamburg. There is no way I will go back to Argentina, and what if I'm not allowed to stay here? Where can I go? What can I do?"

The attorney, Mr. Saddler, listened carefully as Josef explained Lisbeth's dilemma. He examined her passport and visa carefully and nodded calmly. Yes, he explained to them, indeed he could help. He would get in touch with the U.S. Immigration Service and apply for temporary residence status due to the unusual circumstances which were dictating Lisbeth's life. He had no doubt that her request would be granted in view of the fact that she had family who were willing to vouch for her.

Greatly relieved, Lisbeth and Josef left the lawyer's office. There was hope now that she could stay here with the Bauers until the war was over and could make a rational decision about the future. Right now Lisbeth's life was upside down, one shock following another. At the same time she was extremely thankful for the many loving and generous people around her. She offered a prayer for everyone who had been helping her: Mr. Saddler, the immigration officials, and lastly Jim Harding who had been alert enough to help avoid another momentous hurdle in Lisbeth's life.

Arriving back at the house, they saw Jim's car parked in the driveway. As they entered the living room, Anni and Jim looked at them expectantly.

"How did the meeting go?" Anni wanted to know eagerly.

Lisbeth nodded and smiled for the first time in weeks. "Mr. Saddler thinks that I can get an extension to stay here. It will take some time, but he thinks it will be possible. Thank you, Josef, for helping me...and thank you, Jim, for thinking about our welfare. Without all of you, I don't know what I would do."

Lisbeth bent down to hug her children. A great weight had been lifted off her shoulders, knowing that at least one hurdle seemed to be overcome. Now she had been given hope for a safe, although temporary home in the United States. She could remain here with the people who truly loved her. The rest was up to Emilio who, along with Oma-Maria, was her trusted friend and ally in a land she had once called home.

One morning in mid-October, Jim spotted Lisbeth and her children playing behind the old farmhouse. The girls were busy in the sandbox, and Lisbeth sat quietly on a garden bench nearby. Somehow, from deep within him, he found the courage to walk over and sit on the bench with her. Quietly he offered his friendship and sympathy and his help if she ever needed him. Lisbeth was touched by his kindness and tearfully thanked him for his concern. She especially appreciated his affection toward her children who were now happily waving and calling to him. Earlier when he had walked through the gate, they had both squealed with pleasure, running to him and hugging his legs. Lisbeth smiled as she observed their happy play and their joy at seeing Jim.

For a while Lisbeth and Jim sat in silence. The sun still shone warmly, and a gentle breeze ruffled the golden and scarlet leaves of the maple trees. For the first time in weeks, Lisbeth felt a new sense of peace. Looking at her contented children gave her strength and hope for the future.

Jim's voice startled her as he spoke. "Lisbeth, I have been thinking.... You know, you should continue with your driving or you will forget everything I have taught you. Would you like to drive again some evening?"

Somehow Lisbeth found herself laughing again, just a quiet little laugh, accepting this simple offer of friendship. "Yes, Jim, that would be nice. I cannot afford to forget what you have taught me."

FOURTY-FOUR

And so began Lisbeth's gradual healing, her coming out of herself, her acceptance of her fate and new life. The grief and disappointment were still tormenting her, but she began looking forward to the future now instead of wallowing in the pain and despair of the past.

One thing had been on Lisbeth's mind for some time. So far she had been a guest at her aunt's house. But now the situation had changed. It was time to make more permanent living arrangements. One evening after dinner, she timidly approached Anni and Josef with an idea that had been hatching in her brain for several days.

"Would it be possible to move into the little farmhouse near the greenhouse?" All the thoughts tumbling in her head now spilled out. As Lisbeth saw it, she would only need the two bedrooms upstairs, the bath and the small kitchen. Anni certainly could continue the use of the lower rooms for her office. Lisbeth explained her desire to pay monthly rent as she now had money available to her due to the kindness of her Papa. With a pleading look in her eyes, she sat still awaiting their answer.

"What a great idea!" Anni and Josef answered almost in unison. "Of course you can live there as long as you like, although we love having you here with us," Anni added.

"I know, and I am so grateful for all you have done for us. But things are different now, and I must not depend on you forever. My little family—we need our own little place."

Josef nodded. Certainly both he and Anni understood Lisbeth's need to become more independent, to be the head of her family. But then a troubled look clouded Lisbeth's face as she remembered something. "Oh, no! You told me once, Anni, that you had plans for the house. I totally forgot!"

"Oh, that!" Anni laughed. "That is far, far into the future. It will certainly not conflict with your living in the house."

"What did you have in mind?" Lisbeth was curious to know.

"I thought that someday I would open a little shop in the living and dining rooms of that house. You know, small gifts, dried flowers, some of my small antiques and collectibles, maybe some craft items my friends make, hand-knit baby clothes and embroideries, things like that," Anni replied dreamily.

"But for now I am too busy with the office work and my family. Someday, maybe, but for now it would be much better for the farmhouse to be occupied. You and the girls can live there for as long as need be, and we will be able to see each other every day. Someday we'll turn the front part into a gift shop. But right now I have no time for it."

"But *I* would," Lisbeth replied, laughing out loud for the second time in weeks. "We could do it together. My girls are getting older now. Before long Rosalinde will be going to school. And I could knit for you. Everyone at *Bien Cielo* admired the sweaters and scarves I made," Lisbeth bubbled on. The evening suddenly had an upbeat mood to it. Lisbeth was feeling alive again, having something positive, something practical, something real to plan.

"Maybe we could even work on it this winter during the slow time at the garden center. What if we could have it ready by spring when all the customers come to Bauer's?" Lisbeth was so excited that her enthusiasm was infecting Anni and Josef as well.

"Slow down, Lisbeth," Anni laughed. "Let's get the house ready first. Let's get you moved in, and then perhaps in January we can begin thinking about the shop."

"Yes, yes, that's a grand idea. Let's do it that way."

Josef sat quietly, smiling as he watched the two women make plans. How good it was to see Lisbeth participating in life again!

Everyone was satisfied with the new solution, and Lisbeth was filled with a new hope and excitement as she thought of having her own home, a home that for the first time would be her very own domain. With sadness, she realized that even during her marriage to Lorenzo, she had only been a guest in her in-laws' home. This time it would really be her own home.

The next few weeks were filled with work and happy anticipation. With Josef and Jim's help, all the rooms were freshly painted, the floors washed and polished, the old kitchen scrubbed. Anni was busy sewing new curtains for the bedrooms, and in doing so taught Lisbeth how to use a sewing machine. There were so many happy activities surrounding the upcoming move that at the end of each day Lisbeth fell asleep, exhausted but satisfied. No more sleepless nights interrupted by bitter tears and troubling doubts and fears.

Anni had always loved old things, attending many barn and estate sales. Lisbeth's upcoming move gave her the perfect excuse to drive Lisbeth around the area, looking for antiques and interesting things that might fit into the farmhouse. Over the time Lisbeth had spent with her aunt, she too had slowly acquired a taste for the unique and unusual. She truly enjoyed her weekly excursions with Anni, anxious to begin furnishing her new home. She was so absorbed with the project that there were many hours, occasionally even a whole day, when she was able to forget and distance herself from the grief and disillusionment that had so suddenly and shockingly befallen her.

With each week the farmhouse took on a more sparkling face. Soon it would be ready for the new residents. Anni took Lisbeth on several shopping expeditions acquiring the necessities. What surprised Lisbeth the most, was the interest and generosity of Anni's friends who brought all sorts of useful items to furnish the kitchen. One evening Jim surprised them by hauling an old armoire that had been standing useless in his house. His mother had stored her sewing patterns in it, and Jim felt it would be of greater use in Lisbeth's new place. She was totally delighted with the beautiful, ornately carved walnut piece which reminded her of the furnishings in her parents' house.

By November, when Lisbeth first learned about the feast of Thanksgiving celebrated in America, most of the furnishings had been moved in, the curtains hung, the little pantry stocked with food. Her children were well and happy, never asking for their father. They were everyone's total joy. Lisbeth reflected that she had so many reasons for her own thanksgiving. Despite all she had gone through this past year, God had given her the strength and grace to overcome her hurt and bitterness, and she knew that she was beginning to heal.

The spirit of the upcoming Christmas holiday had enveloped her, and despite her heartache, she felt hope. She even found confidence that her loved ones back in Hamburg would safely overcome the dangers of war.

Lisbeth had complied with all of Emilio's requests regarding the divorce and other legal matters. She trusted him completely, knowing that he and the attorney would look out for her welfare. Whatever the outcome, she was ready to accept it. If Lorenzo wanted his freedom, she would not stand in the way. All she wanted was her children, as Lorenzo apparently wanted his new family with Elena.

Whether his financial settlement was generous or nonexistent did not matter to Lisbeth. She had been overwhelmed at the sizeable amount Emilio had transferred from her father's investment and could subsist on that for quite some time. In her heart she hoped that her present living arrangements would be temporary, as returning to Europe after the war was still her fervent hope. But for now, she felt safe and welcomed in the United States. She even included in her daily prayers of thanks the unknown immigration officials who had granted her an extension to her visa!

On her first night in the farmhouse, after Lisbeth had tucked Rosalinde in her own new bed and Angelina in the Bauers' comfortable crib, she sat quietly in the old rocking chair at the foot of her bed. Looking around her new home, the curtains Anni had sewn, the dresser Josef had repainted, the quilt on her bed that one of Anni's friends had made for her, she thought how very lucky she was. On this first night, Lisbeth fell asleep in her new home with a feeling of total contentment and wellbeing.

FOURTY-FIVE

Christmas of 1940 was also approaching in Hamburg, and Marianne was attempting to prepare for the holiday with old family traditions. She baked Pfeffernüsse and Springerle and wished her two granddaughters were here to celebrate St. Nikolas Day. What wishful thinking! There had been no mail from South America or the United States. All she knew was that Lisbeth and the children had visited Anni during the early summer. Whether she was still there or had returned to *Bien Cielo* she did not know, but she prayed they were safe.

"Safer than here anyway," she thought. So far the family in Hamburg had survived the first year of the war fairly well. Thanks to Johann, they had been well supplied with fresh vegetables, and the cellar held a large crop of potatoes for the winter. The basic food supplies were still available, but shortages became more and more apparent each month. All the young men were in the service, and farms and industry were operated by an older, in many cases retired work force or the inexperienced youth of the country, and the earlier optimism about the quick end of the war was waning. Peter wrote regularly to Margarete, and Kurt to Wilhelm. But both refrained from stating their opinions. Peter was still stationed in Poland, Kurt in France. Margarete was still employed at the opera house, singing in the chorus. Marianne and Wilhelm continued to visit with their friends as before, but now the subject matter of their conversations had a different focus.

Hans Birkner had also closed his shoe factory as it was impossible to obtain imported leather, and his work force had shrunk considerably. Instead he had taken a job at a local newspaper, handling circulation and distribution. He was in a unique position, too old for military service, too young to retire. But if this war dragged on, as everyone feared, even his age group might face the draft. For now, that was unthinkable.

Wilhelm still spent much of his time reading the newspapers and listening to the war news. The reports were always glorious, full of national pride and optimism. He was concerned about Hitler's latest alliance with Mussolini who had invaded Greece in October. "Where will it all lead?" Wilhelm wondered. "Will this war eventually involve the whole world?"

Recently he had been at the harbor. He was shocked to see how the area had changed. No more foreign ships flying flags from all over the world; only German warships were visible. There were no pleasure craft to be seen. All had been docked or stored. In peacetime the harbor had always invigorated Wilhelm with its hustle and bustle, its bars and restaurants overflowing with exotic strangers, sailors, tourists and hard-working locals. Now a pall seemed to hang over the area as if waiting for some sort of disaster. And disasters would come, he thought. It was only a matter of time. How thankful he was that his Lisbeth was safely far away!

FOURTY-SIX

As the end of the year approached, Lisbeth wavered between her new-found contentment and her old self-doubt. She remembered the bitter argument she had with Lorenzo during the early weeks of December a year ago. Slowly she put the puzzle pieces together and realized that this was the beginning of his relationship with Elena. How blind she had been in her self-absorbed homesickness and longing for her family! Why had she not paid attention and noticed the warning signs? But, as the saying goes, love is blind. She had observed his lack of interest and devotion to his daughters but had always made excuses for him. "What was it that I did not understand? What did I not see?" Nagging self-doubt alternated with blaming Lorenzo. Had he really ever loved her, or was it a romantic interlude while traveling the world?

"No," she thought again. "I know he loved me, and I really loved him." But something had changed in the last four years. Was it the cultural differences, her homesickness, the war and the uncertainty, two children in rapid succession, coupled with various circumstances that drove her to neglect him?

Perhaps it was just easier for him to be with Elena with whom he had grown up, who spoke his language, who knew him and accepted life as it was. Elena knew only one kind of life, whereas Lisbeth had been constantly comparing her new life with her old. Still it was very painful to think of Lorenzo with another woman with other children and obviously no longer wanting her.

Lisbeth shook her head. Enough of recriminations, enough of brooding of what might have been. She had to accept the facts as they were. Emilio had informed her that the divorce proceedings were in the works and so far had Lorenzo's complete cooperation. Apparently the fact that Lorenzo had married her in a foreign country by a judge rather than in a religious ceremony made the present request for dissolution of marriage much easier in Argentina. Emilio hoped to have everything resolved and finalized within the next six months.

Christmas Eve 1940 was celebrated at Anni and Josef's house with a simple but delicious meal. As Little Joe commented, "Our whole family is here, our Tante Lisbeth, our cousins, and our Uncle Jimmy!"

After dinner the tree was decorated and the family sang some traditional songs. Both Anni and Lisbeth shed a few tears trying to sing *Silent Night* in the original German. Memories of Christmases past came to life again.

In his quiet and relaxed manner Jim coaxed a smile out of Lisbeth by singing *Jingle Bells* while bouncing her children on his knees. The evening ended on a happy note, and it was time to drive Lisbeth back to the farmhouse. On Christmas Day, everyone reconvened at the Bauer house for a special turkey dinner and gift exchange. Lisbeth had knit scarves and hats for all the children as well as scarves for the adults. Jim brought two Raggedy Ann dolls for Rosalinde and Angelina and books for the older children. For Anni and Josef, he had bought a case of wine. But it was Lisbeth who received the most unusual gift of all. The gift was from Jim. Having heard about her mother's famous rose garden, Jim had sketched out a new, much smaller, but carefully thought-out rose garden for Lisbeth. Come spring, he would plant the new rose beds for her. Lisbeth was touched to tears, unable to speak. But her eyes said everything as she hugged everyone, overwhelmed by the kindness and love surrounding her.

With the second glass of wine it was decided that after the holidays the time would be perfect to begin work on the new shop. Josef and Jim would have some free time to build the display shelves, and the two women would start scouting around for small antiques, collectables and craft items for their inventory. Lisbeth would begin knitting baby items, and Anni would make decorative wreaths. Josef suggested Anni talk to her church ladies group, selling the talented ladies' creations on consignment. As they talked, they came up with more and more ideas for the shop—sachets, home-made jams and jellies, old linens, antique glass and household items.

"Stop, stop!" Josef finally said. "There won't be room for half the things you are planning."

But the more they talked, the more involved they became in their new venture; they couldn't wait to get started.

"You'll have to think of a name for your shop. That is very important," Jim interjected. Everyone promised to do their part as they settled on a tentative opening day in mid-May.

FOURTY-SEVEN

As the new year 1941 began, Lisbeth was almost her old self again. She enjoyed living in her own place, cooking for her children and anticipating the opening of the shop. The cold winter months passed quickly. The girls who had never seen snow before were enchanted by it. Little Joe built a snowman beside the front porch as Willy pulled the girls around on the old sled. Lisbeth loved seeing her girls in her homemade hats and scarves and smiled watching them having as much fun as she remembered having as a little girl. It didn't snow very often in Hamburg, but when it did, everything closed down and the children enjoyed frolicking in the snow. She prepared hot chocolate for the five little snowmen, stomping the snow off their boots on the porch. As they warmed their cold little noses, Lisbeth herself felt a warming of her heart with a new feeling of belonging.

Bien Cielo and all the people she knew there were retreating further and further into the past, the pain lessening day by day. The only person she missed and wanted to remain in her heart and in her memory was Oma-Maria, who wrote faithfully, missing Lisbeth and the children a great deal. She was very tactful, not writing about life at *Bien Cielo,* and it was easy to discern that she no longer spent much time there. Instead she wrote of Alma and Juliana, the vineyard and her short visit with Emilio and Paulina in Buenos Aires.

Occasionally the old sadness and melancholy returned. But it was temporary. Lisbeth's life was fuller than it had ever been, as she was totally responsible for her and her childrens' wellbeing. She thought of her parents and Margarete daily, praying for their safety, but not despairing as before. With the support of those around her, she had found strength and purpose.

Lisbeth and Anni were now totally committed to preparations for the new boutique. All their free time was spent creating and collecting various items for sale. Every weekend, sometimes accompanied by Jim, they drove to estate and barn sales and became as excited as children at Christmas each time they found pieces of old glass, linen or artwork. Slowly a sizeable inventory was accumulating, and the display shelves were filling up. A farm table was draped with an old silk shawl, displaying a beautiful orchid plant. Slowly the living and dining rooms of the farmhouse were transformed into an inviting and unique shop with many interesting gifts and treasures. Anni's friends brought a number of handmade quilts and pillows which totally amazed Lisbeth. Never had she thought that ordinary housewives could be so creative and artistic. It gave her a great deal of confidence that she too could contribute and reaffirm her own worth.

One day in March a late spring storm dumped a foot of snow on Springbrook. As Lisbeth looked out the window, Jim appeared in his truck. But instead of going toward the greenhouse, he stopped on the road and began clearing the snow up to her house. Then he cleared the path to the Garden Center. The job finished, Jim returned the shovel to the truck and dragged out a long rectangular package. Just as Lisbeth was opening the door to invite him in for a hot drink, Jim set down the package, ready to ring the doorbell.

"Come in. What have you got there?" she asked.

"Just a little present for you," he smiled shyly, shrugging off his jacket.

"Isn't it enough that you come and clear our snow? You also bring us presents?"

"Well, open it up and see. Perhaps you won't even like it."

"Oh, surely we will," she replied, tearing off the paper. It was a large framed sampler Jim's mother had made many years ago and which had hung in his living room for a long time. It was beautifully done with the finest needle- and petit-point stitches with the sentiment "Home is where the heart is."

"I thought it might bring you good luck too and make people feel good about entering this place."

Then he saw Lisbeth's happy look of anticipation change into a sad and wistful one. "What is it? Don't you like it? You don't have to hang it up if you don't like it," he stammered, red-faced.

"No, no, Jim, it isn't that. This is beautiful. Your mother

must have been quite an artist to have designed and created this wonderful piece. It's just that, well, you know, this sentiment, 'Home is where the heart is'...what does it mean really? I don't know where my home is. I don't know where my heart is. There was a time when I knew where I belonged. I was loved and secure in my parents' home. Then I gave my heart to Lorenzo. I left everything behind to make my new home with him. But it didn't work out."

With a heavy sigh, she continued quietly. "Yes, you know what happened to me. Much as I tried and wanted to have my home and my heart with him, I failed. Now I am here with my dear Aunt Anni, and—please don't misunderstand—I love them and appreciate all they have done for me. They've made me welcome, letting me live here in this house, letting me help them start this business. All that is wonderful. Still I don't know where my heart is. I long to go home to my parents, but you know that's impossible."

Never before had Lisbeth talked so openly to Jim about her situation and her worries. Jim sat quietly, not interrupting her. It was clear to him that she needed to talk, needed to share her thoughts.

She continued, "I'm making my home here, Jim, but I know it can only be temporary as I wait and pray every day for the war to be over. So tell me, Jim, where is my home? Where is my heart?"

By now tears were flowing freely, and both little girls had stopped playing and came snuggling up to their mother.

"Why are you sad, Mommy?" Rosalinde asked as Lisbeth tried to compose herself by blowing her nose and smiling at her daughters.

"It's nothing," she said. "Everything is all right. It's just that sometimes Mommy feels sad when she thinks about her own Mommy who is far, far away. Let's make some hot chocolate for all of us," she said as she rose to enter the tiny kitchen. Jim followed her and without preamble put his strong arms around her shoulders and said kindly, "You'll find your heart and your home again. I know you will. You just wait and see. I know you will, I promise you."

"I hope you are right," Lisbeth sniffled, and to please Jim, she added, "And now, let's hang up your mother's sampler."

FOURTY-EIGHT

On a dreary, rainy day in April, Lisbeth received a large manila envelope by registered mail. A letter from Emilio explained the contents. The enclosed papers were part of the divorce documents and had to be signed and returned to him for the final decree. Lisbeth signed all the marked spaces, not bothering to read the particulars. Her Spanish was not perfect enough to understand the legalities, and besides she trusted Emilio and the attorney implicitly. She could see various sums and numbers within the documents, but it mattered not to her. She returned the papers promptly. The sooner she could return to the business of her present life, the better.

The "shop" as they called it was beginning to take shape. There were pictures on the walls, country-style curtains on the windows, and every available surface brimful with merchandise for sale. The only thing that had not been settled on was the name. A number of suggestions had been made, but none seemed just right. Then one spring evening, both Anni and Josef stopped in to have a word with Lisbeth. They seemed happily excited as if they had a wonderful secret to share with her. Josef settled himself in the only comfortable chair in the room, and with one last conspiratorial look at his wife, he began: "Lisbeth, Anni and I have been talking about the opening of this shop, how hard you have been working at getting it ready, how much happier you are since you became involved in this project, and we have come to a decision."

Lisbeth looked anxiously from one to the other, but Josef held up his hand reassuringly and continued, "Lisbeth, we have decided that this little shop will be yours, yours alone. It was your idea to start it. You have a certain talent in designing and planning this venture, and we want this to be your shop. We even have the perfect name for it." Josef and Anni were beaming.

Lisbeth was speechless. "Why?" she finally stammered. "It was Annie's idea all along, and she has helped all these weeks to get it ready."

"Yes, it was my idea," Anni replied, "but as you know, I am too busy with other things. I love helping you, and I will continue to go scouting for goods with you, but we want this to be your business. We insist, just as you insist on paying us rent for this little old house."

Lisbeth could not believe the generosity of her aunt and uncle. She simply could not grasp or believe what they had just told her. She jumped up, hugging them fiercely. "You are just too good to me! How can I accept this? How did you know that working in this shop makes me so happy?"

"Yes, we know, and we also know that you will be

successful, that you will do very well here. It is also a way of keeping you here with us," Anni joked.

With that, Josef went out to the car, returning with a bottle of wine and three glasses. "Of course, we have to toast this venture," he smiled, "and Anni knows that you only have water glasses," he added, lifting the crystal. "To Lisbeth! May she have success in business and find happiness here forever!"

With the cheerful clink of their glasses, Lisbeth suddenly called out, "And what will we call this new shop?"

Anni and Josef answered almost in unison, "Liesl's Treasures, of course!"

By mid-May when the gardening season began in full swing, "Liesl's Treasures" was ready for business. The veranda was inviting with its swing and two wicker rocking chairs. A large wooden tub filled with geraniums brightened the wide stairs leading to the front door. A hand-painted sign noting the store hours was displayed in the window, and best of all, a large new sign had been installed along the upper railing of the porch. It proudly proclaimed, "Liesl's Treasures" and had been painted by a friend of Jim's. A garland of flowers decorated the border and offered a friendly invitation to stop in.

As customers began arriving at the garden center, it became a must to stop at Liesl's too. In the beginning, Lisbeth was continually amazed at how many people came in, congratulated her, visited with her, and bought her merchandise. Word of Jim's newly designed rose garden for Lisbeth had spread, and many customers were eager to walk out into the back yard to admire its beauty. Lisbeth was very proud of Jim's present to her and was happy to show it off. He stopped early each morning to check on the rose garden's progress and emerging loveliness. Lisbeth was well aware of his daily care and enjoyed sitting on the bench in the cool of the evening. The girls played and Lisbeth basked in the pleasure of home and of the man whose kindness had created this peaceful oasis for her.

She woke every morning with thankful anticipation. Her customers became her friends, and she looked forward to each day. After a busy weekend she also looked forward to Mondays and Tuesdays when Liesl's Treasures was closed. She and Anni continued to scout for merchandise, finding new suppliers of unique, handmade goods. Occasionally Jim invited them to drive to Springbrook where the girls loved riding the merry-go-round in the park. A special treat afterwards was a stop at Mayer's Malt Shop for ice cream cones. There was no time for trips like the previous summer, but Lisbeth didn't mind.

The Bauers were planning an outing to Amish country before school resumed and invited Lisbeth to come along. But Lisbeth laughingly answered, "I have a business now. I must stay here and take care of it." How glad Anni and Josef were to have helped Lisbeth to find a new goal and purpose in life. It was obvious that Liesl was very content.

"You go ahead and have a great trip. I am happy to stay here and take care of the shop. I just love doing it."

Summer turned into fall. More apples and pumpkins were being sold at Bauers' than flowers and plants. Lisbeth had expected her business to slow down with the fall season, but she continued to be busy. Her customers kept coming, ordering knits from her, and buying gifts for all occasions. They were already inquiring what items she might carry for Christmas. She and Anni spent many enjoyable hours on their shopping excursions. There never seemed to be a shortage of estate sales and auctions. Anni taught Lisbeth how to keep her books, and she found that she enjoyed learning the basics of business from her aunt. She had shown a small but steady profit since the opening in May. How proud her father would be, seeing his daughter becoming a businesswoman in her own right!

She thought of her parents daily, wishing she could share with them what had happened to her in the past year, the bad and the good as well. She continued to write letters, but Josef told her it was futile. There was no international postal service to war-torn Germany. Since the opening of the shop, Lisbeth had been too busy to scan the daily papers for war news. She relied on Josef to tell her what he knew or heard. He told her that it seemed Hitler was busy invading one country after another, but apparently there was no actual war zone in Germany itself.

During the summer, German forces had invaded the U.S.S.R., but even that event seemed too distant and remote to affect Lisbeth in any personal way. She had suffered enough private tragedy and had survived it. For the time being, she was too busy with her own life. She put aside the alarming events in Europe, ignoring the effects they would soon have, not only on her, but the entire world.

Suddenly everything changed. On December 7, 1941, the Japanese fleet attacked Pearl Harbor, and the United States was forced to enter the war. Christmas that year was a very subdued affair. Uncertainty and fear of the unknown plagued everyone in the country.

Lisbeth's own family had lived with this fear for over two years already, but the United States had been safe and untouched until now. Jim Harding was one of the first to receive his draft notice with orders to report on February 10. Everyone tried their best to create a festive air at Christmas for the children's sake, but a dark cloud had gathered over the country, and nothing was ever the same again.

The evening before Jim was to leave for the local Army induction center, he stopped by the farmhouse for a last goodbye. As always, Roselinde and Angelina were ecstatic to see their Uncle "Immy." As he had done many times before, he took them upstairs to read them a bedtime story. After begging him to read just one more, it was finally time to say good night and goodbye. He told them as gently as he could that he would have to go away for a while, but he would be back, and they would do all the fun things together again.

As he descended the stairs, he thought how much he would miss those two little dolls! How important they had become in his life! He remembered how he had fallen in love with Rosalinde the day they met when she shyly smiled at him, partly hiding behind her mother's skirt. Angelina too had stolen his heart when she first grabbed at his hair and blown a bubble in his face. How well he remembered that first meeting when Lisbeth had walked into the greenhouse with Anni and the little girls! "I think I fell in love with all three of them on that very first day," he often thought to himself but had never uttered a word to anyone.

In his quiet way, Jim had savored the times he could see her and the children. During their driving lessons, he had been happy just to be near her, although she spoke often of Lorenzo then. Jim kept his feelings to himself, and only after her abandonment had let himself dream that perhaps in time she would come to love him too. But he had never imagined that he would have to say goodbye to her in the way he was forced to now. He was going off to war, to God only knows where, and perhaps he would not return. His heart was full of uncertainties and anxieties, but also of hope and love.

Coming down the stairs, he saw Lisbeth standing at the window, looking out at the dark starless night. As he searched for the right words of farewell, his emotions overflowed, and his words to her took a totally different direction. Putting his hand on her shoulder and turning her gently toward him, he said, "Lisbeth, I'm leaving tomorrow. I don't know if I'll ever see you again. I must..." But Lisbeth interrupted him. She had endured too many painful goodbyes in her young life and was afraid to face another.

"No, no, don't say that. Of course you'll return. Maybe the war will not last long. You will be back, I just know it," she cried.

Jim silently took her into his arms and continued, "Yes, I want to return. I'll do my best to stay alive. But I can't leave without telling you how much I love you. I have loved you from the moment I met you, and if it is possible, I love you more every day. I will carry your picture in my heart and that will help me survive this war."

Lisbeth looked at him sadly as tears welled up in her eyes. She was confused. She could not find the right words to answer him. Perhaps it would be better to leave some things unsaid, especially now at this stressful time. Quietly they both sat down, Lisbeth gently taking his hands into her own.

Looking deeply into his eyes, she began, "Jim, you know how much I care for you, and you know how much we will miss you. You have been the best friend anyone could ever wish for. I can never thank you enough for what you have done for us, for me. I wish I could tell you what you want to hear. I want to, but there is so much... You know I'm only here temporarily. When the war is over I have to go home again..." Lisbeth was crying openly now.

"Yes," Jim replied sadly, "you told me your heart is not here and you want to go home again. But can you understand that I love you with all my heart, and I want you to find your heart and home with me? Just think about it, Lisbeth. I only wanted you to know how I feel about you. This war...we both know how uncertain life is. I simply had to tell you before I have to go."

"I'm confused," Lisbeth muttered. "I have known for some time how you feel about me. All the special things you have done for me and the girls. I'm confused about my feelings. I loved Lorenzo, and you know what happened. I have been fighting the feelings that I have come to have about you...because, you know, I can't stay here..."

Jim sat quietly, letting her talk. He understood her predicament, not wanting to give him false hope. Still he hoped.

"Lisbeth, I love you, and that is all that matters. You love me too. I heard you say it, Lisbeth. That is all I needed to hear. Whatever happens, knowing you care for me, wait for me, I will come home again. We can work out everything later. I will miss you terribly, but with your love I can survive anything."

"Let's wait and see," Lisbeth replied cautiously, not wanting to face the confusing issues that had been brought up by Jim's declaration of love. Still perplexed and uncertain, Lisbeth nevertheless felt a strange excitement. They continued to talk quietly for hours, and with a final kiss they embraced one last time.

"Auf Wiederseh'n," she whispered as Jim smiled broadly, skipping down the steps as if he had not a care in the world.

After Jim left, spring and summer dragged for Lisbeth. She missed him more than she could have imagined. She could not get their last evening together out of her mind. She thought of his beautiful blue eyes, full of love and longing for her. She missed his daily visits looking after her rose garden. Her children kept asking about their Uncle "Immy." As Lisbeth had promised him, she took his car for a short ride each week, usually driving to Springbrook for a ride on the merry-go-round and to Mayer's Malt Shop for ice cream as they had done the previous summer. But it wasn't the same. Somehow it just wasn't as much fun without Uncle "Immy," and the girls missed his playful ways. Lisbeth too missed Jim's calm presence beside her, his kindness and his undeniable love.

At least Lisbeth and the Bauers received letters from him. After basic training, he shipped out to the Pacific theater, but he wrote no details. All they could do was listen to the radio and scout the newspapers for news from both fronts, the Atlantic and the Pacific. Lisbeth prayed for everyone she knew across both oceans. It was truly becoming a war of the world.

FOURTY-NINE

Lisbeth was not the only one dealing with uncertainty and loss. In Hamburg life was becoming increasingly difficult. There were more and more shortages of food, and Johann kept busy in the garden, determined to have another good crop of vegetables. He surprised Wilhelm and Marianne with his ability to wheel and deal, trading his crops for other necessities of life. As gasoline was rationed, it was just as well that the Daimler was gone. He had fitted his bicycle with front and rear baskets and went to market weekly. One never knew what he might bring home, but it was always a welcome surprise.

Sometimes Johann brought home eggs or fruit, other times thread or batteries. He had many friends among the trades people and was tireless in the pursuit, bringing home many necessities to the family. Marianne depended on Johann as much as she needed Wilhelm. Without their help, Marianne would have drowned in her worries, unable to manage her existence. Since the closing of the glass works,

Wilhelm had become a different man. His days were spent reading the papers and listening to news of the war. Quite often when Johann was in the garden, Wilhelm joined him, discussing the latest events, speculating on what might happen next. They were concerned about Peter on the Russian front and Kurt somewhere in France. Their letters were few and far between, without specific information of any kind. Wilhelm's Skat group still met as before, but now they rarely played. It was more important to share ideas and discuss survival plans.

Since America had become involved in the war and Britain's Royal Air Force had begun a major offensive against Germany at the end of May, the men were busy improving their air-raid shelters, stocking them with food, medicine, water and other supplies. By July when the raids became more frequent across the Netherlands and Germany, some of Wilhelm's friends and their families spent their nights sleeping in the shelters. Marianne and Margarete refused to hide in the cellar and "live like rats," as they called it, and Wilhelm did not insist on it. But he was prepared for the worst. He and Johann had done all they could for their little family.

Margarete was still employed at the opera house. But there were rumors that the grand theater would close by the end of the year. Attendance was dwindling, the staff shrinking, the singers unable to perform without the supporting cast. Despite the glorious war reports, the people were afraid. The carefree mood of the country had changed. The population was skeptical despite the victories that were promised.

The Lindemanns worried about Lisbeth and her children. They had not received word from her since her arrival in the United States. They assumed she was back in Argentina but had not received any more communication. Still, they felt she was safe, certainly safer than she would be with them in Germany. It was Margarete they worried about now. She had not heard from Peter in a long while and imagined the worst. By September, when the German forces penetrated an area outside Stalingrad, Margarete had a feeling of foreboding. She was certain that Peter was in that area and that the Russian troops would fight fiercely to save the city. She and her father became obsessed with the news reports and as the number of casualties rose, so grew her fear and despair for him. She prayed daily for a letter and was daily disappointed. The battles around Stalingrad intensified, and Margarete's anxieties turned into panic. There was no way to cheer her up. Peter was her whole life.

Meanwhile across the Atlantic, Josef was working long hours at the garden center, trying to do the work of several men with the help of his family. He especially missed Jim's quiet, reliable presence. Most able-bodied young men had been drafted, and many women had gone to work in shops and factories.

Lisbeth continued to be busy with her shop as well as her constant knitting. The rose garden Jim had planted the previous summer was blooming—a daily reminder of his kindness and love. She tried her best to maintain it with Josef's help and wished Jim were here to enjoy it with her.

She was reminded of her mother who had often said, "The roses will bloom again, even if you are not here to see them. They will bloom for you again next time."

There was so much she wanted to share with Margarete and her parents, and even with Johann. But she had finally accepted the fact that there would be no letters until the end of this horrible war. She was glad to hear from her old friends, the Alvarez family, from Oma-Maria and now from Jim. For the others, only prayers would do.

In September Lisbeth prepared Rosalinde for kindergarten. At five, Rosalinde was a very mature little girl, anxious to start school. She loved reading and was already able to write her name and count to ten in three languages.

"Time is going so fast," Lisbeth said to herself. "Only two years ago I came for a visit, not knowing that I would never return to Argentina or see Lorenzo or Oma-Maria again. Here I am, my little Rosalinde already taking her first steps away from me."

FIFTY

One day the mailman brought a large stiff envelope to Lisbeth's mailbox. When she saw Emilio's return address, she began to shake. The envelope was large and official looking, and her first thought was that Lorenzo had changed his mind and wanted her children. With trembling hands she tore at the paper. A large thick card fell to the floor. Then Lisbeth saw the heavy dark print and black border, indicating a death announcement. She thought her heart would jump out of her chest as she read Oma-Maria's name, Maria Gabriela Ludwig Moncrief. Uncontrollable tears flowed as she sat, stunned, unable to read the accompanying letter.

Drained and exhausted, she finally read the sad news Emilio had been kind enough to send her. As soon as he had received the notice from the Moncriefs, he had sent it on to Lisbeth. Oma-Maria had not been well for some time, but instead of seeing a doctor, had blamed old age for her fatigue and chest discomfort. When she did not appear as usual at *Bien Cielo* for Sunday dinner, one of the men was dispatched to her house. She appeared to have died peacefully in her sleep the previous night, as one of the field hands had seen and waved to her the day before. Great as the shock was for the family, Emilio reminded Lisbeth of Oma's great love for her and the blessing of a peaceful death. By the time Lisbeth received this notice, her beloved Oma had been buried in the warm earth of the Pampas for several weeks. Lisbeth could not stop crying. Her grief for Oma-Maria was almost more painful than her rejection and abandonment by Lorenzo. For days she thought of nothing else but her wonderful memories of Oma's love and acceptance from the very beginning. She remembered the kindness Oma-Maria had shown toward the young bride who had come full of love and hope, only to be hurt and discarded.

As the weeks passed, Lisbeth slowly came to terms with her latest loss. She found comfort in her memories and in her prayers. She cut the last roses from her garden and placed them in a vase next to Oma-Maria's photograph. When another thick envelope from Emilio arrived several weeks later, she was puzzled by the sudden frequency of his correspondence. Besides a letter from him, there was another smaller sealed envelope and a copy of an official document.

"What is all this?" Lisbeth wondered, alarmed. "I thought everything about the divorce had been finalized."

Unable to grasp the meaning of the document, she began to read Emilio's letter first. He informed her that Oma-Maria's last will and testament had been processed and that she, Lisbeth Lindemann Moncrief, was the sole heir and beneficiary of all her worldly goods—her house, its contents, her 200 acres, including the vineyard. The land and vineyard were currently leased to Diego Morales, the lease running another twelve years. At the end of this time the lease could be renewed or the property sold. Meanwhile, Lisbeth was to sign and return the enclosed document for final processing. Emilio was willing to continue to handle her affairs if she so chose, and he would remit quarterly the income to her account in the U.S.A.

Lisbeth was stunned. She could not grasp the enormity of this bequest. Apparently Oma-Maria had written this will a few months after she and her children had left, and had it witnessed by Emilio and an attorney at the bank. She had also enclosed a letter to be given to Lisbeth at the time of her death. Lisbeth's hands were shaking as she opened the small envelope that was addressed to her in Oma-Maria's old-fashioned flowery handwriting:

Meine liebe Lisbeth, liebe Rosalinde, liebe kleine Angelina,

This will be my last letter to you. I do not know when it will be mailed, but I do know it will be after my death. I cannot tell you how heartbroken I have been since your departure and the events that followed. From the moment you came into our family, I have loved you as my own, and you and the girls have been the sunshine of my life. I had not realized how lonely my life was until you came. With you I discovered again the joy of living, the adventure that every day could be. Helping you learn Spanish was great fun, and your help to me, relearning the German language of my youth, was a very special gift. Now you are gone, and the sunshine went with you. Your beautiful, smiling photograph is all I have as a reminder of happier days.

The pain and disappointment in the actions of my grandson are indescribable. How could he, with cunning and malice, engineer a plan to let you go under the pretense of being a loving, generous husband, making a great sacrifice for you? In truth it was only his cowardly and egotistical way to mask his shocking betrayal of you. May God forgive him as I cannot. Still, I do believe that he loved you with all his heart. I think and pray for your welfare every day and know that Tante Anni is looking out for you. I wish I could do something that would take away your pain and rejection and make everything well again. But all I can do now is to ensure your and the girls' future and to make amends in some small way for the suffering my family has imposed on you.

I have instructed Señor Alvarez to handle all the legal papers and when the time comes he will inform you. In my last will and testament, I am leaving all my worldly goods to you. My house and contents, the acreage around it, the vineyard, (Roberto's Folly) and all my assets are yours to do with as you wish. My last wish is that you and the children may have a happy and satisfying life. I give it all to you with love. Remember, Lisbeth, your mother's roses, how you tried to pamper them in foreign soil, and still they never thrived or blossomed. But you, Rosalinde and Angelina, you are my three lovely roses that will bloom in my heart forever.

Auf Wiederseh'n! All my love, Oma-Maria.
Maria Gabriela Ludwig Moncrief

Lisbeth collected the papers around her and slowly replaced them in the envelope. What an incredible woman Oma-Maria was! With her last independent act she had given Lisbeth validation and freedom in her final gift of love.

That night before going to bed, Lisbeth read Oma-

Maria's letter once again. Her mind was churning with old memories, wondering how Lorenzo's once fiery love had turned into the final betrayal. She knew that she was equally guilty, her homesickness and depression had definitely impacted their marriage. "Love conquers all," she had naïvely believed, although she began to understand Lorenzo's dilemma. Yet how could he stoop so low as to forsake his children, to let them go, never to see them again? Were his new sons more important to him than his sweet little daughters? As she was tossing and turning, sleep kept eluding her. Then suddenly she heard a dear and familiar voice, unmistakably Oma-Maria's voice, sweet and clear, whispering to her, *"Schlaf' wohl, mein Schatz, Schlaf wohl..."* And with that Lisbeth finally found peace.

Fall turned into winter, and once again the old melancholy overtook Lisbeth. Jim's departure, coupled with Oma-Maria's death caused a great void in her life. Not only did she miss them, but the joy seemed to have gone out of everything. What kept her going were her children and the activities at the shop. Rosalinde was enjoying school and felt very grown up, getting on the big yellow schoolbus every morning. Angelina, at three and a half, was a busy little person. If she got bored being at home with Mommy, she toddled next door to the greenhouse where she was always welcomed by someone in the Bauer family. There was usually someone to give her a ride in the wheelbarrow or find a special treat for her. She was friendly and outgoing and loved being busy. Often Josef gave her some less than perfect seedlings which she proceeded to plant in a huge pile of topsoil. She loved planting and of course returned home covered with dirt. She would smile broadly, her dark eyes sparkling, announcing what a great help she had been to Uncle Josef. In fact, everyone called Angelina his new assistant.

Liesl's Treasures continued to be successful. More often than not, friends and customers met not only to shop, but also to visit. Everyone had a story to tell as husbands, brothers, sons, neighbors and friends were called up to war. Some of the women had gone to work. Others attempted to run their husband's business. But despite uncertainty and fear, everyone was willing to do what was necessary. Just as Lisbeth's family in Europe prayed for an end to war, her American friends and neighbors prayed for the same here. Nationality did not matter. All were united with the same hope for peace.

Meanwhile the war in Europe raged on. There were daily reports of battles and offensives in places most people had never heard of. Josef read the paper carefully every night, then brought it to Lisbeth on his way to work the next day.

"Thank God, there is nothing about Hamburg," he would tell her. "But I think it's getting worse everywhere else—like Stalingrad—you better read about it yourself."

As Lisbeth read about the air raids over Europe, she could not help but fear for Hamburg. Not knowing what was happening there certainly did not ease her mind. Instead, she imagined the worst. What if Hamburg had been bombed too? What if her family were hungry and cold?

What if...? Firmly she tried to dispel these disquieting thoughts.

She continued reading about a place called Stalingrad as Josef had suggested. Apparently the German forces had many large battalions engaged in fierce door-to-door battles in and around that city. Hundreds of thousands of soldiers on both sides were launching savage attacks and counterattacks with immense losses of life. Lisbeth shuddered, imagining the bloody battles resulting in thousands of casualties. Sighing deeply, Lisbeth folded the paper, throwing it into the wood box. "I shouldn't have read this," she admonished herself. "It's all too terrible. It makes me ill just thinking about it."

What Lisbeth did not know, could not know, was how this particular battle in Stalingrad did affect someone she loved, her dear sister Margarete. Four weeks before Christmas, Margarete's fiancé Peter von Orb, a member of the Sixth Army stationed at Stalingrad, paid the ultimate price in a futile war.

Christmas 1942 came and went without any great celebrations. For the sake of the children, the Bauers and Lisbeth continued the family traditions, but the pall of war that had fallen over the country was felt even by the children. Monika was now a teenager, more interested in herself than in talk of war, shortages and hard times. Willy, still the patriot, was extremely interested in every piece of news he read. He scanned the globe and searched the atlas, looking for the various locations of conflict and places where Uncle Jimmy might be in the Pacific.

Little Joe was not quite as involved as his brother but

even he was aware of the many world crises. His own personal crisis at the moment was that he no longer wanted to be called Little Joe. He was growing tall and sturdy, hoping to surpass Willy. But old habits die hard, and it seemed destined that he would remain Little Joe for some time, if not forever.

As spring 1943 approached, Josef decided to plant more vegetables than flowers at the greenhouse. There were now hundreds and hundreds of tomato plants where before there had been marigolds and dahlias. Everyone was trying to do his part in the war effort by growing vegetables in "Victory Gardens".

Lisbeth continued to work hard at "Liesl's" and the community pulled together in work and prayer. Although certain items were harder to find and gasoline, meat and sugar were rationed, nobody went hungry or worried about their safety at home.

Lisbeth often thought with great admiration of the country she lived in now. How generous the United States had been toward her, allowing her to remain in this country instead of cold-heartedly ordering her to return to her war-ravaged homeland. How generous and humane to let her and her children live in safety! She often declared, "Surely there is no other country in the world like this." When attending various school or community functions, she joined in with all the others as they proudly sang "God Bless America" and truly believed it with a thankful heart.

As 1943 drew to a close, the war continued to rage both in Europe and the Pacific. Daily life for Lisbeth and the Bauers, however, was not interrupted by the war. They did worry when they heard reports of the bombing of German cities. But work and hope were all they could do. The passing of the years was most noticeable on the children. Monika at 16 had become a stunning young woman. Willy at 14 had overtaken both parents in height. Even Joe was no longer little, having grown muscular and strong. The baby cousins were both in school now, Rosalinde in second grade, Angelina in kindergarten. Both had adapted well to school and to American life. The only person they remembered well enough to miss was Uncle "Immy." He and the Bauers were the only family they knew. Despite worries about the people in Hamburg and Jim somewhere in the Pacific, they were holding up well, working together and hoping for a good ending.

FIFTY-ONE

However, during these same war years, life had drastically changed for the Lindemanns and their neighbors in Hamburg. Daily life had become more difficult with shortages of food and medicine, and the daily fear of attack from the air. Since the first heavy air raid on Cologne by the Royal Air Force, the Lindemanns had spent almost every night in their basement shelter. Every day without fail, Johann and Margarete went out "scouting," as they called it. Whenever they saw a line forming in front of a store, one of them joined, hoping that whatever was available was not sold out by the time they reached the door. Everyone had been issued ration cards for basic food, but occasionally they were lucky to get additional supplies. Even if it was something they did not need, they bought it in order to trade with someone else. Thanks to Johann's tireless work in the garden, they were well supplied with vegetables. If nothing else, they always had potatoes. Through his resourceful trading, they also had some flour in their storage room.

So far they had spent their days upstairs in the house and garden, but at nightfall they hurried down into the cellar. Margarete and Johann had brought their bedding and other necessities to make their overnights more comfortable, but Marianne hated "living like rats." She complained daily, wanting back her old life of comfort and security. She could not help wondering how the rest of the family was able to adjust and accept. For Margarete too, life had changed radically. The opera house was closed. Peter was gone, and there was no song in her heart. Her life now revolved around the care of her parents, helping Johann, and trying to survive from day to day. The piano was draped and closed. Margarete had no desire to sing or play. Wilhelm worried greatly about her. There seemed to be no joy in her life.

"Please, Margarete, play something for me, please," her father begged her. "Let's try to forget our troubles for a while. Let's be thankful we have each other."

But Margarete just shook her head. She was not in the mood to sing. It was as if she had lost her voice. There was too much to do just to get through each day.

"When I get the next letter from Peter, when we have something to celebrate, then I'll sing for you, Papa. I promise. Right now, there is nothing to sing about."

Wilhelm knew this was true, but he still longed to hear her clear, beautiful voice. He wanted to put everything aside and simply enjoy a song of beauty, hope and peace. He turned on the radio, searching for some classical music, but every station seemed to be only reporting war news. Finally, through crackling static, he heard the faint sounds of a violin. He closed his eyes, remembering the days when

Margarete's singing and Lisbeth's laughter filled the house with happiness. That time seemed eons ago. Now they lived with constant fear and uncertainty.

When the first bombs were dropped over the city they were thankful they had a cellar to hide in. Every morning at daybreak, they climbed upstairs, hoping to find their home intact. One cold winter morning Johann was outside, sweeping the light dusting of snow that had fallen overnight. When he saw the postman trudging up the street, his heart quickened for a moment. Perhaps a letter, perhaps some good news from somewhere. But there was nothing.

That night one of the bombs that exploded nearby shattered most of the upstairs windows. Johann quietly closed and locked the shutters. After that, even Marianne stopped fretting and settled into their dreary life in the bomb shelter. Throughout all this, Wilhelm continued to read the papers and listen to the radio. He stubbornly held on to the hope that somehow this madness would end and his family be spared. That hope was shattered, however, when Margarete received word from Peter's family that he had been killed in Stalingrad late in 1942. Margarete stared at the letter, at first unbelieving, then, crumpling it in her fist, gave vent to her pain with screams of anger and deep despair.

"Why Peter? Why did it happen to him? He was a good man, never hurt anybody. Why my Peter? Why, why, why?" she sobbed. Wilhelm and Marianne looked on helplessly. There was nothing they could do to comfort their child. There was no answer to her anguished pleas, no explanation. All they could do was to hold her, love her, and support her with their loving arms. With this deep personal loss, the insane horrors of war penetrated the last vestiges of their security. They had lost one of their own forever.

The days and weeks dragged by. Margarete lived in silence, holding in her pain, stoically working alongside Johann to make their life bearable. She busied herself with everyday tasks, concentrating only on survival. It seemed she had buried her loss deep within her soul, put aside for the moment. She could only deal with the challenge of outliving the war, for her parents' sake. She could not bring herself to speak of Peter. But late at night when Wilhelm could not sleep, he heard the dry, hard sobs escaping Margarete's chest.

On July 26, 1943, the first massive bombing of Hamburg left the city burning and in ruins. After that, even Johann did not venture out daily to scout for supplies. No longer only nights were spent in the shelter. More and more daylight hours were spent hiding and watching. Wilhelm become more despondent with each disturbing broadcast of events. When the Americans coordinated with the British, resulting in round-the-clock bombing, he hung his head and cried, "We will not survive this war. It is all around us and we have no chance. What a waste, this terrible war!" he whispered to himself. But as bad as it was, it would become worse. By now they were practically prisoners in their bomb shelter. Relentless nightly air raids continued over Hamburg, destroying the harbor. One day Johann ventured out of the neighborhood and turned back in horror, having seen smoking ruins and survivors wandering aimlessly. He returned, unable to describe the devastation he had seen. Wilhelm's face looked gray and ashen. He felt tight around his chest, almost unable to breathe. He popped one of his little pills under his tongue and reclined on his pallet, closing his eyes. But sleep eluded him as the weight on his chest grew heavier.

Several nights later, during another thunderous raid over the city, Wilhelm suffered a second heart attack, and this time it was fatal. There was no first aid of any kind, no ambulance, no doctor, and Wilhelm died peacefully in Marianne's arms. Shocked beyond tears, she held on to Wilhelm's cold, lifeless body until the loud crashes of the devastating bombs, the wailing of sirens, and the shaking of the earth around them began to wane with the gray morning light.

This tragic loss affected the family in a disastrous way. Papa, who had always taken care of everybody and everything, was suddenly gone from their midst. It fell to Margarete to make decisions. For once, Johann did not know what to do. Wilhelm had been his pillar, his guide, his idol and his friend. Johann was numb with grief, looking to Margarete for help and guidance. Marianne was unable to speak, not fully comprehending the finality of his death. Surrendering to anguish, she left everything in Margarete's hands.

In a calm and stoic manner, Margarete managed with the help of an elderly clergyman to have her father buried in the family plot. She had lost two of the dearest people in the world in a matter of months, and yet standing at her father's grave she could not shed a tear. She felt cold and numb, paralyzed with grief and fear. She stared unknowingly at the few friends and neighbors who had come to the funeral.

Johann stoically held up Marianne, as she moaned and sobbed in despair. The pastor's consoling words of peace and hope were lost on the two women. Only Johann clung to his comforting words.

Quietly everyone stood at the grave, unable to believe that their dear father, husband and friend had left them forever. Each was lost in thought and remembrances. Margarete felt a deep stab of pain and regret. She had never fulfilled one of her father's rare wishes. If only she had sung for her dear Papa when he had asked her to forget the war for a while and be happy they had each other. But she had denied him. Quietly she began singing the *Ave Maria* as her last farewell. Johann and Marianne looked up in surprise, but they understood. Margarete hoped that her father understood too.

In the weeks and months that followed Wilhelm's death, Marianne had begun ailing, not from physical deprivation, but from grief and lack of hope. She simply gave up. She refused to eat, barely spoke, and lost her desire to live, lost in the sadness of old memories and total hopelessness. It was all Johann and Margarete could do to keep her alive with loving and comforting words, warm blankets and the thin soup and bread which they could still provide. Her only sustaining thoughts were of Lisbeth and her granddaughters, hoping that they were well and safe. Little did she know that Lisbeth, although safe, had suffered her own devastating blows.

Christmas 1944 was the bleakest holiday ever. Johann had been able to find a few sacks of coal so that they could fire up the small stove. He had also traded some apples and potatoes for a few scraps of meat and bones from the butcher. Their Christmas dinner consisted of soup, thick with potatoes, carrots and kohlrabi. There was also a fresh loaf of bread and a box of dry biscuits. Marianne did not eat much. She had developed a cold and a dry cough. She turned her pale face against the wall and cried herself to sleep. Margarete and Johann made a feeble attempt at conversation, remembering other Christmases, happier times. But it was impossible. The loss of Peter and Wilhelm was still too raw and painful, and so they sat helplessly by, thinking of the bleak days that lay ahead. They both knew they would soon lose another loved one. It would not be long before Marianne would join Wilhelm in the loving embrace of God.

Part Four

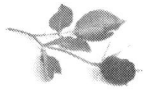

Journey Home

FIFTY-TWO

Another spring arrived, the spring of 1945. Once again the Bauers toiled in the greenhouse, getting ready for the new planting season. As in the last three years, there were more tomato plants than tulips. Everyone missed Jim, his calm ways and his friendly smile. Where was he in the vast Pacific? They had not heard from him in many months but still remained optimistic. Josef tried to reassure everyone. "As long as we receive no notice of bad news, he is alive and well. Jim knows how to take care of himself." The family fervently clung to that hope. One day was like the one before: work, pray for our boys and hope. That was the motto everyone seemed to live by.

On a warm April day, Lisbeth spent the day with Anni's help cleaning up "Jim's rose garden," as she called it. Remembering her mother and her roses, Lisbeth began to cry. Were her mother's roses still there in Hamburg? Was her mother working in her rose garden as she was doing now? Then another disturbing thought crossed her mind. She remembered the two rose bushes her mother had lovingly packed and sent with her when she left Germany to make her new home with Lorenzo. What had happened to them back at *Bien Cielo*? Hard as Lisbeth had tried, those rose bushes had never found their roots in the Moncrief garden. They did not die, but they never thrived. They had never bloomed. What had happened to them since she left five years ago? Had they died of neglect and lack of love, as Lorenzo's love for her had died, shriveled petals blown away by a cold wind? Lisbeth shook her head sadly and dried her eyes. "What is past is past. I must look forward, not back. Jim will be coming home one of these days, and I want his roses to bloom and welcome him home. Please, God, let Jim return when the roses come into bloom," she prayed.

As if Anni knew what had been going through Lisbeth's mind, she stopped working and looked at her. "I know what you are thinking. I thought about it too. Jim will be so proud of you when he comes home and sees how well you have taken care of the roses."

"If he ever comes home. Oh, I do want him to come back soon. I really want to see him again."

"Be brave, be strong. He'll be back, you'll see," Anni said. Both women continued working. There was no time to brood. "Liesl's Treasures" kept Lisbeth occupied, and her children needed a different kind of attention now. They had homework to do, loved visiting the library, drew pictures and wrote letters to Uncle "Immy." Their works of art graced the walls of the stairwell, leading up to the bedrooms.

"Soon Uncle 'Immy' will come home again, and he will see how much we missed him," Rosalinde proclaimed as Angelina added, "And how much we love him."

Lisbeth smiled, in her heart agreeing completely with the sentiment of her innocent children. If only it were so, she thought to herself. If only he will come home again!

But when you least expect it, something wonderful can happen. Finally the day the world had been hoping for arrived. On a bright May morning, Josef came running breathlessly to Lisbeth's door, waving the newspaper. He had heard the news on the radio already and was ecstatic. His hands were shaking as he unfolded the paper and showed her the headline: "War ends in Europe! Germany Surrenders!"

"Thank God, thank God!" Lisbeth cried, hugging him. Happy tears streaming down her face, she called out, "Now we will find out how my family is."

They danced around the porch like two carefree children, hardly believing and absorbing the good news.

Church bells were ringing, drivers were honking their horns and children were dismissed early from school. Everyone was suddenly in a party mood. Lisbeth too felt the relief. Bright banners and flags of all sizes were fluttering in the warm spring air, and there was literally dancing in the streets.

"But when will Jim be coming home?" Lisbeth asked herself, at the same time wondering how she would receive him. She suddenly realized that very soon, perhaps only months from now, she would have to leave the United States. When she voiced her concerns to Anni and Josef, they were quick to respond that it would take considerable time before anyone could travel back to Germany. Its cities had been destroyed, that was clear to all of them. Surely it would be impossible to return at this time. She realized that it would take weeks or months before even the American troops would be able to return.

"Just relax and be glad it's over," they advised her. "But for now you are here with us where you are safe."

"You're right. Let's just rejoice the European war is over at least. Maybe we'll hear from Margarete and my parents. Just knowing they are safe would be enough for me."

"Let's just wait and see," Josef advised. "There is still much to be done before there is a real and lasting peace."

Lisbeth knew he was right, but she didn't want to let go of the feeling of relief and thanks that was flooding her at this moment.

"*Deo gratias,*" she prayed. "The European war is over and thank God all will be well again soon."

She found herself in a sort of happy turmoil, waiting for Jim, yet not knowing exactly how she would feel when she actually saw him again. Rosalinde and Angelina also felt the feverish excitement all around them, constantly asking how soon they would see Uncle "Immy" again. Soon, soon, they were told, although there was still no word from him.

Lisbeth realized that the war in the Pacific was far from over. As they devoured the news regarding the end of the European war, they understood just how destructive this ravaging war had been at the cost of millions of lives. As they read about the continuation of the war in the Pacific, a pall fell over their initial joy. Throughout most of the summer, they eagerly listened to the radio until they heard the final good news. Once again Josef came by Lisbeth's farmhouse waving the paper and shouting, "It's over. It's finally over. A day to remember! Japan has surrendered. August 14, 1945! They have surrendered, and now our Jim will finally come home."

The country once again erupted in celebration. The troops from Europe were returning home, but there was no news of Jim. They had no idea whether he had survived or just where he was. Lisbeth and the Bauers continued to hope and pray, never giving up.

Eventually word reached the Bauers that James Harding, although wounded, was recovering in a hospital in Hawaii. Knowing Jim would be returning to them soon, Anni and Josef began making plans for his homecoming. He had no other family. They were his family. Lisbeth was touched by her children's excitement as they drew pictures for him, waiting to be with Uncle "Immy" again. Although still feeling somewhat nervous and unsure, Lisbeth also could hardly contain herself with happiness and anticipation.

Finally a telegram arrived, informing them of his release and homecoming. Anni started cooking, and Josef began washing and decorating the car for Jim's ride home. Everyone was thrilled at the news, and all of Springbrook was happy for him. When the day of his arrival came, half the town was waiting for him at the train station, carrying balloons and flowers, waving huge banners to welcome home their hero.

Anni and Lisbeth and all the children stayed at the farmhouse waiting for Jim and Josef. The road to Anni's house passed the greenhouse and the farmhouse, so they had decided to welcome him there. The children were anxious and impatient, wishing they had been able to see him at the station. But this was the plan—a private welcome for him with just the people he loved most. Anni was nervously happy, sending one of the children to the mailbox, looking down the road for their car. Lisbeth's heart was beating wildly, happy and yet afraid. She had put on her very best Sunday dress, pale yellow with tiny red roses, and had unbraided her pretty blonde hair. Angelina and Rosalinda were running around happily, yelling, "Uncle 'Immy' is coming, 'Uncle Immy'...!"

At last, followed by a cloud of dust, Josef's car came down the road. As Josef drove slowly past the garden center, Jim saw the banner the children had made and taped across the entrance: "Welcome Home, Jim! We love you! Welcome!"

Jim's eyes filled with tears and even before Josef had come to a complete stop, he jumped out of the car. Despite his limp, he started running toward the family waiting for him. Seeing the entire group assembled on the porch, he let out a loud whoop: "Hi, everybody! I'm home. I'm home," he cried. Everyone screamed for joy, crowding around him and showering him with hugs and kisses. Josef stood by the side of the car, watching the wonderful welcome for his dear friend and partner. Over the years Jim had become a true member of the family and never had he felt more loved and cherished than he was at this moment. As he looked up, he saw Lisbeth standing on the top step with her not-so-little girls, watching the boisterous demonstration of love before her. With a big grin, Jim disentangled himself from the cheering little crowd. Smiling and crying at the same time, Lisbeth came down the steps and fell into his arms.

"Oh, Jim, you are home. You are finally home. We've missed you so," she cried as he held her in his tight embrace.

"I love you," Jim whispered into her ear over and over as Rosalinde and Angelina tugged at his pant legs.

"Uncle 'Immy!' Hi! We've missed you. Are you home to stay now?"

"Yes, yes, I'm home to stay now, and I will never leave you again," he told them as he bent down and swept up both little girls into his arms. They clung to him, not wanting to let go. As Lisbeth watched, her own happiness welled up within her, and she joined them in a family embrace. Finally the girls slid down and went off in search of other adventures with the Bauer kids.

Once again Lisbeth's arms encircled Jim and, catching her breath, she was finally able to say the words that had given Jim hope during his darkest and most dangerous moments, the words he had been longing to hear forever: "I love you too, Jim. I'm so happy you came back to us. I have finally figured out some things."

"What have you figured out, my darling girl?" Jim teased. Neither he nor Lisbeth had noticed that the Bauers had slowly walked back to their car, letting them savor the happy moment of homecoming alone. Glancing back, they saw Lisbeth's arms around Jim, and they knew Jim was home at last.

Between breathless kisses, Jim was finally able to ask again, "What is it, Lisbeth? What have you figured out?"

Beaming with happiness, without a doubt in her mind, she was eager to tell him, "Dearest Jim, I have finally figured out where my heart is. It is here. My home and my heart are here with you."

As they kissed again the five children came running around the corner, stopping in surprise, then cheering and applauding the happy couple.

Jim looked fervently at Lisbeth. Never had he seen her more beautiful, more desirable. Lisbeth too, looked at Jim through new eyes. He had grown thinner. There were new lines along his face. He had been in a war, but he had come back to her. She felt happy, totally his. Both felt a gratitude, a blessing such as they could never have imagined.

It had been a homecoming beyond all expectations. Not only had Jim returned from a gruesome war that day, but finally his darling Lisbeth had come home too.

Behind the house, in the garden that Jim had so lovingly planted for her, and that Lisbeth had carefully tended for him, the roses bloomed in full splendor and glorious beauty. They would always bloom for the love of the people within who had finally found each other forever.

FIFTY-THREE

After a long and difficult winter, spring finally came to Hamburg. Not only in the sense of warm sunshine and budding trees, but also in the hope of a new day, a new beginning. On a very ordinary day on May 7, 1945, the German High Command finally surrendered all forces unconditionally at Reims, France, and the war ended officially at 12:01 a.m., the next day.

Huddled in their shelter, Johann and Margarete heard the final radio broadcasts. Both of them had known that the war was lost. They had prayed daily that it would soon be over. But now that it had been declared so, they could not totally believe it.

"You mean, we can go upstairs into our house? We can go into the garden? There will be no more bombs, no more nightly sirens?" Margarete asked ecstatically. The old man and the young woman passed from anguish to disbelief to joy in a matter of minutes.

"The war is over. It's all over. Thank God, it's over,"

Johann cried. Now for the first time in many months, Margarete could cry, cry for all she had lost. Cry for Peter, cry for her parents, cry for all the hardships and deprivations they had suffered. While the hot tears cleansed her soul, she suddenly heard her dear Papa's voice. "Don't cry for us, Margarete. Dry your tears and be happy. You have been given your life again. You have hope and youth and strength. You will rise up from these ashes and build your life again. You will make me proud of you. You will sing again and be happy."

Margarete looked up from Johann's frail shoulder and marveled at this revelation. "Johann," she asked quietly, "did you hear someone talking just now? I thought I heard something...a voice..." But old Johann only shook his tired head, answering, *"Nein, nein."* Her father's words filled her with an unexpected strength and energy as she took Johann by the hand.

"Let's leave this dark cellar. Let's go outside and breathe the fresh air. Let's look at the world again." Pulling Johann up the stairs, Margarete continued her lively chatter. "Come, Johann. We have much work to do. We must rebuild. We must reclaim what once was. And we will never have to be afraid and sleep in the cellar again."

Johann almost ran up the steps with her as his heart leaped with joy at her young and hopeful face, knowing that the sun would truly shine on them again.

The weeks passed in frenzied activity as Margarete and Johann began to restore a semblance of order in their house as well as their lives. There were still great shortages and ration cards to deal with, and as it was spring, they had nothing from the garden to trade. One day Margarete opened her father's safe. Johann looked at her questioningly. "Are you sure your father would...?" But she stopped him. "Papa wants us to stay alive, Johann. What good is silver when we are starving? Take these coins and see what you can do with them. Please, we can't give up now."

Johann wheeled his old bicycle out of the garage and set off to the countryside. Perhaps he would be lucky and find a butcher or a farmer who could still afford to sell him some meat, some eggs or some grain for the hard coins jingling in his pocket.

So began a time of a different kind of trading for survival. Once he traded Wilhelm's winter coat for a small can of smoked ham. Another time several pairs of Marianne's shoes bought them some flour and a little butter. With each trade came painful memories, but there was no other way.

An overall depression had fallen across the land as the population slowly dealt with the humiliation of losing the war, the pain at the loss of human life and the destruction all around them. Most cities lay in shambles, homes and schools, businesses and factories, theaters and parks, reduced to smoking rubble. The presence of the British occupation forces was evident everywhere in Hamburg, as they began to restore order in the chaos.

Margarete often accompanied Johann, seeing for herself the incredible destruction and waste in the city. Homeless people had dug out small spaces in the ruins, trying to find shelter. Miraculously the opera house was still standing, its broken windows gaping holes, staring as if in shock. It was impossible to get to Lindemann's Glass Works as many streets were covered with the wreckage of fallen buildings. But at the moment, getting to her father's factory was not a priority for Margarete. Johann was forever optimistic. Unless the buildings had taken a direct hit, Johann was trusting that there would be a future for them.

Despite the many difficulties and hardships facing the people, despite their losses and deprivations, they found the strength to pick up the pieces of their lives again, grateful to have survived and relieved that the war with all its dangers was finally over. With an amazing spirit of hope, they found the energy and willpower to go on. Men, women and children were busy from daybreak to dusk, cleaning up the rubble, stone by stone, determined to rebuild their lives. The great uncertainty remained, however, about the many who had been killed or lost or maimed in the past six horrible years. It would take many more years before these uncertainties could be laid to rest.

For Margarete and Johann it was a lonely time. Every day there were reminders of Wilhelm and Marianne who had lived their entire married life and died in this house. Whenever tears and sadness overwhelmed Margarete, she held on to the words she knew she had heard her father speak to her on the last day of the war. His encouragement, faith and confidence in her, his conviction that life was worth living, gave her the needed strength to hope and to persevere. For his sake, she vowed to rebuild their existence into a vibrant life again.

Marianne's rose garden, neglected for so many years, was still miraculously producing roses despite the lack of care. To Johann and Margarete they were reminders of steadfast endurance, a work of beauty in the midst of chaos. "One of these days we will plant your mother's roses again where we made the vegetable garden during the war," Johann said. "I'm glad your mother did not allow us to dig up all of her roses," he mused, remembering the discussion he had had with Marianne at the beginning of the war.

"Yes, I am glad too. Looking at her roses I feel she is still with us, watching us, making sure that we take care of them," Margarete said wistfully. How she missed her mother who, despite all her worrying, was the soul of their family. And her dear father, how he had always made sure they had everything they needed, and then some. Even beyond the grave, Margarete felt that Papa was with them, helping and guiding them. Much as she missed them, in some ways she was grateful her parents had been spared much pain and many sorrows.

Her thoughts also traveled to Lisbeth. Since the spring of 1940 there had been no word from her. The last they knew, she had undertaken a daring voyage with the two little girls to visit Tante Anni in New Jersey. Surely she had returned home safely to Lorenzo before the United States had become involved in the war. Although missing her sister greatly, Margarete was confident that Lisbeth and her family were safe. It would only be a matter of time before she heard from her again. She remembered the excitement when she and her parents were planning their trip to Argentina. Then, like a bolt of lightning, the war began and tore their family apart forever. She thought lovingly about Rosalinde and Angelina who would never know their precious grandparents. Rosalinde would be close to eight years old, and Angelina around six. How Margarete longed to see her sister again, to hold them all in her arms.

She glanced over at Johann, still working near the roses. He was all she had. He was her family now, and she was grateful for that. She had lost everyone else in just a few short years. She thought of Peter with an aching tenderness and of her parents and the distress they had endured. She also thought of Kurt, whom her father had respected and loved as one of his own. Where was Kurt now? Had he survived? There had been no news from him for two years. A quick prayer for him formed in her heart. "Let him be safe. Please God, at least let him come home."

One warm September day as Johann was again toiling in the garden, he heard a sound he had not heard in years. Through the open door he could hear someone playing the piano, hesitantly at first, but gaining confidence. Johann straightened up, his heart filled with happiness as he heard Margarete's beautiful clear voice ring out in triumph and joy. "She is finally singing again. She is singing for her Papa, for all of us. We will overcome everything. I know it now. Our wonderful Margarete is singing again." Quietly Johann stepped up on the veranda and, leaning against the open door, smiled in deep gratitude.

That day was a turning point in both their lives. There was a new spring to Margarete's step, a new lightness radiating from her. In finding her music, she had regained an inner balance, a new acceptance of life as it was now. Through her music she could put aside her sadness, her loss, and sing to hope, to life, to the future.

"We will make it now," Johann thought to himself. "Wilhelm was right. She will sing again, and she will be happy."

A few weeks later, on a cool fall afternoon, as Margarete was helping Johann rake leaves, she felt a piercing look behind her. Turning slowly, she saw a tall, haggard stranger walking past the house, up the garden path toward her. "I wonder who that can be," she asked herself. "Could it really be?"

Suddenly his cap flew off his head and with a few quick steps, Margarete found herself looking into the bluest eyes she had ever known. The eyes of Kurt Walter, set deeply in a thin, lined face, eyes overflowing with joy. It was Kurt who had survived the tragedies of the war by keeping Margarete's lovely face in his heart, hoping, willing himself to return to her one day. The day had come, and here she was, alive and well. And here was Kurt, no longer the shy young man who had not dared approach Wilhelm Lindemann's daughter, but a mature man with purpose and resolve. Whatever her decision, Kurt would try to win Margarete's heart.

"Kurt! Is it really you? Where have you come from?"

Wordless, he held Margarete in his arms. Astounded by this unexpected miracle, Margarete folded herself into his embrace, feeling a strange calm and comfort spreading through her, a feeling of coming home, and his love waiting there for her.

"Kurt, it is you! You came back! I'm so glad you are home!" Kurt simply held her in his arms, kissing her wet face, her eyes, her mouth, as she clung tightly to him.

"You are the only one who came back. Papa and Mutti have died. Peter was killed at Stalingrad! But you came back!" Margarete was able to exclaim between kisses.

Kurt looked lovingly into her eyes and spoke hoarsely, "Finally it's over, it's over. I'm so sorry for all your losses. I was determined to live to see you again. I wanted to hold you in my arms and never let you go."

Margarete suddenly realized how much she had hoped and prayed for his safe return. How often her thoughts had wandered to him, not knowing whether he was alive or dead. An unbelievable happiness flooded her, seeing him before her eyes, and holding him in her arms.

"Kurt, when did you come home?" she asked.

"Today, today. I have come home to you today. I have walked and walked across the border from France. I don't know how long. And I would walk to the ends of the earth for you, my Margarete. I love you, Margarete. I love you."

She stared at Kurt, barely able to believe what he was trying to tell her. She looked into his weary eyes, smiled, and with a deep kiss she answered all his unspoken questions.

Perhaps her sister had been right after all when she used to tease Margarete that Kurt was in love with her. They continued to hold each other, their hearts beating wildly, almost unable to contain the happiness they both felt.

"Oh, Kurt, I love you too," Margarete whispered. "I just didn't know it until now, until you came back to me. But I know it now. Believe me, I know it now."

Johann sat on the bench observing their tender reunion and their final long kiss. He said to himself, "I can't believe it happened. My prayers have been answered. I'm so happy

Kurt came back to us. He is such a good man. Now Margarete will never be alone again. She will have a good life with him. I'm sure of that. I'm tired now. I'm old. My work is done here. We survived the war, thank God, and we saved Margarete for Kurt. Wilhelm would approve; he would be so relieved and at peace. Just look at the happy couple, holding each other. What more can I ask for now? All is well. If the Lord calls me today, I'm ready to go." Johann leaned back and sighed contentedly.

Finally Margarete and Kurt realized that they were not alone, that Johann was in the garden with them. Joyfully they ran toward the old man, embracing him, all three rejoicing in the happiness of the reunion.

Kurt took both of Johann's old and gnarled hands in his own, thanking him over and over for his loyalty and his unceasing care of Margarete and her family. As Margarete watched this moving scene, she knew without any doubt that her heart belonged to Kurt. The tears running down her cheeks now were no longer tears of sadness and despair, but tears of happiness.

"Why did I not see it before? How could I not have felt Kurt's love for me before the war?" she wondered. "How could I not know until today that I actually loved Kurt? Why does it take a frightful war and tragic loss to open my eyes and see clearly the wondrous possibilities right before us?"

Carefully Kurt helped Johann get up from the garden bench, and together, like a family, they walked into the house. "Let's celebrate your homecoming, Kurt. Johann, please see what is left in Papa's wine cellar. We must toast this happy day." As Johann disappeared, Margarete set about preparing some kind of meal for them. There were enough potatoes and vegetables from the garden as well as a can of herring which they had been saving for a special occasion. Well, Kurt's homecoming was certainly the happiest day in many years.

Late into the evening they sat, sharing stories over the simple meal. When asked about his war experiences, Kurt became very quiet. "It's difficult to talk about all that right now. Everything is still so fresh and painful in my heart," he replied sadly. "Perhaps it will become easier with time. Seeing my comrades fall, so many young men dying, the pain and hopelessness of it all, in some way I am still in shock. When I was taken prisoner, I was almost relieved to be out of the midst of carnage. But I had no idea how degrading it is to be a prisoner of war, alone and scared and humiliated in defeat."

With a deep sigh, Kurt continued quietly. "For weeks we were held in an enclosed outdoor arena, suffering from heat and cold and lack of food and water. Later we were housed in an abandoned building, and things improved slightly. But aside from the physical hunger, there was this emotional hunger for home, for family and a normal life, for the end of this horrible war."

Margarete and Johann sat in stunned silence. "Oh, Kurt, how much you have suffered during these dreadful years!" Margarete stammered, only imagining his despair and pain, but thankful for his wondrous survival.

Finally Kurt continued, "But you two have endured just as much as any soldiers at the front. The losses you have suffered right here in this family, I almost cannot believe it.

That both your parents died, Margarete, and Peter, the man you loved, dead in the massacre at Stalingrad. I can't even fathom your suffering and loss."

As Margarete's tears welled up again, Kurt rose and put his arms around her shoulders, kissing her gently on the head. "I'm so sorry, I'm so sorry. I wish..."

"Yes, we all wish, we wish this war had never happened. We wish they were still here with us. But it was not meant to be. We did the best we could, didn't we, Johann?"

"Yes, we did. We did," Johann nodded.

"And we must do as Papa said," Margarete added.

"What did your father say, Gretl?" Kurt asked. He was puzzled by the special look that passed between Margarete and the old man. She smiled and explained: "On the last day of the war, I knew I heard Papa's voice speaking to me. He told me to stop crying and to be happy again. Never did I believe then that I could be as happy as I am today. Papa told me to be strong, to rise up from these ashes and to rebuild my life and my future. It is as if he knew that you would come back to us, Kurt, and that together we could build a new life."

Kurt nodded in agreement and understanding. "Your Papa was right. We have survived so far, and we will survive from now on too. For your father's sake, we will build up all that has been destroyed. For him and for us we will start up Lindemann's Glass Works again. You will see. We can do anything together."

Johann smiled and nodded in happy consent. "And, don't forget, Margarete, you will sing for Kurt again, won't you? You will sing for all of us again, for your parents, for all that was lost and for all that is to come."

"Yes, Johann, singing for Kurt will be easy. I will sing again for all of us."

Kurt was beaming now. For the moment, all the pain of the past had vanished. He had found his love and he was not afraid. "Margarete, I know, I have just come home today, and perhaps I am speaking too soon. But after all we both have been through we have no time to waste." Looking deeply into her eyes and holding both of her shaking hands, Kurt asked formally, "Margarete, my darling, will you walk with me along life's path? I have waited so many years for this moment. Margarete, will you marry me? I promise to do all I can to make you happy and to keep you singing."

"Yes, yes, I will marry you, Kurt. Together we can do anything." With another kiss they sealed their promise as Johann laughed out loud, applauding as he had at Margarete's recital, feeling happier than he had in years.

"Yes, Kurt, we can do anything together," Margarete repeated, "but it will not be easy. Everything is destroyed, perhaps even the factory. People are struggling for daily survival. Who will buy fancy mirrors and crystal chandeliers from Lindemann's even if we can start again?"

But Kurt looked up at the broken windows all around him and replied full of confidence, "Trust me, Margarete, trust me. There is always window glass! Everybody will need window glass!

"This is our future: window glass!!

"Let's drink to window glass."

Raising their glasses, the old man and the young couple understood. Together they would build a new life again. After years of sorrow, slowly and cautiously, peace, hope, laughter and even song, could be theirs again, at last.

ACKNOWLEDGMENTS

My deepest thanks to my editors and proofreaders, Katharine and William McLaughry, for their endless patience, their insight, their enthusiasm and encouragement. Without their outstanding help, this novel would still be a stack of typewritten papers in a shoe box.

I also thank Patricia Cox, author and writing teacher at The Academy, for her sage advice and practical suggestions. It was her inspiration that led me to pursue publication of my work.

My sincerest appreciation and thanks to Angela Keane, of Story Preserves, who did the formatting and design of the manuscript for publication.

Patricia Grassfield was the only person outside of family whom I trusted to read my early manuscript. Her positive comments pushed me into action. Thanks, dear friend!

Lastly, my heartfelt thanks to my husband Franz for his devotion, common sense, understanding and support. (And … he never laughed at me.)

I thank all of you from the bottom of my heart, and can only repeat in three languages:

Danke schön! Gracias! Thank you!   EKH.

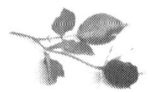

APPENDIX

Farewell Song

Wo die Nordseewellen schlagen an den Strand
Wo die gelben Blumen blüh'n ins grüne Land,
Wo die Möwen schreien, schrill im Sturmgebraus
Da ist meine Heimat, da bin ich zu Haus.
Wind und Wellen sangen mir mein Wiegenlied
Hohe Deiche waren mir, das "Gott behüt"
Merkten all mein Sehnen, und mein heiss' Begehr
In die Welt zu fliegen, über Land und Meer.
Wohl hat mir das Leben meine Qual gestillt
Und mir das gegeben, was mein Herz erfüllt.
Alles ist verschwunden, was mir leid und lieb
Hab' mein Glück gefunden, doch das Heimweh blieb.
Heimweh nach dem grünen Marschenland
Wo die Nordseewellen schlagen an den Strand.
Wo die Möwen schreien, schrill im Sturmgebraus
Da ist meine Heimat, da bin ich zu Haus.

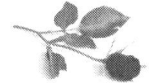

English Translation

Where the North Sea waves crash along the strand
Where yellow flowers bloom in green marshy land
Where the seagulls shriek during raging storms
There is my homeland; that is where I am at home.
Wind and waves sang for me my cradle song
Protected by high dikes and God's care
The waves knew all my longings, my deep desire
To fly out into the world, over land and sea.
Life has calmed my fears and expectations
And has given me what fulfills my heart
Everything has vanished, the pain and the love
Though I have found happiness, the homesickness remains.
I'm homesick for the beautiful green marshes
Where the North Sea waves still crash along the strand
Where the gulls are shrieking during raging storms
There is where my home is; there I will always belong.

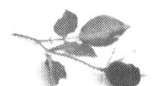

ABOUT THE AUTHOR

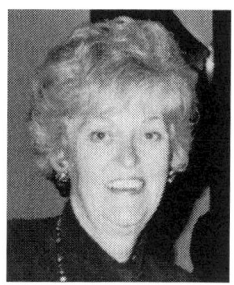

Elsa K. Hummel grew up in Bavaria, Germany, and was a young child when World War II ended. Educated at a private boarding school at Frauenchiemsee, she was instilled with a love for faraway places and adventure. As a teenager she and her family emigrated to the United States. Like Willy, in her novel, she is a patriot and truly loves America. She earned a Bachelor of Arts Degree from Loretto Heights College in Elementary Education and French. She taught in the Denver Public Schools, and after raising her family, embarked on a second career in Travel. This allowed her to follow her dream of seeing the world. *Home at Last* is her first novel. The original draft was written in German many years ago. Later, she rewrote the manuscript in English, adding insight and life experience. She and her husband, four married children, and ten grandchildren all live in Denver, Colorado.

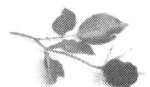

Made in the USA
Charleston, SC
16 June 2012